LIFE-SPAN PERSPECTIVES ON
HEALTH AND ILLNESS

LIFE-SPAN PERSPECTIVES ON HEALTH AND ILLNESS

Edited by

Thomas L. Whitman
Thomas V. Merluzzi
Robert D. White
University of Notre Dame

Lawrence Erlbaum Associates, Inc., Publishers
10 Industrial Avenue
Mahwah, NJ 07430

Cover design by Kathryn Houghtaling Lacey

Library of Congress Cataloging-in-Publication Data

Life-span perspectives on health and illness / edited by
Thomas L. Whitman, Thomas V. Merluzzi, and Robert D.
White
      p. cm
    Includes bibliographical references and index.
    ISBN 0-8058-2771-4 (cloth). — ISBN 0-8058-2772-2
(paper)
    1. Health promotion. 2. Life cycle, Human. 3. Devel-
opmental psychology. I. Whitman, Thomas L. II. Merluzzi, Thomas V. III. White, Robert D.
    [DNLM: 1. Human Development. 2. Life Change
Events. 3. Aging—Psychology. 4. Socioeconomic Factors. BF 713L7224 1998]
    RA427.8.L54 1998
    613—dc21
    DNLM/DLC
    for Library of Congress   98-21788
                                                    CIP

10   9   8   7   6   5   4   3

Contents

Preface

UNTIL RECENTLY, psychology and medicine have existed to a great extent as parallel universes. However, with the emergence of the behavioral medicine and health psychology fields, the recent research on the critical connection between mind and body, the emphasis on holistic medicine and health promotion, and the recognition of the importance of psychosocial aspects of illnesses, there have been unprecedented interdisciplinary efforts by two disciplines to collaborate on the treatment of disease and maintenance of health. As a consequence, psychology has progressed from playing an ancillary role in medicine to one that is more integrated into the comprehensive treatment of illness, particularly chronic illness, and the promotion of health and wellness.

The goal of this book is to expand this integration of psychology with medicine by placing these disciplines into a life-span developmental context. The life-span approach presents a broad conceptual perspective for viewing human development. When medicine is viewed in this framework, the development of biological, psychological, and social systems can provide a new way of contextualizing health and illness. This developmental context provides information that has significant implication for medical and psychological treatments and outcomes. With a life-span developmental perspective as the guide, this book examines the changing influence of biological, psychological, and social factors on health and illness during infancy, childhood, adolescence, and adulthood.

The first section of the book (chapters 1–4) introduces the life-span model. Chapter 1 traces the historical relation between psychology and medicine. In addition, models for examining the connections among biological, psychological, and environmental factors and health are described, with particular attention in childhood health. Chapter 8 examines how the unique cognitive, emotional, and behavioral characteristics of adolescents place them at risk for specific health problems. It emphasizes that adolescents are basically biologically healthy but might become vulnerable because of social, lifestyle, and psychological factors as well as risky behavior.

Chapter 9 examines the diverse impact of childhood illnesses, particularly those that are more chronic in nature, on the adjustment of affected children. Conceptual models for understanding child adaptation to illness are described, giving special attention to the influences of illness-related parameters, child characteristics, and socioenvironmental factors. The need for research that examines factors that moderate and mediate the influence of chronic illness on child adjustment is discussed at length.

The next four chapters examine health issues during the adult years. Chapter 10 explores the biological, socioenvironmental, and psychological changes that occur during adulthood and how these changes influence health and illness. A conceptual framework for studying health during this period is examined. Chapter 11 examines psychosocial attributes that promote stress resistance and resiliency in later life and identifies factors that are important elements in intervention and prevention programs for older people. Chapter 12 examines the health effects of caregiving on the care receiver and caregiver. The influence of care receiver and caregiver characteristics and social support are explored along with implications for the development of intervention programs. The last chapter (chapter 13) in this section explores death and dying in our society. The causes of death across the life span are reviewed in a gender and race/ethnicity framework. Changing attitudes toward death as aging occurs are described. Attention is also given to how individuals cope with death and how family and society cope with its dying members and the dying process. Finally, the aftermath of death, specifically grieving and bereavement, is examined in a life-span framework.

Using the life-span developmental conceptual framework described in chapter 1, chapter 14 integrates the materials from the other chapters as well as presents a process-oriented model of health influences and health outcomes. The model describes individual, social, and environmental factors that affect coping processes that, in turn, affect health outcomes.

ACKNOWLEDGMENTS

Special thanks are in order for numerous individuals, specifically to chapter authors who generously spent extra time revising their contributions in order to create a more dynamically integrated book; to Pauline Wright, who assisted with word processing; and to the staff at Lawrence Erlbaum Associates, who have been very helpful throughout the process of compiling this work. Finally, we express our gratitude to the Center for the Study of Children and Memorial Hospital of South Bend for their active support of this project.

—Thomas L. Whitman
—Thomas V. Merluzzi
—Robert D. White

⁂ ❖ ❧

This book is dedicated to the memories of Karen Whitman,
Bernadette Merluzzi, and many prematurely born babies.
Karen, born with a congenital heart problem, died
early in her life journey, when she was 20 years of age.
Bernadette—wife, mother, and professional—died of cancer
in the prime of her life. Their lives and deaths, along with the babies
who could not be saved, have helped us appreciate the importance
of health and life as well as to find meaning in death and dying.

⁂ ❖ ❧

PART I

Background

I

Conceptual Frameworks
for Viewing Health and Illness

Thomas L. Whitman
University of Notre Dame

FROM AN historical perspective, patterns of health and illness have undergone extensive change. In contrast to earlier centuries, people are, on average, living much longer and are afflicted by quite different types of illnesses. Whereas in earlier times people were likely to die of infectious diseases (e.g., smallpox, diphtheria, yellow fever, and influenza), today deaths are more commonly due to noninfectious and sometimes chronic degenerative illnesses, particularly heart disease, cancer, and stroke. The types and causes of "modern" illnesses have also been expanded with the advent of new viruses, toxic substances, and problematic lifestyles. Because people are staying alive longer, they are giving considerable attention to disease prevention and health maintenance. Accompanying this emphasis has come the realization that psychological and socioenvironmental factors play vital roles in the creation and treatment of medical problems.

This chapter examines historical and current concepts of the causes of health and illness. The terms *health* and *illness* have been referred to as concepts on opposite ends of a continuum (Antonovsky, 1979; Sarafino, 1994), with *health* indicating a positive state of physical well-being that varies in degree from illness. *Illness*, at the other end of the spectrum, is characterized by signs, symptoms, and disabilities varying in severity. Whether health and illness are in fact quantitatively different, as this continuum suggests, or qualitatively different, can be debated. An alternative concept emphasizes that although biological, psychological, and environmental factors play a role in both health and illness, the specific types and pattern of factors that increase or maintain healthy states are different from those that produce illness. Moreover, the impact that these various determinants have on health and illness changes in profound ways across the life span as people grow older. A unique contribution of this book lies in its emphasis on a life-span perspective.

Although a life-span approach to the study of human development is no longer as novel a conception as it was several decades ago, psychologists have been slow to adopt this framework for studying and understanding health and illness. As Peterson (1996) pointed out, "too little attention has been directed toward development as a dynamic force that shapes health behaviors" (p. 155). She suggested that health psychologists have viewed age as a static variable, like gender and ethnicity, rather than as a shifting background against which illness and interventions are placed. As individuals grow older, profound biological, cognitive, socioemotional, and behavioral changes occur, along with equally dramatic shifts in the environments in which the developing person resides. Little is known, however, about how these changes, when viewed normatively as well as from an individual difference perspective, influence patterns of health and illness. Peterson (1996) compared the literature in health psychology to "a series of isolated snapshots" of persons of a particular age rather than as a videotape that captures the "rich dynamics of changes" (p. 155).

Ironically, even though developmental changes occur most rapidly during childhood and adolescence, health psychology has focused to a large extent on adults (Peterson, 1996). Moreover, until recently, researchers have paid comparatively little attention to the study of older adults, a developmental period in which occurs rapid change that varies considerably among individuals. As this book points out, researchers seldom examine questions relating to health and illness through the use of either age-comparison or longitudinal designs; instead, they tend to focus on cross-sectional studies of a specific age group. Health psychologists, not unlike developmental psychologists, are generally inclined to focus on one age group to the exclusion of others. Peterson (1996) suggested that even among scientists who identify themselves as developmentalists, few are prepared through training or experience to work with both children and adults. As a consequence, many models of health and illness have limited external validity, in that they are age-restricted, paying minimal attention to the relations between changes in developmental processes and changes in health status.

The first section of this chapter examines some of the historical ways that philosophers, biologists, psychoanalysts, psychiatrists, and psychologists have thought about the causes of illness and more generally the relation between the mind and body. The next section summarizes specific models for conceptualizing how biological, psychological, and environmental factors influence health or illness. The chapter concludes with a discussion of a life-span perspective on health and illness.

HISTORICAL BACKGROUND

An intimate relation between psychology and medicine has existed since ancient times, even before their inception as modern scientific disciplines. For example, the Greeks (Hippocrates, ca. 460–ca 370 B.C., Galen, 129–ca. 199) proposed a humoral theory of illness in which specific personality types were associated with specific temperaments, which, in turn, were associated with a mixture of body fluids—blood, black bile, yellow bile, and phlegm. Illness occurred when these fluids became out of balance. Although many early philosophers speculated about the relation of physical and psychological components of human beings, formal consideration of the connection of the mind and the body was catalyzed by the French philosopher René Descartes (1596–1650). Historically, philosophers' views have varied on the nature of this connection and whether the mind and body are part of the same system or are two separate systems.

Descartes is often credited with formulating the mind–body problem. This problem, which postulates the existence of two distinct components of human action, the mind and body, is concerned with how these entities interact. A variety of resolutions to this problem has been suggested by philosophers, biologists, and psychologists, including dualistic solutions (e.g., psychophysical parallelism and interactionism) and monistic solutions (idealism and materialism). Psychophysical parallelism accepts the dichotomy of mind and body, postulating that their activities can be explained by completely separate principles. For example, the actions of mind have been related to the existence of innate ideas or the "will," whereas the actions of the body have been explained by a variety of naturalistic (biological and environmental) causes. An interactionistic resolution to the mind–body problem suggests variously that the mind causes bodily action, the body influences mental activity or that the mind and body influence one another (reciprocal interactionism). Descartes suggested that involuntary motor responses could be explained by physical (hydraulic) principles, whereas intentional action was produced by the mind. Although Descartes seemed to favor the position that the mind and body were separate systems, he allowed for the possibility of the mind's controlling the body through the pineal gland.

In contrast, monistic solutions to the mind–body problem do not accept the basic proposition of dualists such as Descartes, advocating either that only the mind exists (idealism) or that only the body exists (materialism). Although these monistic positions have often been characterized as extremist, they are represented, in more moderate forms, in modern day psychology by proponents of constructivism and physiological psychology. Constructivists suggest that our conceptions (perceptions) of our environment are mental constructions that are innately determined as a function of the structure of the mind. These constructions might or might not correspond with more objective views of physical reality. In contrast, physiological psychologists reduce mental as well as physical activity to neurobiological events that are naturalistically (biologically and environmentally) determined.

With the advent of psychology as a discipline, early psychologists in the late 19th and early 20th century were concerned more with the activities of the mind (psyche) than the body. Employing introspective methods, they focused on understanding the composition of the mind (structuralism) as did Wilhelm Wundt, or they focused on examining how ideas emerged and the purpose they served (functionalism), as did William James. Essentially, proponents of the these positions left the study of the body mostly to the biologists. Other psychologists, such as Wolfgang Koehler, showed some interest in the body but viewed the mind and body as basically separate and noninteracting entities (gestaltism). With the advent of behaviorism, a reductionistic and monistic type of solution to the study of the mind–body problem emerged.

John Watson, the father of behaviorism, suggested that the mind, if it indeed existed, could not be scientifically studied, and that the focus of psychology should be on the naturalistic study of behavior, which was composed of motor and glandular responses. Watson stressed that learning and development occurred as a consequence of environmental influence on behavior, which was basically reflexive in orientation. He was greatly influenced by Russian physiologists including Sechenov, Bekhterev, and Pavlov. Sechenov argued that all behavior—whether animal, human, physical, psychological, conscious, unconscious, voluntary, or involuntary—was biological and reflexive in nature and that biologists should study the problems of psychology through objective experimental methods. Bekhterev further suggested that even social behavior could be explained through a "collective reflexology." Pavlov demonstrated how reflexive behaviors could become associated with new stimuli through the process of associative learning, specifically, via classical conditioning. Thus, for Watson and the Russian physiologists, psychological functioning was reduced to biological and environmental events.

In contrast to the biological and reductionistic orientation of early behaviorists such as Watson, Freud, although a physician, acknowledged the importance of mind and body. He suggested that some biological symptoms, such as hysterical paralysis, have their roots in underlying psychological conflicts which have social and historical origins. Freud's theory emphasized the importance of both biological (the id), psychological (ego and superego), and environmental influences on personality development and psychopathology. His theory stands in marked contrast to that proposed by many of his fellow physicians who adhered to a medical model of behavior. According to a strict medical model, biological as well as many psychological symptoms occur as a consequence of an underlying biological (disease) processes, with the treatment of choice for both types of symptoms, not surprisingly, also being medical or biological in orientation.

Several developments attenuated the influence of the medical model as a way of understanding physical illnesses. First, due in large part to the emergence of psychoanalysis and psychiatry, the field of psychosomatic medicine evolved, catalyzed by the formation of the American Psychosomatic Society and the publication of *Psychosomatic Medicine* in 1939. Research and theory in this area suggested psychological causes, particularly emotional conflicts, for health problems including ulcers, asthma, high blood pressure, and migraine headaches. As a consequence of this movement, a limited number of medical problems were seen as psychologically influenced. One criticism of the psychosomatic movement, however, was that it underestimated the range of medical disorders influenced by psychological factors (Taylor, 1995).

Behavior medicine, which emerged as a subarea of behavior therapy in the 1970s, further diminished the dominance of the medical model. During the 1970s, the *Journal of Behavioral Medicine* was founded and the Society of Behavior Medicine was formed. In contrast to psychosomatic medicine, which emphasized the underlying psychological (cognitive and emotional) roots of some diseases, behavior medicine viewed biological responses, both normal and pathological, as behaviors that were environmentally as well as psychologically influenced via principles derived from classical conditioning, operant conditioning, and social learning theory. Diverse problems, including alcoholism, pain, nausea, headaches, epilepsy, and cancer, were asserted to be, at least in part, socially or environmentally caused. A variety of behavioral therapeutic procedures, such as biofeedback, aversion therapy, extinction, positive reinforcement, and cognitive behavior therapy, were developed to treat somatic symptoms. Moreover, many of these procedures were also directed at maintaining and enhancing health behaviors.

Matarazzo distinguished between the fields of behavior medicine and behavior health in an article in the *American Psychologist* (Matarazzo, 1980). According to him, "behavioral medicine is the interdisciplinary field concerned with the development and integration of behavioral and biomedical science knowledge and techniques relevant to health and illness and the application of this knowledge and these techniques to prevention, diagnosis, treatment and rehabilitation" (p. 812). In contrast, "behavioral health is an interdisciplinary field dedicated to promoting a philosophy of health that stresses individual responsibility in the application of behavioral and biomedical science knowledge and techniques to the maintenance of health and the prevention of illness and dysfunction by a variety of self-initiated individual or shared activities" (p. 813).

Thus, from a behavioral perspective, health and illness in general, not just the specific diseases suggested by proponents of the psychosomatic medicine, are influenced by a diversity of factors that are psychological, social, environmental, as well as biological in nature. Behavioral therapists not only directed their attention to the development of specific treatment and prevention techniques but also considered more generally the roles of other factors, such as self-regulatory processes, the patient–practitioner relationship, patient knowledge and attitudes about disease, conditioned emotional responses, and the physical features of medical treatment environments, as determinants of health and illness.

Another movement, closely related to that initiated by behavior therapists, emerged in the late 1970s, marked by the formation of the Division of Health Psychology (Division 38) in the American Psychological Association and the development of a new journal *Health Psychology*. Joseph Matarazzo (1980), the first president of Division 38, defined *health psychology* as "the aggregate of specific educational, scientific, and professional contributions of the discipline of psychology to the promotion and maintenance of health, the prevention and treatment of illness, and the identification of etiologic and diagnostic correlates of health, illness, and related dysfunction" (p. 815). Historically, the health psychology movement differed from the behavioral medicine movement in its more exclusive psychological orientation, the extent of its emphasis on the promotion and maintenance of health and the prevention of illness, and in the diversity of the psychological models (e.g., social, cognitive) it employed for understanding and promoting health. Moreover, the health psychology movement also focused at a more molar level on how medical delivery systems and social policies affect health and illness.

In summary, when viewed from a historical perspective, a panorama of conceptions regarding the interrelationship of psychological and biological processes and the determinants of health and illness have been put forth. Increasingly, the influence of psychological and environmental factors on physical functioning, health maintenance, illness, and recovery from illness have been stressed. For a more extensive discussion of the mind–body problem and historical perspectives on the relations between psychology and medicine, the reader is referred to Brennan (1991), Leahey (1992), and Taylor (1995).

MODELS FOR VIEWING HEALTH AND ILLNESS

In this section, I examine more explicitly dominant conceptual frameworks for understanding health and illness. In an attempt to explain how people become sick, researchers and practitioners have emphasized to varying degrees the importance of biological, psychological, and environmental factors. Earlier conceptual models tended to be more univariate in nature, suggesting simple casual explanations, whereas recently more complex multifactorial models have been put forth. Four of these models are described briefly here, including a biomedical, a psychological, and an environmental model as well as a hybrid of these three models—a biopsychoenvironmental model.

Biomedical Model

The biomedical model has dominated the way society has conceptualized health and illness for the past century. As Taylor (1995) pointed out, the biomedical model is reductionistic, defining illness in terms of biological processes, such as hormonal imbalances and neurophysiological abnormalities, rather than considering the role of psychological and social factors (see Fig. 1.1). Since the development of the microscope and modern laboratory techniques, evidence has been provided for the view that illness is caused by underlying disease processes. Literally hundreds of pathogens have been isolated as causes of illnesses, such as smallpox, mumps, measles, rabies, influenza, polio, and malaria. Researchers have also discovered the genetic bases of a multitude of physical anomalies, such as Down syndrome and phenylketonuria, as well as advanced our understanding of the

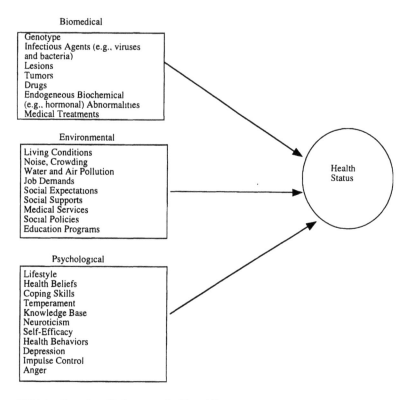

Biomedical

Genotype
Infectious Agents (e.g., viruses
and bacteria)
Lesions
Tumors
Drugs
Endogeneous Biochemical
(e.g., hormonal) Abnormalities
Medical Treatments

Environmental

Living Conditions
Noise, Crowding
Water and Air Pollution
Job Demands
Social Expectations
Social Supports
Medical Services
Social Policies
Education Programs

Psychological

Lifestyle
Health Beliefs
Coping Skills
Temperament
Knowledge Base
Neuroticism
Self-Efficacy
Health Behaviors
Depression
Impulse Control
Anger

Health
Status

FIG 1.1.   Domains of influence on health and illness.

genetic foundation of such traits as intelligence and temperament. The Human Genome Project, a federally funded project now in progress, promises to yield a highly specific map of genetically caused disorders. In addition, developmental biologists have provided considerable information concerning how embryological and fetal development can be disrupted by teratogenic agents, such as alcohol and rubella.

Testimony to the success of the biomedical model is the multitude of potent diagnostic techniques (e.g., magnetic resonance imaging and position emission tomography), medications, vaccines, and surgical procedures that have been developed. As a consequence of these developments, many diseases have been virtually eradicated (e.g., smallpox), prevented (e.g., rubella and tetanus) or successfully treated. The biomedical model has also provided insights into a range of psychological problems (e.g., mania, depression, dementia, and hyperactivity). Although the biomedical model has been indisputably successful, it has paid little attention to the influence of psychological and environmental factors on illness. Moreover, because of its disease orientation, it has tended to view health as the absence of disease rather than as a state that can be actively promoted.

Another aspect of the biomedical model is that it emphasizes the importance of maturational factors in physical development, a process, genetically influenced, which, under favorable environmental circumstances, is more or less automatic and sequentially invariant in its unfolding. Physical development involves a variety of changes, for example, in general stature (weight and height), organ structure (brain, heart), skeletal, muscular and neurological features, hormonal production and reproductive capabilities. Moreover, physical development is associated with a unique pattern of biological risk and protective mechanisms which have implications for health and illness. These are discussed in chapter 2.

The Psychological Model

The psychological model is in part an outgrowth of the psychosomatic medicine, behavioral medicine, and health psychology movements discussed previously. Whereas the biomedical model emphasizes the biological substrates of illness, the psychological model stresses the role of the cognitive, emotional, and behavioral systems in the development of illnesses (see Fig. 1.1).

The cognitive system includes sensory, perceptual, memory, thought, reasoning, and language processes. With growth and development humans acquire new cognitive capabilities, such as an increase in knowledge and the ability to think abstractly. They also show new capacities for monitoring and thinking about issues relating to health and illness. The psychological model recognizes that people's knowledge, beliefs, and attitudes about issues such as their susceptibility to illness, their role in producing and treating illness, the nature of their illness, their prognosis, the medical personnel who treat them, and the medical procedures used in their treatment programs, can influence whether they engage in health-promoting behaviors, contract a disease, comply with a treatment regimen, or recover from an illness.

The psychological model also postulates a critical relation between people's emotional status and the state of their health. People who are in poorer emotional health have more physical problems and need greater medical care (Taylor, 1995). Considerable research has demonstrated the connection between emotional states, such as anxiety and depression, and the incidence of physical illness. Personal stress has also been related to disorders such as arthritis, asthma, back pain, cancer, cardiovascular disease, diabetes, glaucoma, headaches, hypertension, leukemia, pregnancy complications, stroke, and ulcers.

Finally, in the psychological model, the role of personal behavior in health and illness is stressed. Healthy people are more likely to eat right, exercise frequently, refrain from smoking and excessive alcohol use, get appropriate amounts of sleep, and go to the doctor for routine checkups. People who are sick are more likely to get well if they take appropriate steps to receive medical treatment and comply with prescribed treatment regimens. In contrast, individuals who do not engage in these health-engendering behaviors are at increased risk for becoming and staying ill.

More generally, characteristics that distinguish the psychological model from the biomedical model include its greater emphasis on health, prevention of illness, and the critical role that people play in maintaining their own health. People are viewed as bearing at least partial responsibility for their illness and recovery rather than as being passive recipients of pathogens and medical care. Utilizing a psychological conceptual framework, researchers have developed a range of educational and therapeutic options to assist people with health problems, including cognitive therapy, behavior modification, stress management, and lifestyle management programs.

The Environmental Model

Whereas the biomedical and psychological models emphasize the relation of characteristics intrinsic to the individual and health or illness, the environmental model stresses how social and physical surroundings can affect a person's physical status (see Fig. 1.1). These environmental factors include diverse agents such as chemical pollutants, noise, lighting, radiation, biotoxins, sanitation, neighborhood, peer groups, parents, schools, job settings, day-care facilities, television, medical services, and natural disasters. For example, individuals learn healthy and unhealthy behaviors and attitudes from significant others, such as parents, teachers, and friends, both through the examples set and through the information they provide. Moreover, social environments influence the health of individuals through the mass media (television, radio, magazines, newspapers and the Internet). The media can promote or hinder healthy behaviors through editorials, advertisements, and movies that deal directly or indirectly with topics such as dietary habits, exercise, sexual behavior, seat belt usage, smoking, drinking, reckless driving, and physical violence. This model also acknowledges the effect that government policies, such as those regarding pollution, crime, health care, education, the economy, and welfare, can have on a citizen's health. Local, state, and national governments, along with other community organizations, promote health through enactment of laws, law enforcement, agency funding, and educational programs.

Biopsychoenvironmental Model

This model is built on the assumption that biological, psychological, and environmental factors all combine to influence health and illness. Some authors refer to this as the *biopsychosocial* model (e.g., Taylor, 1995). The descriptor *environmental,* in contrast to *social,* is employed in this chapter because it recognizes the critical role that nonsocial as well as social factors play in health and illness. Different versions of this model can be generated based on how these three factors (biological, psychological, and environmental) exert their influence. One variation is that each of these factors plays a distinctive and independent role in determining a person's health (an additive model—see Fig. 1.1). Another variation, and one that health psychologists generally prefer, is that these factors operate interdependently and interactively as part of a complex system. That is, each of the components in this system, including an individual's health status, exerts, in a reciprocal fashion, influences on the other components (see Fig. 1.2). Ultimately, the psychological, environmental, and biological components manifest their effects through a biological substrate to produce health and illness. Health and illness not only are biological states but also psychological and social ones. These states in turn exert influence on the entire system through their continuing impact on each other.

To articulate this model further, a brief overview of systems theory, risk–resiliency, and stress–coping conceptualizations are examined. Each of these conceptualizations provide insights into the dynamic interplay of the components in the biopsychoenvironmental model and the manner in which they affect physical health.

Systems Theory. Miller and Miller (1992) defined a *system* as "a set of interacting units with relationships among them in which the state of each unit is constrained by, conditioned by or dependent upon the state of other units" (p. 11). The units of a system can sometimes be thought of as subsystems, which, in turn,

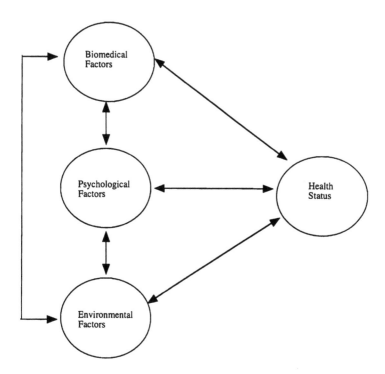

FIG 1.2.   Reciprocal influences operating in a biopsychoenvironmental model.

can be broken down into their own separate interactive components. The systems perspective stands in distinctive contrast to conceptions that suggest that the components of an object depend little on one another and that these components can be examined in isolation and then reintegrated in a summative fashion to understand the object of study.

When health and illness are viewed within the context of a biopsychoenvironmental system, a person's biological condition, psychological status and surrounding environment not only exert direct influences on health, but, in addition, each of these components in turn may influence one another and thereby indirectly affect health (see Fig. 1.2). For example, a person who perceives (psychological component) his co-workers in a job setting (environmental component) as unsupportive, feels stressed and consequently misses work (a psychological component), then experiences increasing stress as a consequence of avoiding work (psychological component), and manifests a state of high physiological arousal (biological component) that over time leads to an ulcer (health outcome). Another example shows a quite different relation among these components: a person drinks too much at a party (psychological component), has a hangover the next day (biological component), consequently is inattentive (psychological component) at work (environmental component), and gets his hand caught in a machine and is injured (health outcome).

As mentioned previously, each of the components in the biopsychoenvironmental system can be broken down further into subcomponents to form subsystems. As suggested in earlier examples, a variety of transactive relations might exist in the psychological subsystem (a person's cognitions, emotions, and behaviors) and between this subsystem's components and the other components of the system to influence a person's health. To illustrate further, a man who perceives himself as incompetent (cognitive subcomponent) at work (environmental subcomponent) becomes depressed (emotional subcomponent) and does not eat properly (behavioral subcomponent). Consequently his immunity (biological component) is reduced, leading him to be susceptible to a cold virus brought home by his son who caught it at day care (environmental component), and as a result the man catches a cold (health outcome).

Risk, Resiliency, and Health. Conceptualizations concerning risk and resiliency provide another way of thinking about the *systemic* relationship of the components of the biopsychoenvironmental model and how they influence health and illness. Why are infants and older adults at greater risk of getting sick than younger adults? Why do some older adults seem to have more health problems than others? Some insight into these issues can be gained by considering the notion of risk and resiliency.

Coie et al. (1993) indicated that the salience of specific risk factors might vary with development, with some risk factors operating to a greater extent during a particular period of development. The authors also suggest that a combination of risk factors have cumulative "exposure effects" (p. 1014), with populations that manifest multiple risk characteristics more likely to experience adverse health outcomes than populations displaying one risk characteristic. For example, persons who are exposed to a cold virus generally are at even greater risk for developing a cold if they are eating inappropriately, are not getting enough sleep, and are under stress at work. In general, an age group might be considered at risk for illness to the extent that the individuals in that group possess characteristics (biological, psychological, or environmental) that are associated with adverse health outcomes. For example, preterm infants are at increased risk for medical problems, such as bronchopulmonary dysplasia (lung damage) and intraventricular hemorrhage (bleeding in brain), because of factors such as immature lung and vascular development (biological component), limited self-regulatory behaviors (psychological component), and environmental stressors, such as bright hospital lighting. As another example, older people are at greater risk for broken bones because of calcium deficiencies and reduced muscle mass.

Although some populations, such as preterm infants, are at increased risk for adverse health outcomes, specific individuals in such populations do not always manifest these outcomes. These individuals are often referred to as *resilient*. Resiliency has been referred to as "the process of, capacity for, or outcome of successful adaptation despite challenging or threatening circumstances" (Masten, Best, & Garmezy, 1990, p. 426). Resiliency has been used to describe (a) favorable outcomes despite high risk status, (b) sustained competence under threat, and (c) recovery from trauma (Masten et al., 1990; Werner, 1994). Research on resiliency is generally directed at isolating protective factors that moderate the effects of a person's vulnerability to risk. Protective factors are associated with positive outcomes in members of a population, which, because of its high risk status, often experiences negative outcomes. That is, protective factors can serve to make an individual who is at risk more resilient. Both personal characteristics (e.g., healthy lifestyle) or characteristics of the environment (e.g., availability of social supports) can serve a protective function. Rutter (1987) suggested that the crucial difference between risk and protective factors is that risk factors lead directly to a disorder, whereas protective factors operate via their interaction with risk factors. Many factors can serve variously as either protective or risk agents. For example, good social supports can act as protective factors moderating the adverse effects of job stress on health. Conversely, poor social supports can act as risk factors by not providing assistance to an individual experiencing job stress.

Whereas Rutter (1987) suggested that risk factors lead directly to a disorder and that in certain instances risk factors might be moderated by protective factors, it also is likely that the influence of risk factors may sometimes be mediated by protective factors. For example, the extent of influence of a flu virus on a person's health may depend on the person's immune system and its ability to fight the virus, with people with better immunity being better able to ward off the virus and its adverse effects on health. Generally, mediational explanations provide insights into specific processes through which a risk factor exerts its influence. In this regard, Baldwin, Baldwin, and Cole (1990) distinguished between distal and proximal risk factors. Distal risk factors, such as low socioeconomic status, do not affect a child directly. Their effects are mediated by proximal risk factors, such as inadequate diet and poor health care. For another discussion of mediating and moderating variables, the reader is referred to chapters 7 and 9 in this volume.

Many of the factors in Fig. 1.1 can be thought of variously as either protective or risk factors. For example, persons who have good eating habits (diet) might be protected from getting a cold, whereas if their eating habits (diet) are poor, they might be at risk for getting a cold. Individuals often have a mixed profile of risk and protective factors. The constituents of a protective factor also depend on the nature of the risk situation. For example, psychological factors can influence whether one gets a cold but have no or little effect on determining the course of a lethal genetic disorder. Finally, it is also possible for certain factors to serve simultaneously a protective or risk function. For example, a jogger, through the aerobic benefits of running, may be at less risk (protected) for developing high blood pressure, but may be a greater risk for developing knee problems.

Masten et al. (1990) pointed out that although resiliency research has yielded descriptive information concerning the factors that allow individuals to adapt in problematic situations and place them at risk for negative outcomes, it has yielded little insight into the underlying processes that influence adaption. Some of these insights are provided by a closely related research area that examines how people cope with stressful situations.

Stress and Coping. A stress and coping framework shares many similarities with risk–resiliency conceptualizations, however, it provides another perspective for viewing the interrelationship of the factors in Figs 1.1 and 1.2, which can be variously thought about as potential stressors or coping resources. In this framework, impairments to health are postulated to be a consequence of an organism's inability to cope with internal and external stressors. *Stress* is typically defined in terms of a situational demand and a negative emotional experience accompanied by cognitive, biological, and behavioral responses. Most definitions of stress emphasize the relation of a person experiencing stress to an event that acts as a stressor. These stressors vary widely and include such diverse events as divorce, family illness, job loss, birth of a child, leaving home, noise, and bright lights. Events in the individual, such as fatigue, disease, hormonal changes, or low self-esteem can also serve as stressors. Although certain events are stressful for most people (e.g., a death in the family or major surgery), the degree to which individuals actually experience specific events as stressful varies considerably. For example, individuals might react to a particular stressor differently (such as getting the measles), depending on their ages and age-related characteristics.

According to Lazarus and Folkman (1984), for individuals to experience stress they must evaluate an event as harmful or threatening (primary appraisal) and their coping resources as insufficient to overcome this event (secondary appraisal). The assumption that cognitive appraisal is always necessary for an event to be experienced as stressful, however, has been challenged (Repetti, 1993). For example, preterm infants who have no formal appraisal capabilities often show physiological signs of stress when exposed to bright lights or noise.

Selye's work (1956) provides insight into the ways stress leads to physical illness. Selye suggested that organisms confronting a stressor go through several characteristic stages. They become physiologically mobilized, then attempt to try to cope with the stressor, and finally, if coping is unsuccessful, experience exhaustion. Continuous exposure to a stressor along with prolonged exhaustion can lead to biological damage and disorders, such as hypertension, ulcers, or coronary heart disease. From a physiological perspective, stress might influence physical functioning through different pathways, specifically through the actions of sympathetic-adrenomedullary, pituitary-adrenocortical, peptide, and immune systems; for example through the release of a variety of agents, including catecholamines and corticosteroids. Some individuals appear to be more reactive to potential stressors than others, a temperamental trait strongly influenced by genetics. Individuals also vary concerning the organ systems that are most affected by stress (Taylor, 1995).

Ultimately, whether individuals experience stress depends in large part on their coping characteristics. These coping characteristics, which can be personal or social in nature, dictate how much stress is actually experienced. Common personal coping characteristics cited in the literature include hardiness, optimism, internal locus of control, high self-esteem, high self-efficacy, and religiousness. Although these general characteristics do not constitute specific behavioral coping mechanisms, they relate to an attitude about the world, for example, that life's stressors are manageable, that personal effort can be effective, and that things will turn out all right. In addition to such characteristics, effective coping often involves having specific problem-solving skills, knowledge regarding the nature of the stressors, strategic knowledge about how to handle stress, behavioral skills, and experience. Such personal resources serve to buffer the adverse effects of stressors. Similarly, people with good social resources (e.g., family, friends, co-workers, church group, and social agencies) are often more effective in coping with stress because they are provided with emotional, instrumental, and physical assistance. Physical illness often results if a person's social, psychological, and biological resources for coping with a stressor are overtaxed.

Summary. Comparisons of the risk–resiliency and stress–coping conceptualizations of health and illness reveal many similarities. Events that place a person at risk for health problems, such as violent environments or viruses, are potential stressors. A person's resiliency in dealing with a stressor depends on his or her coping resources, which in the risk–resiliency framework are referred to as protective mechanisms. When viewed within a systems framework, risk factors and stressors

along with coping resources and protective mechanisms, are transactionally related to one another and in conjunction influence health and illness. Both stressors
(risk factors) and coping resources (protective mechanisms) can be biological,
psychological, or environmental in nature (see Figs. 1.1 and 1.2).

LIFE-SPAN DEVELOPMENTAL
CONCEPTUALIZATIONS OF HEALTH

This book considers risk–resiliency, stress–coping, as well as other conceptualizations of health and illness in a life-span context. More specifically, biological,
psychological and environmental influences on health status are considered for
the major periods of human development from both normative and individual
difference perspectives. That is, characteristic functioning and common health
problems are described in major age groups, along with the role that individual
differences in age-related characteristics play in health and illness. Through this
presentation, I show how changes in biological and psychological functioning
across the life span, as well as in the environments surrounding the developing individual, can create a unique pattern of risk and protective factors, stressors and
coping mechanisms that differentially influence health and illness.

Overview

Life-span developmental theory is directed at understanding how individuals
change through the course of their lives, that is, how they develop. As Baltes and
Graf (1996) pointed out, "development is a lifelong process and . . . each stage of
aging is not only the result of age specific but also of life-span precursor conditions" (p. 431). In other words, aging is influenced by current and past events. They
also emphasized that with development, both positive and negative changes occur
in behavior and its underlying structure. As these changes transpire, new processes
are mobilized, with behaviors selected that allow for optimal adaption to new circumstances. Because development goes on from birth to death, life-span theory
does not emphasize any one age period over any other.

Hoyer and Rybash (1996) stressed that aging (and development) not only is
multidirectional but also multidimensional, with "variability in [both] the rate
and direction (gains and losses) of change for different characteristics within the
individual and across individuals" (p. 65). Development is influenced by age-
related normative (e.g., the maturational processes), history-related (e.g., the
Great Depression and the Vietnam War), as well as nonnormative idiosyncratic
factors (such as an automobile accident) that vary from individual to individual.
Sometimes the adaptive process reflects compensations for deficiencies in a particular domain of development. Thus, aging is a complex phenomenon and often is
not uniform across different domains of development, varying substantially de-

pending on biogenetic processes and historical–cultural conditions and generally less optimized in later life.

Nevertheless, there is plasticity and resiliency throughout the life span as individuals age (Hoyer & Rybash, 1996). *Plasticity* refers to an individual's potential for change and adaption in the presence of a changing environment, biological challenges, and social demands. Staudinger, Marsiske, and Baltes (1993) described resilience as one type of plasticity, involving either a person's maintenance of functioning and normal development in the face of internal or external stressors or risk factors or recovery of function if development is interrupted. Another type of plasticity involves a person's growing beyond a normal level of functioning. The extent of plasticity is a function of a person's protective mechanisms and coping resources or what Staudinger et al. (1993) referred to as *reserve capacity.* Protective factors not only help maintain functioning in a person at risk because of internal or external challenges but also allow the person to grow in spite of (or because of) these challenges. Coping resources are directed at helping a person maintain or recover functioning when stressed.

As a person enters his or her later years or when an individual is confronted with intense stressors (such as a serious illness), personal resources are more likely to be directed at maintenance or recovery of functioning than to growth. When an individual is faced with multiple, intense, or sustained challenges, coping resources might become depleted. Coping resources and protective mechanisms are social, cognitive, emotional, and biological in nature, as are the developmental domains they influence, and have developmental trajectories that change as a function of age-related, history-related and nonnormative influences. As Hoyer and Rybash (1996) pointed out, there are "age-related differences in the extent to which the individual is or can be active in determining the course of aging" (p. 67). They distinguished between primary and secondary aging. *Primary aging* is a relatively predictable process that occurs in the absence of disease and that ultimately affects all systems of the individual. This "normal" developmental process can, however, be sped up by factors such as stress and disease, thus resulting in *secondary aging.* Not surprisingly, the study of development from a life-span perspective is multidisciplinary involving both the biological and social sciences (see Baltes, 1987; Baltes & Graf, 1996; Hoyer & Rybash, 1996; and Staudinger et al., 1993, for a more complete discussion of these characteristics of life-span development).

Health Perspectives

When examined within a life-span framework, health can also be viewed as a developmental construct similar to other personal characteristics. It is a lifelong process that is multidirectional, involves gains (growth) and losses (decline), and is multidimensional, sometimes involving greater change in one domain of health (e.g., skeletal–muscular) than another (e.g., cardiovascular). Nevertheless, change in one domain often, if not inevitably, has implications for change in other domains. Changes in physical functioning can be viewed as moving progressively toward a positive end of a continuum (health) or toward a negative end (illness, death). As a dynamic process, health changes occur as a result of adaptation to changing biological, psychological, and environmental and cultural conditions.

Protective mechanisms (e.g., a good diet) allow a person to maintain or improve health. Health, similar to other developmental domains (e.g., cognition), is an outcome influenced not only by concurrent factors (such as sleep, exercise, and eating patterns) but also by historical (e.g., early medical care) factors. Personal health is also influenced by the cultural context and changes in this context, such as the advent of health maintenance organizations (HMOs). Cultural attitudes affect individual attitudes and the value placed on health programs and specific health-engendering behaviors. As health deteriorates (e.g., in old age or because of chronic disease), individuals engage in efforts to cope with structural and functional changes in behavior. Sometimes when recovery from a health problem is not possible, they compensate for such changes by directing their efforts elsewhere (selective optimization). For example, an older person who can no longer engage in activities such as tennis and basketball might take up golf or walking or spend more time reading. Although it is debatable whether health actually develops the way other biological and psychological processes do, changes in health certainly occur as a consequence of development in these domains. As indicated in Fig. 1.2, health is embedded in a complex system in which the individual components dynamically change and develop over time.

The question of whether one age group might be considered healthier or more at risk for illness than another age group is an interesting one. For example, it could be argued that infants are healthier than adults because the catabolic processes that gradually erode body structures and processes have had less time to operate. Conversely, it is known that infants and young children are more at risk for many illnesses than adults because their immune system processes are still developing. Closer examination of this question points out that general statements about health or illness are overly simplistic, given that different biological (and psychological) systems have different developmental trajectories (see chapter 2, this volume). Just as different age groups might have unique and complex constellations of health indicators, so too do individuals within age groups. A system perspective suggests that even though a person might be healthy at a particular time, a specific problem (e.g., diabetes), if uncontrolled, can have adverse generalized effects on functioning.

As development occurs, the types of biological, psychological, and environmental events (e.g., school, puberty, job, marriage, retirement) that serve as stressors change. Similarly, coping resources change, as the child or adult becomes more self-regulatory and independent of parental supports; as sensory, motor, cognitive, and socioemotional competencies evolve; and as biological systems, such as the neurological and immunological, mature and later begin to deteriorate. For some individuals, the intensity and range of stressors might be greater due to the envi-

ronments they live in and their coping resources less adequate due to biological defects and inadequate socialization. The health implications of these types of individual differences have yet to be fully explored.

When health and illness are examined from a life-span developmental perspective, a myriad of questions, such as the following, are generated: How do patterns
of health and illness vary across the life span with molar variables including social
class, ethnicity, race, and gender? How do genes influence health and illness across
the life span? How do brain development and hormonal changes affect health?
Why are some individuals in an age group healthier than others? How do parents
and peers influence health attitudes and behaviors? How do the changes that accompany the development of the motor, cognitive, and psychosocial systems influence health? To what extent is age of patient taken into consideration in developing
medical prevention and treatment programs? Do our government programs and
social policies take age into consideration in addressing health issues?

This book is dedicated to examining these types of questions, to showing how a
life-span developmental framework can provide new insights into the factors that
influence health and illness, to suggesting new approaches to formulating prevention and intervention programs, and to generating a different type of research
agenda. The biological, behavioral, socioemotional, and cognitive characteristics
of different age groups (infancy, childhood, adolescence, and adulthood) are examined, along with their environments, to improve our understanding of how
age-related characteristics influence specific patterns of health and illness. Moreover, this volume addresses how types of health problems, causes of illness, and
challenges to health vary. Two underlying assumptions are developed in this book:
First, to understand health and illness both in and across age groups, individual
differences in biological, psychological, and environmental characteristics must all
be considered. Second, the factors that determine health status across the life span,
although sometimes similar, also differ considerably depending on a person's developmental status. Thus, we attempt to provide insights into the reasons that patterns of health and illness are different across age groups and the reasons that
health status varies across members of specific age groups.

Specific chapters examine how the major biological systems of the body develop and change from conception to old age and why different age groups have
a different pattern of health risks (chapter 2); the influence of genetic factors on
physical development and health across the life span (chapter 3); the effects of
poverty on the health of different age groups (chapter 4); the types of illnesses that
occur and the factors that influence health status during different major age periods, specifically during the embryonic and fetal stages of development (chapter 5);
infancy (chapter 6); early and middle childhood (chapter 7); adolescence (chapter
8); and adulthood (chapters 10 and 11). The effects of chronic child illness on the
sick individual and his or her family also are discussed (chapter 9). Also examined
is caregiving for chronically ill adults in later life (chapter 12) and the influence of
individual and social factors on the death and dying process (chapter 13). Finally,

patterns of health and illness, causes of illness and prevention or intervention programs are examined more globally from a life-span perspective in the final chapter
and recommendations made regarding age-appropriate treatment programs and
future research (chapter 14). Throughout the book, emphasis is placed on understanding how risk factors, stressors, coping resources, and protective factors,
which vary across individuals and age periods, operate to influence health and
illness.

REFERENCES

Antonovsky, A. (1979). *Health, stress and coping.* San Francisco: Jossey-Bass.
Baldwin, A. L., Baldwin, C., & Cole, R. E. (1990). Stress-resistant families and stress-resistant children.
  In J. Rolf, A. S. Marsten, D. Cicchetti, K. H. Neuchterlein, & S. Weintraub (Eds.), *Risk and protective
  factors in the development of psychopathology* (pp. 257–280). New York: Cambridge University Press.
Baltes, P. B. (1987). Theoretical proposition of life-span developmental psychology: On the dynamic
  between growth and decline. *Developmental Psychology, 23,* 611–626.
Baltes, P. B., & Graf, P. (1996). Psychological aspects of aging: Facts and frontiers. In D. Magnusson,
  T. Grentz, T. Hokfelt, L. G. Nilsson, L. Terenus, & B. Winblad (Eds.), *The lifespan development of individuals: Behavioral, neurobiological, and psychosocial perspectives* (pp. 427–460). New York: Cam-
  bridge University Press.
Brennan, J. F. (1991). *History and systems of psychology* (3rd ed.). Englewood Cliffs, NJ: Prentice-Hall.
Coie, J., Watt, N., West, S., Hawkins, D., Asarnow, J., Markman, H., Ramey, S., Shure, M., & Long, B.
  (1993). The science of prevention: A conceptual framework and some directions for a national research program. *American Psychologist, 48,* 1013–1022.
Hoyer, W., & Rybash, J. (1996). Life span theory. J. E. Birren (Ed.), *Encyclopedia of Gerontology* (Vol. 2,
  pp. 65–71). New York: Academic Press.
Lazarus, R. S., & Folkman, (1984). *Stress, appraisal, and coping.* New York: Springer.
Leahey, T. H. (1992). *A history of psychology: Main currents in psychological thoughts* (3rd ed.). Engle-
  wood Cliffs, NJ: Prentice-Hall.
Masten, A. S., Best, K. M., & Garmezy, N. (1990). Resilience and development: Contributions from the
  study of children who overcome adversity. *Development and Psychopathology, 2,* 425–444.
Matarazzo, J. D. (1980). Behavioral health and behavior medicine: Frontiers for a new health psychol-
  ogy. *American Psychologist, 35,* 807–817.
Miller, J. G., & Miller, J. L. (1992). Cybernetics, general systems theory, and living systems theory. In R. L.
  Levine & H. E. Fitzgerald (Eds.), *Analysis of dynamic psychological systems* (Vol. 1, pp. 9–34). New
  York: Plenum.
Peterson, L. (1996). Establishing the study of development as a dynamic force. *Health Psychology, 15,*
  155–157.
Repetti, R. L. (1993). Short-term effects of occupational stressors on daily mood and health complaints.
  Health Psychology, 12, 125–131.
Rutter, M. (1987). Psychosocial resilience and protective mechanisms. *American Journal of Orthopsychi-
  atry, 57,* 316–331.
Sarafino, E. P. (1994). *Health psychology: Biopsychosocial interactions.* New York: Wiley.
Selye, H. (1956). *The stress of life.* New York: McGraw-Hill.
Staudinger, U. M., Marsiske, M., & Baltes, P. B. (1993). Resilience and levels of reserve capacity in later
  adulthood: Perspectives from life-span theory. *Development and Psychopathology, 5,* 541–566.
Taylor, S. E. (1995). *Health psychology.* New York: McGraw-Hill.
Werner, E. E. (1994). Overcoming the odds. *Developmental and Behavioral Pediatrics, 15,* 131–136.

2

Biological Development and Health Risk

Kathleen J. Sipes Kolberg
University of Notre Dame

THE CAUSES of death change across the life span. Perinatal data, which includes that of stillbirths and neonatal deaths up to 28 days of age, indicates that mortality during this period is predominately associated with congenital anomalies, organ function deficiencies (especially lung, cardiovascular, and digestive), and infectious disease (Guyer, Strobino, Ventura, MacDorman, & Martin, 1996). During infancy and childhood, primary causes of death are accidents and adverse effects,[1] followed by congenital anomalies, cancer, and homicide (Rosenberg, Ventura, & Maurer, 1996). Accidents are also the leading cause of death for individuals aged 15 to 24 years, but homicide and suicide push ahead of cancer as the next most prevalent causes of death. Acquired immunodeficiency syndrome (AIDS) has become the leading cause of death in adults aged 25 to 44 years, followed by accidents and cancer. In the 45-to-64-year age range, death from cancer and heart disease become more frequent than lethal accidents and AIDS. For individuals who reach age 65 and older, accidents fall to the seventh leading cause of death, whereas organ system function problems (cardiovascular, lung, or pancreas), cancer, and infectious disease (non-HIV) become more prevalent again (Rosenberg et al., 1996).

Why do the causes of death change so drastically across the life span? Differences can be attributed to life-span changes in organic, environmental, and psychological risk and resiliency factors. This chapter examines the role of biological factors, specifically the ways various biological systems change with development and how these changes can either protect or place the individual at risk for illness and death.

---

[1] *Adverse effects* covers an array of circumstances including motor vehicle accidents, drowning, fire, firearm accident, falls, choking, neglect, starvation, dehydration, desertion, accidental poisoning, suffocation, adverse effects from medical procedures or drugs, and weather or geologically related incidents.

Some biological models of aging, influenced by nuclear transplantation, cell culture, and programmed cell death research, suggest biological limits of the cellular life span. Other models (e.g., epigenetic model of development) view development and senescence as a dynamic outcome of an interaction between the genotype and the environment, including all gene–environment interactions that have taken place in the life span. From this perspective, development does not occur as a pretimed genetic program that simply unfolds but occurs as a conditional program that depends on the preceding steps and the nature of current environmental inputs. (For further reading on this subject see Michel & Moore, 1995.)

In considering physiological function across the life span, changes previously believed to be simple outcomes of time are viewed in the context of changing cultures and changing environments. For example, there has been widespread belief that muscular atrophy occurs in a biologically automatic fashion as people age. However, research has shown that older adults can retain and regain significant muscle mass with appropriate exercise (Fiatarone et al., 1990). There are, however, differences in the tissues' ability to recover from insult, such as disuse or reduced oxygen supply. For example, nerve tissue is relatively easily damaged by a low oxygen supply and has a limited capacity to regenerate. Other tissues, such as skin, liver, blood, and intestinal and lung linings, can regenerate and recover from acute insult. These high-growth tissues, however, carry another risk—errors in uncontrolled growth (i.e., cancers; Rensberger, 1996). Thus, individual differences seen in many physiological or developmental outcomes depend on lifestyle, biological, and hereditary factors.

As diseases affecting major organ systems are examined, a few basic patterns of disease incidence become apparent (see Table 2.1). Examples of such patterns in-

TABLE 2.1
Patterns of Disease Prevalence as They Pertain to the Life Span
(Derived From Fry & Sandler, 1993)

Pattern	Frequency	Example
Diseases of childhood	Decrease with age	Childhood infectious diseases
Diseases of aging	Increase with age	Coronary artery disease Lung cancer
Diseases of adulthood	Most frequent in early to mid adulthood	Work related injuries Migraine headache Pregnancy complications
Diseases of young and old	Most frequent in infants and elderly	Stroke Infection Immobility Injury from abuse
Persistent	Occur in similar frequency across the life span	Common viral infections Chronic diseases

clude diseases of childhood, which decrease with age, such as childhood infectious diseases; diseases of aging, which increase with age, such as coronary artery disease; diseases of adolescence or adulthood, such as sports injuries or pregnancy complications; and diseases shared by the very young and very old, such as serious infection, intracranial hemorrhage, lack of mobility, and vulnerability to abuse. There are also persistent diseases, which affect all ages groups consistently, such as common viral infections and chronic diseases such as diabetes. Many of these patterns are related to changes in biological systems that occur with development.

The following sections review the ways major organ systems change across the life span, including the bone, muscle, nervous, cardiovascular, endocrine, immune, gut, lung, and urinary systems, and how these changes are associated with disease risk.

BONE DEVELOPMENT

Calcification of the bone begins to occur rather late in fetal development, with bones remaining soft and pliable at birth. In the fluid-filled environment of the uterus, weight-bearing demands on the fetus are minimal and soft bones provide sufficient support for fetal movement. Problems with bone deformations can occur, however, if the uterus constricts the fetus too tightly, as in cases of oligohydramnios (low amniotic fluid volume), premature amniotic sac rupture, multiple fetuses, or a large infant in a small uterus. These bone malformations most commonly occur in the feet or legs and are often treatable with postnatal manipulation, splinting, or casting.

The normally soft fetal bones can constitute a problem for the preterm infant removed from the fluid-filled environment. In premature infants, orthopedic problems in the hip and shoulder girdle have been common, caused by the effects of gravity on the soft bones and lack of support by the underdeveloped muscles and ligaments. However, with the advent of nursing practices in newborn intensive care units (NICUs) that emphasize proper positioning, the severity of this complication of prematurity has been reduced.

For children, high activity levels, accidents, and physical abuse leading to broken bones are a significant source of morbidity, accounting for about 15% of all pediatric injuries. Although this prevalence is often related to psychological factors of the child and caregiver, the severity and complications are related to biological factors. The long bones of children and adolescents have cartilaginous ends, with an epiphyseal growth plate and a thicker layer of surrounding connective tissue, which causes the fracture patterns to be different from adults. Fractures outside of the epiphyseal growth plate tend to heal well, but because bone growth occurs from extension of the epiphyseal plate, fractures in the area of the growth plate are associated with growth arrest and vascular complications within the bone tissue. These complications are most common when the epiphyseal plate is transected and crushed. Fractures of the growth plate account for about 15% of all pediatric fractures (Berkowitz, 1996).

During adolescence, sports-related injuries are a common source of orthopedic injury. Among 13-to-19-year-olds engaging in organized sports, 7% to 11% are injured, with 20% of these sustaining significant injuries. Among adolescents and young adults, considerable force is required to produce a fracture. Males have more fractures than females, and boys tend to have upper body injuries related to football, basketball, and soccer. Overuse injuries of the knee and ankle, often associated with gymnastics, are common in girls (Berkowitz, 1996).

Because of rapid bone growth, adolescents are also vulnerable to orthopedic difficulties other than fractures. For example, idiopathic scoliosis (abnormal lateral curvature of the spine) and slippage of the capital femoral epiphysis (a displacement of the femoral head from the neck of the femur through the area of rapid growth) occur most commonly during adolescence. Also, the onset of bone-based cancers, such as osteogenic sarcoma, is most common during puberty.

Diet is particularly important in the years preceding puberty because bone mass increases most rapidly during this period. Approximately 30% of the vertebral skeletal mass is accumulated in the 3 years surrounding puberty. Disturbances during this critical period of bone deposition may have serious consequences in later life. Anorexia nervosa, affecting both diet and estrogen levels in adolescent women, is associated with deficits in bone mass, particularly in the spine. Although there are few studies regarding anorexia recovery, it appears that bone mass might not fully recover even when normal diet is resumed (Slemenda, 1994).

Once the epiphyseal plates have closed, signaling the end of long bone growth in early adulthood, bone continues an active state of remodeling. Bone is resorbed (dissolved and absorbed) and formed continuously, with rates generally balanced to maintain a stable bone mass in early adulthood. Bone mass peaks at age 30, and after age 40 bone resorption exceeds formation. Bone mass decreases at an average rate of 1% to 2% per year. For women in the first 6 years after menopause, bone loss averages 3.9% per year. Moreover, women at any age have less bone mass than men.

Osteoporosis, a pathological lack of bone matrix (protein of the bone tissue on which the minerals are deposited), not merely low calcification, was once considered an automatic aspect of aging in women. Numerous factors contribute to bone loss, only some of which are related to age. These factors include low estrogen levels (normal in older women and common in anorexic women), smoking, low body weight (thin women have less bone), lack of weight-bearing activity, malnutrition, low levels of growth hormone, ethnicity, diet, very high levels of glucocorticoids, and family history of osteoporosis. With the loss of bone tissue, fractures occur more easily. In contrast to fractures in younger patients, which occur more frequently in males, most fractures in the elderly are seen in females. The common sites of fracture are vertebral, femoral neck (near the end of the femur), and the distal radius (near the wrist).

Treatments of osteoporosis, directed primarily at women, have consisted of additional calcium in the diet pre- and postmenopause, estrogen replacement therapy (ERT), increased exercise during the pre- and postmenopausal periods, and smoking cessation. ERT in postmenopausal women has been found to increase calcium absorption in the intestine, reduce calcium excretion, and increase calcitonin (a hormone that inhibits osteoclast activity and production). One year of progressive resistance exercise at 2 days per week in postmenopausal women reversed the decline in bone density in the lumbar spine and neck of the femur (Nelson et al., 1994).

MUSCLE DEVELOPMENT

Muscular problems in pediatric populations are often environmentally produced by immobilization or trauma and are related to insufficient nervous control and coordination of muscles, such as occurs in cerebral palsy and Erb's palsy. Cerebral palsy is linked to brain bleeds, such as those discussed in the nervous system section, and periventricular leukomalacia, especially in infants with very low birthweight. Erb's palsy, an injury to the upper brachial plexus (spinal nerves C5, C6, and C7), is generally due to a birth injury of large infants who are difficult to deliver because of their size. Erb's palsy can involve shoulder, arm, and diaphragm control, but 70% to 92% recover from the injury completely by age 2 (Brann & Schwartz, 1992).

In contrast, direct muscle tissue disorders (defects in the muscle tissue itself, rather than its control) in childhood are mainly a consequence of genetic abnormalities of the muscle fiber, such as the muscular dystrophies and congenital myopathies. These conditions can affect muscle tissue as it develops and can be progressive in nature, worsening over time. The most common, Duchenne's muscular dystrophy, occurs in 1 out of every 1,700 to 3,500 male births. Inactivity worsens the disability and care involves provision of orthopedic support structures to maintain activity, predisone to stabilize muscle strength, aggressive treatment for respiratory infections, and diet for complications of intestinal motility.

After adolescence, a gradual loss of muscle mass is common. This loss of muscle mass (sarcopenia) was, until recently, considered a natural part of the aging process. Sarcopenia is associated with decreased muscle strength and can result eventually in problems such as limitations in mobility (walking or rising) and inability to perform household lifting. These handicaps are a chief reason why geriatric patients become dependent on others for their welfare. There is also evidence of an association between loss of muscle mass and medical problems, such as hypertension, insulin sensitivity, osteoporosis, and obesity (for a general review see Timiras, 1988).

Recent studies find that sarcopenia is largely preventable and reversible even in the oldest individuals. Regular strength training (2 or 3 days per week) has been found to produce increased muscle mass and strength gains in women and men age 60 to 96 (Fiatarone et al., 1990; Frontera, Meredith, O'Reilly, Knuttgen, & Evans, 1988). For example, an exerise regimen of 3 days per week increased leg strength in men age 60 to 72 by an average of 227% for knee flexor and 107% for knee extensors. Total muscle area increased 11.4% (Frontera et al., 1988). Even nursing home residents, age 87 to 96, showed an average of 170% increase in leg strength after only 8 weeks of resistance training (Fiatarone et al., 1990). Similar results have been seen in postmenopausal women (Nelson et al., 1994). Thus, although sarcopenia is associated with advancing age and can result in a variety of medical problems, it is highly influenced by the environment.

NERVOUS SYSTEM

The role of the nervous system in health is complex and includes physiological regulation, management of physical and psychological stress, control of voluntary musculature, control of hormonal levels, sensing inputs from the environment, and relating these inputs to appropriate behavioral outputs. The functional ability of the nervous system depends on sensory stimulation, healthy central tissue and effectors, and appropriate tissue support (blood supply, oxygenation, etc).

Common medical difficulties associated with the nervous system are associated with problems in physiological control, motor control, cognitive deficits, or behavioral abnormalities. The health of the nervous tissue can be evaluated through assessments of motor and cognitive functioning. It is not clear, however, what constitutes normal declining function as a stage of development and what is pathogenic loss of function; that is, there are no milestones for loss of memory, motor skills, and so on. The pronounced variability in function among the elderly makes determinations of what is "normal" difficult. Imaging techniques, which involve more direct observation of brain tissue, have been helpful in assessing tissue health and have led to advances in the understanding of nervous system functional losses, such as dementia and stroke.

Structure

Development in the brain proceeds prenatally and postnatally with many brain structures developing at different rates. Although the brain proceeds through organogenesis (layout of the brain chambers and spinal cord) very rapidly, the histogenesis (the arrangement of differentiated cells within the tissues) and acquisition of function in the brain occurs more slowly. Postnatally, the brain of the neonate is still undergoing dendritic sprouting and arborization, synapse formation, neuronal pruning, and myelination. These processes continue for years after birth and are influenced greatly by inputs from the environment.

Fetal and infant brain development relies on environmental interaction. Appropriate sensory stimulation is necessary for normal histogenesis of the brain and the development of the sensory nerves. Motor experience also affects the developing nervous system. Areas of histogenesis affected by environmental interaction include production and stability of dendritic spines, dendritic branching, connection with target tissues, and neuronal pruning (the death of excess neurons). The number of cortical synapses and their connectivity is particularly sensitive to input from the environment. Deprivation experiments in animals have shown a decrease in dendritic arborization and an increase in neuronal pruning (Diamond, 1990).

Experiments involving reduction or increase in stimulation have supported the importance of stimulation in sensory development. For example, removing neonatal rat whisker postsynaptic receptors prenatally led to a reorganization of the sensory cortex, eliminating a specific type of cell, which is usually responsible for the cortical sensory function of the whiskers (Woolsey, Durham, Harris, Simons, & Valentino, 1981). Similarly, studies of visual stimulation deprivation have been found to produce visual cortex atrophy in kittens and rhesus monkeys (Hubel & Wiesel, 1963; Kennedy et al., 1981). Studies of stimulation-deprived children show that brain development might be similarly restricted, leading to reduced school success or mental retardation (Coates & Lewis, 1984; Herber & Garber, 1975). In contrast, extra stimulation of specific digits on the owl monkey's hand has been found to increase representation of those digits in the cortical map (Jenkins, Merzenich, Ochs, Allard, & Guic-Robles, 1990) and numerous studies have demonstrated correlation between physical and social stimulation and achievement on cognitive tests (for a review see Tamis-LeMonda & Bornstein, 1987).

In the fetus, sensory modalities become functional at different times, proceeding through touch and vestibular, smell and taste, auditory, and finally visual. At full-term birth in humans, sensory development is fairly complete, although the visual system will continue to mature through infancy. Auditory response at a physiologic level occurs in the second trimester of prenatal development; cortical processing of the auditory stimulus occurs later in the third trimester. This two-step maturation actually can be a problem for younger preterm infants, with loud noises producing a full-body physiological startle that causing problems with breathing, heart rate, and blood pressure, which sometimes requires clinical management (Als et al., 1994). By the third trimester, higher sensory cortical processing enables more physiologic stability when older preterm and full-term infants are exposed to loud noises. Management of appropriate sensory exposure is likely important for further brain development.

The neural tissue structure in the fetus and neonate differs from that found in the brain of an older child or adult. The cerebral cortex of the newborn and later fetus has a higher numbers of neurons but fewer dendrites and mature synapses. The neuronal membranes are more easily depolarized. There is less isolation of output tracts, resulting in a more global response to stimulation. Instead of a specific response to an object or action, premature and newborn infants show full body reactions (with premature infants also having an adverse basic physiological response in heart rate and respiration). By full term, neuronal function is closer to mature function, but it still has incomplete isolation of response.

Major structural changes take place again in the latter portion of the life cycle. With advanced age, brain weight decreases, neuronal number decreases, and the number of glial cells rises. Neuronal degeneration is also seen in decreased numbers of dendrites. This dendritic loss has been shown in normally aging study participants, but is less severe with diverse and extensive environmental stimulation (Scheibel, Lindsay, Tomiyasu, & Scheibel, 1975). However, in individuals with senile dementia, dendritic counts are very low (Scheibel & Tomiyasu, 1978).

The role of stimulation in healthy older adults is currently being researched. Lack of use or loss of a sensory organ, such as an eye, has been related in adults to atrophy of central neurons (lateral geniculate) specific to that eye. Some of the cellular changes in this disuse atrophy are similar to those seen in brains of older adults. There has been particular interest in the use of activity and stimulation in the treatment of individuals with forms of dementia, such as Alzheimer's disease (AD). Stimulation experiments in rats have resulted in the retention of the thicker cortex characteristic of younger rats (Diamond, 1990). Although clinical management of elderly with AD and other types of dementia related to aging have included stimulation programs, the efficacy of these programs has not been well documented (Williams & Trubatch, 1993). Although reversal of the base neurological difficulty associated with dementia has not been generally demonstrated, activity and stimulation seem to prevent excess disability and reduce stress-related behavioral problems (Mace, 1990). Data from animal studies show that there are regional decreases with aging in protein synthesis, lipid synthesis (especially membrane phospholipids), oxygen uptake, glucose utilization, tissue water content, and cerebral blood flow. Problems with neurological function reported in older adults include reduced sensory effectiveness, sensory processing, visuospatial discrimination, memory, cognition, and motor coordination. Despite these changes, the aged patient shows fewer deficits than would be expected given the changes in metabolism and cell structure (for a review, see Cummings & Benson, 1992).

Vascular Influences on Tissue Integrity

One of the main reasons neurological morbidity and mortality occurs in brain tissue is altered blood flow to the brain. Alterations occur because of hypotension or blockage (related to the risk of hypoxic-ischemic tissue damage) and cerebral hypertension (related to vessel rupture). The neuronal tissue of the brain is among the most sensitive to injury from lack of oxygen. It is 7.5 times more metabolically active than the other tissues of the body at rest and has no mechanisms for extended anaerobic metabolism after the newborn period (Guyton, 1991). Lack of oxygen is associated with cellular damage or destruction within minutes (4–5 minutes in adults and 8–10 minutes in newborns at room temperature).

These oxygen-deprived nerve cells, which die through a process different from programmed cell death, leave behind enzymes that cause inflammation and result in continuing damage. Dead neurons cannot be replaced after the fetal period and might result in functional deficits depending on the extent and location of the damage. Once cerebral circulation is mature, there are physiological mechanisms for maintaining cerebral blood flow steady at mean arterial blood pressures from 60 to 140 mm Hg. Blood vessels in the mature brain resist rupture via their structural integrity and support by the glial cells. However, at both extremes of the age continuum, the control of flow and blood vessel integrity are vulnerable, increasing the risk for stroke and brain injury among very young infants (especially the fetus and premature newborn) and older adults.

Brain hemorrhages are common in premature infants, particularly in those weighing less than 1000g, but are relatively uncommon in full-term newborns. The type of brain bleed most commonly seen in premature infants is periventricular or intraventricular hemorrhage (IVH), which involves rupture of blood vessels adjacent to the ventricles, particularly those of the germinal matrix layer or in the choroid plexus. Clinically significant IVH occurs in approximately 10% to 15% of premature infants weighing less than 1000 g at birth who are discharged from NICUs (R. White, personal communication, July 30, 1997). The vessels of the germinal matrix are susceptible in preterm infants because vessel walls are immature and the surrounding connective tissue provides little support. By full term, the germinal matrix layer involutes with development. The pattern of involution correlates with the pattern of bleeds seen in premature infants (Papile, 1992).

Stresses such as noise and handling commonly cause alteration in heart rate, respirations rate and blood pressure, thereby increasing the risk of hemorrhage in young preterm infants who lack the protective mechanism for controlling cerebral blood pressure. This risk diminishes as the infant becomes more neurologically mature. Current nursing practices in NICUs are directed toward reducing and controlling stimulation that causes stress, thereby preventing conditions that promote hemorrhage. Such environmental controls not only reduce medical risk but also have been shown to foster growth (Als et al., 1994)

Long-term consequences of IVH range from the negligible to the lethal. The severity of the sequelae largely depends on the extent of the bleed. Bleeding may cause damage to the germinal matrix itself, which can decrease the number of neurons or glia produced. Additionally, IVH can cause bleeding into the ventricles associated with inflammatory response along the lining of the ventricles and the arachnoid tissue. If the bleeding is severe enough, clots may form in the ventricles and interrupt flow of cerebrospinal fluid in the infant's brain, specifically because of the small size of the aqueducts between ventricular chambers. About one third of infants surviving with IVH will have some dilatation of the ventricles, which can resolve spontaneously or result in hydrocephalus, a buildup of cerebrospinal fluid in the brain. The most serious IVH involves bleeding into the white matter, which is the sequela of an infarct (obstruction) and can produce additional tissue damage that might result in loss of motor function or cognitive function or in seizures, depending on the location and severity of the bleed.

The brains of full-term infants and young children are susceptible to damage from trauma, because their heads are large relative to their bodies, weak neck muscles, fragile blood vessels, and high water content in the brain. This vulnerability is most evident in cases of shaken infant syndrome. The back-and-forth shaking of an infant, causing rapid acceleration and deceleration of the head on a poorly controlled neck, can lead to cerebral hemorrhage, retinal detachment, and spinal cord injury. The sequelae of this syndrome range from nominal to severe mental and physical incapacitation to death. Most damage occurs from birth to 4 years of age because of the force needed to injure very small children is very small.

During later childhood and early adulthood, the brain is at reduced risk for medical problems from a biological perspective, although brain injuries can occur due to infections (meningitis, encephalitis), accidents, and violence. With advancing age, the brain again becomes more vulnerable. As opposed to those of premature infants, adult strokes occur in mature systems. Vascular pathologies, such as atherosclerotic narrowing of blood vessels, pose a serious threat to the brain. Atherosclerosis results from an accumulation of fatty plaque material accompanied by changes in the wall of the blood vessel. Arteriosclerosis occurs when the plaque-covered arterial walls calcify. The rate of plaque deposition depends on genetic factors, stress, and diet. If the occlusion is in the renal arteries, reduced perfusion of the kidneys activates the renin and angiotensin system to increase systemic blood pressure. With increased blood pressure and weakened blood vessels, rupture of the vessels can occur.

Rupture occuring in the brain is called a *stroke*. Strokes can also occur from complete occlusions of blood vessels caused by clots forming on plaque (thrombosis) or loose atherosclerotic clot or blood clot migrating until it becomes lodged in a small or narrowed vessel (embolism). Clots can occur for a variety of medical reasons, including infection, arteriosclerosis, trauma, and inactivity (especially in bedridden individuals; Guyton, 1991). Disturbed vascular supply to the brain may also result in dementias through several means, including cerebral hemorrhage, local vascular occlusion causing local ischemia, chronic underperfusion due to vascular insufficiency of the vessels in the brain, or underperfusion caused by cardiac insufficiency (watershed injury; Schulz & Einhäupl, 1996).

SENSORIMOTOR DEVELOPMENT

Once the sense organs are developed, they show relatively stable function through young adulthood. Visual accommodation begins to decline in the teens and continues to decline to a minimum in early senescence (from 14 diopters in childhood to 2 by age 45 or 50). This reduced accommodation results in a fixed focal length and the need for bifocal or trifocal glasses to enable sight at set focal lengths. This decline is due largely to changes in the lens itself. Other changes associated with age-related visual deficits include increased corneal thickness and decreased curvature, atrophy of radial dilator muscles of the iris (leading to a 40% reduction in pupillary diameter by age 90), macular degeneration, decreased retinal thickness, loss of rods, and loss of retinal nerves. Disruption of the flow of intraocular fluids is also more likely to accumulate over time, leading to increased risk of glaucoma. Less is known about the aging of central visual mechanisms.

Other sensory systems decline in function over age. Auditory function also begins to decline in the teens and regresses until age 50 or later. More than one third of the aged population has diagnosed hearing difficulty. Hearing loss is especially evident for higher frequency sounds, with men more affected than women. Olfactory function is much less acute in the elderly. This loss may not seem to have a role in health until the link between olfaction and diet, poison avoidance, and accident avoidance is considered. For example, the elderly are 10 times less sensitive to the smell of mercaptans added to natural gas for warning. Decreased gustatory sensation, which mirrors olfactory deficits, can play an important role in the development of poor dietary habits in the elderly.

These reductions in sensory discrimination are often mirrored in the atrophy of sensory cortex. Thus, senescence is associated with deficits in all the sensory modalities. Some changes, such as that of the lens of the eye mentioned earlier, are more direct effects of development (continued deposition of protein), whereas others result from cumulative environmental insult. Hearing loss, for example, is accelerated in populations that experience high levels of environmental noise and in individuals with elevated blood lipids.

Motor control is also reduced during infancy and old age. In infancy and early childhood, developing connections and incomplete isolation of neural signals cause lack of or poorly controlled mobility in infants. Many childhood accidents occur because of children's immature motor control, inexperience, inadequate compensation for rapid growth, and children's immature judgment. Caregivers must continuously re-evaluate infants' motor skills to apply appropriate safeguards, such as "babyproofing." Normal exploration, even in safe environments, leads to falls and bruising. These accidents become less frequent as the motor tracts mature and are myelinated. As children develop, their muscle control increases progressively, particularly in rapid sequenced movements such as typing or dancing, which are refined on the cerebellar level. Learning also reduces the risk. Accidents still occur in later childhood and adolescence, but these accidents tend to be based more on the types of activity and risk-taking behaviors associated with this population.

During adulthood, coordination and muscle control undergo a gradual decline. Deficits in motility, ranging from minor to severe and including a decrease in speed of skilled movements, are common complaints among the aging population. Posture problems appear, which can be related in part to abnormal contractions of skeletal muscles and alteration in the speed of movements (accelerated or delayed). In turn, these changes can lead to difficulty in walking and partially explain the increase in injuries due to falls in the elderly. Some gait changes are due to fear of falling. These problems with ambulation are due at least in part to altered central control of motor function, muscle weakness and increase in resting tone. Deficits at the sensory level, the cortical level, and the cerebellar and basal ganglia level can also lead to these deficits in walking and posture. Actual involution of peripheral nerves and the spinal cord are seen in aged individuals. Exercise can delay these changes, leading to the conclusion that some loss of function is due to atrophy associated with disuse.

CARDIOVASCULAR SYSTEM

The main function of the cardiovascular system is to supply a controlled amount of oxygen and nutrients to the tissues and to remove their metabolic waste products. The cardiovascular system responds to local tissue demand and central neurologic command, responding physiologically to increases and decreases in demand by regulating heart rate, stroke volume, vasodilatation, and vasoconstriction. The ability for this system to respond depends on the individual's developmental stage, general health at the time of the challenge, typical response to stress, and environmental experience.

The cardiovascular system is the first organ system to function in the embryological phase of development. By the fourth week after conception, the heart has formed a functional pumping structure providing unidirectional flow to the aorta and umbilical arteries, thus allowing the embryo to be supplied with oxygen and nutrients and to have waste removed. The main risk for prenatal cardiovascular function relates to organogenesis (organ formation). Eight of every 100 liveborn infants have a congenital cardiovascular defect (Clark, 1997), most of these being sublethal embryonic malformations. Common defects include incomplete separation of chambers of the heart, valve defects, narrowing of major vessels, or persistence of fetal circulation. These problems are often respond to corrective or palliative care. Serious congenital cardiac problems still account for a large proportion of infant mortality.

Control of blood pressure and integrity of the blood vessels are critical at all developmental stages. Bleeding in the brain not due to direct trauma is a common cause of morbidity and mortality in the fetus, premature infant, and older adult populations. Normal blood pressure increases with age and weight. Newborns have a systolic pressure of 50 to 70 mm Hg, rising through childhood to 90 to 120 mm Hg by age 10. This normal rise in blood pressure is due to physical parameters such as increased length of blood vessels, heart growth, and increased cardiac output. Normal parameters for diastolic blood pressure are relatively stable over the adult period but increase for the systolic blood pressure (Timiras, 1988).

Cardiac function generally decreases with age, whereas the risk of cardiovascular disease increases. Cardiac output per unit of body surface decreases in adults, falling 30% between the ages of 30 and 80 years. Moreover, atherosclerosis, in addition to its role in stroke, is a major cause of damage to the heart and other vital organs (Timiras, 1988).

Many of the adverse changes seen in cardiac function with aging (reduced cardiac output and increased systolic blood pressure and peripheral resistance) might be diminished through exercise. Changes in cardiac function similar to those in aged individuals are seen in younger individuals who are sedentary or in astronauts during extended stays in reduced gravity. These changes can be reduced in the younger population with renewed exercise. Even atherosclerotic plaques may be managed through diet, elimination of smoking, and increased exercise.

ENDOCRINE SYSTEM

The effect of hormonal levels on health is a large issue that we can only partially examine. Interested readers should refer to a text on endocrinology, such as that by Hadley (1996). The endocrine system affects every system in the body, affecting metabolism, growth, availability of nutrients, diurnal cycles, immune function, sexual function, cognitive function, and emotion. In this chapter, I examine one class of products of the endocrine system—estrogens. Estrogens have a widespread role in women's health. From puberty to beyond menopause, they have effects on multiple organ systems and the perception of overall health. No other endocrinological treatment receives as much popular attention as ERT during and following menopause.

Estrogens are produced at very low levels in childhood, but at puberty they increase by approximately twentyfold. This rise in estrogen is responsible for many of the changes seen in the internal and external sexual structures. Estrogens are responsible for the general enlargement of the sexual organs and an additional level of histogenesis (such as the maturation of the vaginal lining, important in preventing trauma and infection). Of course, the most well-known effect of estrogen is on the normal menstrual cycle. Several common complaints are associated with menstruation, including dysmenorrhea (painful menses), primary and secondary amenorrhea, breast pain, dysfunctional uterine bleeding (excessive or prolonged), and premenstrual symptoms (headache, edema, mood changes; Carr & Wilson, 1994).

Estrogens also affect nonreproductive tissues. Fat deposition under the skin and in breast, buttocks and thighs is facilitated by estrogen. Skin thickens, but remains soft. Estrogens promote pigmentation in the nipples, labia minora, and linea alba. Estrogens can cause some retention of water and sodium by the kidney (usually minimal except during pregnancy). Estrogens produce lower body temperature (progesterones are thermogenic). Estrogens stimulate the liver to increase production of several proteins including angiotensin, which plays a role in hypertension.

As mentioned in the section on bone, estrogens also affect bone tissue, increasing osteoblast (bone-building cells) activity and facilitating the union of the epiphysis (growing end regions) with the shaft of long bones.

Estrogens play a role in medical management of fertility and side effects of menopause. One in four women in the United States under the age of 45 uses oral contraception based on combinations of synthetic estrogens and progestins or progestins only. The exogenous estrogens, especially at higher doses, have been related to hypertension, headaches, and vascular effects such as thrombosis and embolism. These risks are higher for older individuals and smokers. Oral contraceptives are also associated with increased cholesterol and reduced salts in the bile (increasing risk for gallstone formation). Tamoxifen, a weak agonist–antagonist of estrogens, is used in the treatment of breast cancers bearing estrogen receptors. Estrogen replacement therapy (ERT) is also a common treatment for problems associated with menopause. The treatment is associated with increased risk for breast cancer, endometrial carcinoma, and gallstone formation. Beneficially, ERT has been shown to reduce or reverse the loss of bone mass leading to osteoporosis. ERT also reduces the risk for cardiovascular disease, presumably via alterations in blood lipids and lipoproteins (Miller, Larosa, & Muessing, 1990). It has also been useful in controlling the hot flashes that some women experience in early menopause and in reversing urogenital epithelial atrophy. Recent studies suggest ERT also reduces the incidence of AD (Kawas et al., 1997) and is related to higher cognitive function in AD patients (Doraiswamy et al., 1997).

IMMUNE SYSTEM

Like other systems, the immune system functions differently across the life span. Premature and newborn infants are at particular risk from infection due to an inexperienced and incompletely functioning immune system. Much of their protection comes from maternal antibodies passively acquired across the placenta during the third trimester of pregnancy. Since the advent of antibiotics and vaccinations, children and adolescents have had fewer serious infections (with the exception of HIV). However, infectious disease mortality, from illnesses such as AIDS, pneumonia, and influenza, rises after the age of 25 (Galpin, 1981). There is also an increase in cancer and autoimmune diseases from younger to older adulthood.

Immune system effectiveness is affected by developmental, behavioral, and environmental factors. Protection of the body from infection begins with the maintenance of physical barriers, such as skin and mucous membranes. If these barriers fail, the internal systems (innate and acquired) provide critical defenses against infection. The innate system functions throughout the body (in circulation and in tissue) in response to foreign organisms or matter, using basic recognition systems to destroy intruders. As a system, it is unchanged by the encounter with the foreign body—the goal is to restore homeostasis.

In contrast to the innate system, the function of the acquired system is altered with experience. Mature immune competence is a product of repeated varied exposures to pathogens that build a repertoire of responsive cell populations. This acquired system is the target of vaccinations, which provide exposure to either weakened, dead, or portions of pathogens. The inexperience of young immune systems is one reason infectious disease is so prevalent in the pediatric population. The immune system, once thought to be autonomous, has been shown to be sensitive to physical and psychosocial stress, diet, hormonal levels, and exercise (Roitt, 1994).

Prenatal and neonatal infections continue to be one of the leading causes of fetal death and neonatal morbidity and mortality. Several factors play important roles in this increased risk, such as the maternal environment and incompletely competent immune systems. Premature infants are prone to infection because of incomplete barrier systems such as thin skin and low levels of mucous production, the experience of invasive procedures that can bring pathogens past the barriers, and an immature immune system. Even full-term infants are susceptible to serious infections during the first weeks of postnatal life. A partial explanation of this susceptibility is the fetal environment. The fetus, sequestered in the uterus, has low exposure to pathogens, making newborn systems naïve. Another explanation is the immature functional development of certain components of the immune system. Except in cases of intrauterine pathogen exposure, the spleen and lymph nodes are underdeveloped at term, although the infant does have the ability to respond to antigens and reject grafts or transplants.

Fetal levels of antibodies are quite different from those of the adult. Fetal immune cells are generally fewer and functionally less mature than those found in children. These numbers rise steadily with a dramatic burst at birth, producing peak levels 12 to 24 hours after birth and dropping to stable newborn levels by 3 days (Yoder & Polin, 1992). The 2- to 4-month old infant has low antibody immunity as maternal antibodies are broken down and infant antibodies slowly replace them, but the infant is supported environmentally by breastfeeding. Colostrum and breastmilk also provide passive immunity via IgA (antibodies found in barrier secretions, such as mucous) and nonspecific antimicrobial factors. The IgA produced in breastmilk is largely specific to gut bacteria, providing protection from gut infections and allowing colonization of normal gut bacteria to proceed in a controlled manner. By the end of the first year, infants have antibody levels that are more than half of adult levels, except for IgA (20% of adult levels). As the immune system begins to function in childhood, its developing efficacy is dependent on maturation and environmental inputs, such as hormonal changes of the pubertal period, physiological changes accompanying senescence, nutrition, psychosocial stress, and acute challenges that stimulate the immune system, such as vaccinations and infections.

The incidence of infectious disease in children is due not to defects in their immune systems, but mainly to the fact that their systems have not yet formed memory cells from prior experience with pathogens. Their exposure to pathogens is high, because they are routinely exposed to peers who also have no prior exposure. For example, there is less herd immunity in a class of kindergarten children than among adults in an office. Historically, this lack of memory cells had a considerable adverse impact on child health until the advent of vaccinations.

As the immune system matures there differential function occurs based on gender. The effect of sex hormones on immune tissues was demonstrated in gonadectomized rats at the turn of the century. Current clinical findings show that females have higher levels of cell-mediated immunity, higher immunoglobulin titers, and increased primary and secondary responses to several pathogens. There is also increased risk of autoimmune disease, such as rheumatoid arthritis and systemic lupus erythematosus in women. Lupus symptoms increase and decrease in severity with the menstrual cycle, with the worst symptoms occurring during the luteal phase of the cycle (following ovulation). Rheumatoid arthritis symptoms are generally less severe during the luteal phase in cycling individuals and as well as in pregnant women. The exact mechanisms producing these effects are unclear (Roitt, 1994).

During adulthood, immune function decreases with increasing age. Immune suppression in young adults has largely been blamed on stress—physical and psychosocial. Stress has been shown to decrease function in lymphocytes and macrophages (Chancellor-Freeland et al., 1995), but stress can also have positive effects on the immune response and is important in controlling the immune response. This positive role of the stress response in immune function is illustrated by studies in which animals that are unable to produce corticosteroid stress hormone are exposed to a normally nonfatal respiratory infection. These animals cannot mount a controlled and effective response to the simple infections and succumb (Kapcala, Chautard, & Eskay, 1995).

Aging is also associated with deficits in immune function. For instance T-cell (killer or helper cells of the acquired system) function drops by more than 75% in the elderly (Rowe, 1992). This reduced immunity leads to an increased susceptibility to infectious diseases, such as influenza and pneumonia. It is also responsible in part for the rise in cancer rates. The aging of the immune system is more complicated than just a wearing out of the bone marrow or thymus (the site of production and maturation of immune cells). For example, implantation of younger marrow and thymus does not fully rescue the immune function in aged animals. The immune system is a complex system dependent on the interaction with other systems.

GASTROINTESTINAL SYSTEM

The gastrointestinal (GI) system, extending from the mouth through the rectum, plays an important role in health and perception of well-being. It is also a source of significant difficulties, accounting for one quarter of patient complaints (Fry &

Sandler, 1993). In this section, several components of the GI system and their relative risk across the life span are discussed briefly. Common problems, in order of prevalence, include acute infections, general abdominal pain, upset stomach or nausea, dental and mouth disorders, other stomach disorders, and irritable bowel. Like the skin and lung, the gut surface is mitotically active (dividing) to replace cells damaged by environmental insult. This mitotic activity over time is associated with increased risk of cancer. Eleven percent of deaths are caused by GI disease, the majority due to cancer. Age-related changes in GI system function vary considerably across individuals and components of the system. Much of this variation is due to the amount of environmental and behavioral damage accumulated over the course of the life span and differences in nutrition. Some of the changes, such as the loss of teeth, might interfere with eating, whereas others, such as preterm infant gut immaturity, require special feeding protocols and a vigilance against infections of fragile gut tissue.

All stages of swallowing are affected by development and aging. Difficulty in swallowing is a frequent problem among the very young and the very old. The swallowing functions include voluntary muscle control, reflexes, and smooth muscle peristalsis. These functions must be coordinated with breathing to maintain oxygen supply during feeding and to prevent choking. Young preterm infants do not have adequate coordination of the oral components for swallowing or proper timing with breaths to feed orally. These functions are under moderate control in the healthy full-term infant, but the lack of teeth plus the small diameter of the pharynx puts infants and young children at risk for choking. Older adults, at the other end of the age continuum, may experience weakness of voluntary and smooth muscles and decreased reflexes that might cause difficulty with coordinated swallowing. Mild difficulty in coordinated swallowing leads to increased choking and discomfort, but more severe forms of swallowing difficulty in aging adults are usually related to some other pathology.

The stomach, with its high acid production and proteolytic-enzyme-rich environment, is at risk for inflammation. Children often report and experience stomach upset, with vomiting being one of the most frequent complaints. Such complaints are often associated with gastroesophageal reflux (GER), infections, ingestion of nonedible material, and motion sickness, among others.

GER is a stomach-related malady that can occur in infants, children, and adults. The infantile form is generally self-limiting, resolving by 18 months in most cases. Adult GER, which can show up in childhood, is not by nature self-limiting and might require intervention. Children with lung disease are at higher risk for GER. GER is often caused by high intra-abdominal pressure, such as coughing, strain with bowel movement, or pregnancy. Other stomach problems, such as peptic ulcer and gastritis, are common in the adult population and increase in both incidence and severity with age. Numerous agents are associated with general gastritis and ulcers, including aspirin ingestion, alcohol and tobacco use, and increased stress levels.

The small intestine is the site of major nutrient absorption. Diseases of the small intestine occur across the life span. Efficient nutrient absorption is especially critical in young, growing children. Decreased efficiency of nutrient absorption in the aged is associated with specific nutrient deficiencies, including calcium and vitamin D.

The large intestine is generally functional in the young infant, although control of the timing of defecation with voluntary control of the anal sphincter does not develop until the late infancy or toddler stages. Control begins to be an issue again in middle adulthood for females and later adulthood for males. Rectal muscle tone and anal sphincter strength decrease in older individuals, sometimes enough to cause fecal incontinence. Trauma, such as childbirth, can accelerate this deficiency. Other problems associated with the large intestine relate to the speed at which contents move through and are expelled. As toilet training commences for children, voluntary inhibition of indiscriminatory defecation can lead to inhibition of defecation reflexes and constipation. Defecation becomes painful and can produce further inhibition. In older adults, a frequent cause of constipation is misuse of laxatives, which decreases natural reflexes, leading to constipation. Too-rapid movement through the colon, diarrhea, is present across age groups and has multiple etiologies, such as infection, stress, and inflammatory disease. The primary concern with diarrhea is the risk of dehydration in infants, the elderly, and those with certain disease processes.

LUNG

Lung pathologies are common in the very young and again as adults approach middle to old age. The respiratory (oxygen–carbon dioxide exchange) system involves the gas exchange organ (the alveoli and capillary bed of the lungs), the pump (the respiratory muscles), and central control (central nervous system [CNS] centers and the nerve tracts). Some lung pathologies, such as asthma, can occur at any point in the life span. There is considerable individual variation in asthma onset and duration: Some children who develop asthma "outgrow" it by adolescence; in other cases, onset of asthma occurs at puberty. Often, lung problems are associated with immaturity or damage to the respiratory mechanism, which is not fully mature until around age 20, with the most rapid growth occurring in the first 8 years. After age 25, pulmonary function begins to decline. Although some of this decreased function is due to changes in lung tissue, muscle strength, and CNS control centers, the environment plays an important role in reducing lung function. Infections, smoking (passive and active), pollution, and altered immune responses imperil the lung over the course of the life span. Also, inhalation of high oxygen concentrations can lead to damage via the formation of oxygen free radicals, especially in premature infants.

More generally, preterm infants have immature lungs, which place them at risk for survival or permanent disability. The preterm lung tissue is thicker yet more fragile. It requires more work to inflate and allows less efficient passage of oxygen. Surfactant, a complex phospholipid–protein compound that decreases surface tension in the lung, is critical for effective function of the lung. Infants with reduced surfactant production must fight against high surface tension to inflate the lungs. Pressures required to inflate the lung might exceed the tensile strength of the lung tissue leading to tearing and long-term scarring and decreased respiratory function. In recent years, surfactant supplementation has reduced the risk of lung damage, improving outcomes for premature infants.

Older adults experience several changes that decrease function in the respiratory system. The alveolar ducts and bronchioles are enlarged and the alveoli are shallower, leading to a decrease in relative gas exchange area by 4% per decade (Thurlbeck & Angus, 1975). The lungs become less elastic and more fibrous, producing less elastic recoil. Age has also been associated with calcification of the intercostal joints and with wasting of respiratory musculature. Even though total lung capacity remains constant, except in abnormal disease states, vital capacity (maximum amount of expired air after maximal inhalation) decreases, and residual volume (the air left in the lung at exhalation) increases with age.

Lung diseases of the older adult, such as emphysema, are pathological extensions of these trends of decreased respiratory function. Emphysema, most highly associated with cigarette smoking, involves a loss of alveolar septa, distention of alveoli, local inflammation, and loss of pulmonary elasticity far in excess of that of normal aging, leading to reduced oxygen uptake. Although heavy smoking is the most common cause, silicosis, chronic bronchitis, or inherent defects in the elastic tissue or enzyme systems of the lung can also lead to these changes. Individuals with emphysema experience chronic coughs, difficulty in breathing, and severe responses to respiratory infections. They compensate for reduced oxygen uptake efficiency by increasing the effort to breathe by using additional thoracic muscles, which leads to a barrel-shaped chest. Hypoxia, associated with lung disease, also triggers increased production of red blood cells, hypertension, and an enlarged heart (Guyton, 1991; Timiras, 1988).

URINARY SYSTEM

The urinary system includes the kidneys, ureters, bladder, urethra, and the function of the muscles controlling bladder emptying. Renal function in the fetus is an important component of amniotic fluid formation. Although it matures relatively early, the system is susceptible to damage, especially in infants and young children undergoing critical care. There are several causes of acute renal failure including dehydration, shock, hypoxia, burns, obstructions, or infections. Mortality due to acute renal failure is uncommon.

Complaints regarding the urinary system in general decrease in later childhood and adulthood. The most common problems are urinary tract infections, especially among female patients. In young females, this is due in part to the short urethra, but in adults, infections are frequently associated with sexual activity and pregnancy. Other renal problems seen in young and middle-aged adults include acute nephritis and malignant hypertension.

Renal function decreases with age; from the age of 30 to 60 years, the glomerular filtration rate (amount of plasma filtered by the kidney in 1 minute) drops by half (Timiras, 1988). Renal problems in older age groups are associated with infections, diabetes mellitus, dehydration, and drug usage, in particular in the elderly due to the widespread and extended use of multiple pharmacological treatments. Inadequate fluid intake as well as overuse of diuretics and laxatives, common in the elderly, can also precipitate acute renal failure. If the drugs used rely on renal excretion, excessive strain is placed on the kidneys, thereby increasing the risk for renal intoxication. Infections also rise, as a result of lower urine outputs (especially among males) and obstructed flow from prostate enlargement.

Incontinence is a problem, again, for both children and older adults. Because control of urinary flow is a complicated process that involves cognitive centers, appropriate sensory inputs from the bladder, gross and fine motor coordination, normal urinary tract function, control of and coordination of bladder musculature and urethral outlet, and lack of barriers to flow (e.g., enlarged prostate gland), it does not develop in children until after the first year. Although not connected to mortality, incontinence is often a concern among older adults. Because of the social stigma associated with this disorder, affected individuals and their families often view it as a threat to independent or home-based living. Incontinence, urinary or fecal, is conservatively estimated to occur in 10% to 15% of older adults living at home and in 50% of older adults living in monitoring facilities.

Incontinence is related to trauma such as childbirth, inactivity, reduced cognition, prostate enlargement in men, a weakening of the pelvic floor associated with low estrogen in women, infection, and other health problems. There are several subtypes of incontinence: stress, urge, overflow, and functional. Stress incontinence involves insufficient strength in the pelvic floor to resist abdominal pressure produced by coughing, sneezing, or straining. Urge incontinence involves the inability to stop flow once the full sensation is sent from the bladder, common after a stroke or with mild outflow obstruction. Overflow incontinence occurs when an overfilled bladder reaches the maximum stretch and leaks by mechanical forces. Functional incontinence occurs when the patient is unable or unwilling to reach the toilet before emptying, due to either inadequate timing of urge signals or inattention to the signals (Timiras, 1988).

SUMMARY

Each stage of life has a level of biological risk. The early and later stages of life tend to have the highest risk for medical problems, in particular because of infections and organ failures or insufficiencies. Dependence occurs at both ends of the developmental continuum due to lack of development, loss of mobility, and inability to self-care. Dependence also makes these populations vulnerable to injury from accidents, abuse, and neglect. Certain acute onset stress-related symptoms, such as stomach pain, headaches, and insomnia, show up in mid-childhood and are prevalent complaints through adulthood. In later adulthood, the psychological response to stressors dampens, providing a type of resiliency against "daily hassle" type of stressors and a decrease in stomach pain and headache. Injuries associated with risk-taking behaviors (e.g., accidents and violent trauma) are associated most highly with adolescence. Risks associated with sexual activity, such as sexually transmitted diseases and complications of pregnancy, are particularly prevalent during adolescence and young adulthood. Some diseases are associated most highly with advanced age as a result of wear and tear and cumulative insult over the life of the organism, such as coronary artery disease, lung cancer, emphysema, and basal cell carcinoma (skin cancer). Recovery in the elderly is further complicated by a ripple effect in which reduction of functioning in one organ places additional stress on other organs (e.g., cardiac insufficiency leading to reduced renal flow and to watershed ischemia in the brain). The aged are the most heterogeneous of the age groups with respect to degree of health. This heterogeneity can be due to genetics, accident, or cumulative damage associated with specific life experience. With appropriate stimulation, exercise, diet, management of toxin exposure (e.g., cigarettes and pollutants), cumulative damage can be reduced to improve immune function and organ function, which can change our view of normal health for the aged and perhaps across the life span.

REFERENCES

Als, H., Lawhon, G., Duffy, F., McAnulty, B., Gibes-Grossman, R., & Blickman, J. (1994). Individualized developmental care for the very-low-birth-weight preterm infant: Medical and neurofunctional effects. *Journal of the American Medical Association, 272*, 853–858.

Berkowitz, C. D. (1996). *Pediatrics: A primary care approach.* Philadelphia: Saunders.

Brann, A. W., & Schwartz, J. F. (1992). Central nervous system disturbances: Assessment of neonatal neurologic function. In A. A. Fanaroff & R. J. Martin (Eds.), *Neonatal-perinatal medicine: Diseases of the fetus and infant* (pp. 691–700). Chicago: Mosby.

Carr, B., & Wilson, J. (1994). Disorders of the ovary and female reproductive tract. In K. Isselbacher, E. Braunwald, J. Wilson, J. Martin, A. Fauci, & D. Kaspar (Eds.), *Harrison's principles of internal medicine* (13th ed., pp. 2017–2036). New York: McGraw-Hill.

Chancellor-Freeland, C., Zhu, G., Kage, R., Beller, D., Leeman, S., & Black, P. (1995). Substance P and stress induced changes in macrophages. *Annals of the New York Academy of Science, 771*, 472–484.

Clark, E. (1997). Congenital heart disease. In R. Hoekelman, S. Friedman, N. Nelson, H. Seidel, & M. Weitzman (Eds.), *Primary pediatric care* (3rd ed., pp. 1253–1259). Chicago: Mosby.

Coates, D. L., & Lewis, M. (1984). Early mother–infant interaction and infant cognitive status as predictors of school age performance and cognitive behavior in six-year-olds. *Child Development, 55*, 1219–1230.

Cummings, J., & Benson, D. F. (1992). *Dementia: A clinical approach* (2nd ed.). Boston: Butterworth-Heinemann.

Diamond, M. (1990). An optimistic view of the aging brain. In A. Goldstein (Ed.), *Biomedical advances in aging* (pp. 441–449). New York: Plenum Press.

Doraiswamy, P., Bieber, F., Kaiser, L., Krishnan, K., Reuning-Scherer, J., & Gulanski, B. (1997). The Alzheimer's disease assessment scale: Patterns and predictors of baseline cognitive performance in multicenter Alzheimer's disease trials. *Neurology, 48,* 1511–1517.

Fiatarone, M. A., Marks, E. C., Ryan, N. D., Meredith, C. N., Lipsitz, L. A., & Evans, W. J. (1990). High-intensity strength training in nonagenarians. Effects on skeletal muscle. *Journal of the American Medical Association, 263,* 3029–3034.

Frontera, W. R., Meredith, C. N., O'Reilly, K. P., Knuttgen, H. P., & Evans, W. J. (1988). Strength conditioning in older men: Skeletal muscle hypertrophy and improved function. *Journal of Applied Physiology, 64,* 1038–44.

Fry, J., & Sandler, G. (1993). *Common diseases: Their nature, presentation and care* (5th ed.). Boston: Kluwer.

Galpin, J. (1981). Immunity and microbial diseases. In M. Kay & T. Makinodan (Eds.), *Handbook of immunology in aging* (pp. 141–159). Boca Raton FL: CRC Press.

Guyer, B., Strobino, D. M., Ventura, S. J., MacDorman, M., & Martin J. A. (1996). *Annual Summary of Vital Statistics—(1995). Pediatrics,* 98(6), 1007–1019.

Guyton, A. C. (1991). *Textbook of medical physiology.* Philadelphia: Saunders.

Hadley, M. (1996). *Endocrinology* (4th ed.). Upper Saddle River, NJ: Prentice-Hall.

Herber, R. F., &. Garber, H. (1975). The Milwaukee Project: A study of the use of family intervention to prevent cultural-familial mental retardation. In J. Hellmuth (Ed.), *Exceptional infant: Vol. 3. Assessment and intervention.* New York: Brunner/Mazel.

Hubel, D., & Wiesel, T. (1963). Receptive fields of cells in striate cortex of very young, visually inexperienced kittens. *Journal of Neurophysiology, 26,* 944–1002.

Jenkins, W., Merzenich, M., Ochs, M., Allard, T., & Guic-Robles, E. (1990). Functional reorganization of primary somatosensory cortex in adult owl monkeys after behaviorally controlled contact stimulation. *Journal of Neurophysiology, 63,* 82–104.

Kapcala, L., Chautard, T., & Eskay, R. (1995). The protective role of the hypothalamic-pituitary-adrenal axis against lethality produced by immune, infectious, and inflammatory stress. *Annals of the New York Academy of Science, 771,* 419–437.

Kawas, C., Resnick, S., Morrison, A., Brookmeyer, R., Corrada, M., Zonderman, A., Bacal, C., Lingle, D. D., & Metter, E. (1997). A prospective study of estrogen replacement therapy and the risk of developing Alzheimer's disease: The Baltimore Longitudinal Study of Aging. *Neurology, 48,* 1517–1521

Kennedy, C., Suda, S., Smith, C., Miyaoka, M., Ito, M., & Sokoloff, L. (1981). Changes in protein synthesis underlying functional plasticity in immature monkey visual system. *Proceedings of the National Academy of Science, USA, 78,* 3950–3953.

Mace, N. (1990). *Dementia care: Patient, family and community.* Baltimore: Johns Hopkins University Press.

Michel, G. F., & Moore, C. L. (1995). *Developmental psychobiology: An interdisciplinary perspective.* Cambridge, MA: MIT Press.

Miller, V. T., Larosa, J. C., & Muesing, R. A. (1990). Lipid and lipoprotein changes due to estrogen replacement therapies and their association with prevention of cardiovascular disease in postmenopausal women. In A. Goldstein (Ed.), *Biomedical advances in aging* (pp. 531–536). New York: Plenum Press.

Nelson, M. E., Fiatarone, M. A., Morganti, C. M., Trice, I., Greenberg, R. A., & Evans, W. J. (1994). Effects of high-intensity strength training on multiple risk factors for osteoporotic fracture. *Journal of the American Medical Association, 272,* 1909–1914.

Papile, L. (1992). Central nervous system disturbances: Pt. 4. Periventricular-intraventricular hemorrhage. In A. A. Fanaroff & R. J. Martin (Eds.), *Neonatal-perinatal medicine: Diseases of the fetus and infant* (pp. 719–728). Chicago: Mosby.

Rensberger, B. (1996). *Life itself.* New York: Oxford University Press.

Roitt, I. (1994). *Essential immunology.* Boston: Blackwell Scientific Publications.

Rosenberg, H. M., Ventura, S. J., & Maurer, J. D. (1996). Births and deaths: United States (1995). *Monthly vital statistics report 45*(3, Suppl. 2), 31.

Rowe, J. (1992). Aging and geriatric medicine. In J. B. Wyngaarden, L. H. Smith, & J. C. Bennett (Eds.), *Cecil's textbook of medicine* (19th ed.). Philadelphia: Saunders.

Scheibel, M. E., Lindsay, R. D., Tomayasu U., & Scheibel, A. B. (1975). Progressive dendritic changes in aging human cortex. *Experimental Neurology, 47,* 392–403.

Scheibel, A. B., & Tomayasu, U. (1978). Dendritic sprouting in Alzheimer presenile dementia. *Experimental Neurology, 60,* 1–8.

Schulz, J. G., & Einhäupl, K. M. (1996). The vascular dementias and cerebrovascular involvement in Alzheimer's disease. In J. D. Turner, K. Beyreuther, & F. Theuring (Eds.), *Alzheimer's disease: Ernst Schering Research Foundation workshop 17* (pp. 17–48). New York: Springer.

Slemenda, C. W. (1994). Development of vertebral skeletal mass during childhood and adolescence. *Spine: State of the Art Reviews 8*(1), 83–90.

Tamis-LeMonda, C., & Bornstein, M. (1987). Is there a "sensitive period" in human development? In M. Bornstein (Ed.), *Sensitive periods in development: Interdisciplinary perspectives* (pp. 163–182). Hillsdale, NJ: Lawrence Erlbaum Associates.

Thurlbeck, W. M., & Angus, G. E. (1975). Growth and aging of the normal human lung. *Chest, 67,* 3s–7s.

Timiras, P. S. (1988). *Physiological basis of geriatrics.* New York: MacMillan Publishing Co.

Williams, J. K., & Trubatch, A. D. (1993). Nursing home care for the patient with Alzheimer's disease: an overview. *Neurology, 43*(Suppl. 4), S20–S24.

Woolsey, T., Durham, D., Harris, R., Simons, D., & Valentino, K. (1981). Somatosensory development. In R. Aslin, J. Alberts, & M. Peterson (Eds.), *Development of Perception: Vol. 1. Audition, somatic perception and the chemical senses* (pp. 259–292). New York: Academic Press.

Yoder, M. C., & Polin, R. A. (1992). The immune system: Developmental immunology. In A. A. Fanaroff & R. J. Martin (Eds.), *Neonatal-perinatal medicine: Diseases of the fetus and infant* (pp. 587–617). Chicago: Mosby.

3

Physical Health Across the Life Span: A Behavioral Genetic Approach

Julia M. Braungart-Rieker
C. S. Bergeman
University of Notre Dame

BEHAVIORAL GENETICS is a theory and a set of methodologies that assesses the etiology of individual differences in a population. Behavioral genetic methodologies can answer questions about why some children develop diabetes or why some individuals are more prone to heart attacks or high blood pressure, but the approach is less relevant to questions regarding group differences, such as why women on average live longer than men. In other words, this theory is applicable to individual differences in behavioral characteristics but can provide little information about the average differences between groups (e.g., differences between males and females or between members of different cultures). Although the focus of research in this area is often on genetic influences on health and behavior, the theory is also useful for describing environmental sources of variance that contribute to individual differences. Thus, the label of behavioral *genetics* is misleading, because the theory and methods are as informative about environmental influences on characteristics as they are about genetic factors.

This chapter discusses the contribution of behavioral genetic research to the understanding of individual differences in health from infancy to old age. The chapter begins with an overview of the behavioral genetic perspective followed by a brief summary of the designs and statistical analyses that are used to assess the etiology of genetic and environmental influences. Next, the behavioral genetic research that focuses on health issues across major developmental life stages is reviewed, and the chapter concludes with a discussion of its implications for theory, future research, and intervention.

It is important at the onset to emphasize that this chapter does not focus on single-gene phenomena such as Huntington's Chorea or chromosomal abnormalities such

as Down syndrome. It is certainly the case that single-gene defects and chromosomal abnormalities serve as major contributors to health problems, especially ones
that are severe or life-threatening, and molecular genetic techniques, such as linkage
analysis, have produced a rapidly expanding human genome map that will no doubt
result in the identification and cloning of many single-gene disorders. The new
frontier for behavioral and molecular genetic research, however, lies with common
and complex diseases central to behavioral medicine (Plomin, 1995). Thus, the primary focus of this chapter is limited to a discussion of behavioral genetic research
on complex health traits that are largely due to multiple genes *and* environmental
factors, of varying effect, which contribute additively and interchangeably to health.

A quantitative genetic approach, which considers the influence of many genes
as well as environmental factors, is important for studying normal variation in the
development of complex characteristics (Plomin, 1986). Because of the complex-
ity of most health-related problems, it is unlikely that just one direct cause contributes to individual differences. Additionally, it is important to remember that
there are no "genes for health." Genes are simply blueprints for the assembly and
regulation of proteins, which are the building blocks of the human body. Each gene
codes for a specific sequence of amino acids that the body assembles to form a protein. The proteins then interact with other physiological intermediaries (e.g., hormones or neurotransmitters) or environmental factors. Therefore, when genetic
influences on health are discussed, the reference is to indirect and complex paths
between genes and health via proteins and physiological systems. Although the information coded in DNA can ultimately influence behavior in certain directions,
it is important to keep in mind that the paths are indirect, and genetic influences
are indeed just influences—propensities or tendencies that nudge development
in one direction rather than another. It is also important to avoid the mistaken notion that genetic influences are immutable. Genes do not determine one's destiny;
they do not turn on at conception and proceed undeterred until death. Thus, even
though research has indicated that genetic differences among individuals can contribute to phenotypic differences, *genetic influence* does not imply that the environment is not necessary for development, nor does it imply genetic determinism
in the sense of a direct relation between genes and their effect on behavior.

ESTIMATING GENETIC
AND ENVIRONMENTAL INFLUENCES

Heritability is a descriptive statistic that is defined as the proportion of phenotypic
variance in a population that is due to genetic variance, which in turn can be parti-
tioned into two types—additive and nonadditive.[1] *Additive genetic variance* is the

---

[1] Behavioral genetic studies often differ in their presentation of results. Heritability can be presented
as a percentage (e.g., 40% of the variance) or as a statistic (e.g., $h^2 = .40$); these numbers are interpreted
in the same manner. Studies that examine concordance rates on typically dichotomous characteristics

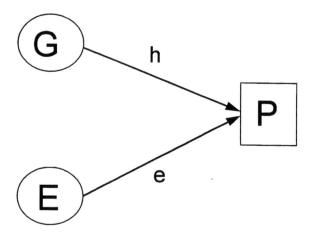

FIG. 3.1.   A path diagram representing the basic quantitative genetic model; *G* is the genotypic value, *E* is the environmental deviation, and *P* is the observed phenotypic value; *h* is the square root of heritability (h^2) and *e* is the square root of the corresponding environmental component (e^2).

extent to which genotypic values add up linearly in their effect on the phenotype, whereas *nonadditive genetic variance* represents genetic influences due to dominance (interactions between alleles at a single locus), as well as the variance due to the higher order interactions, called *epistasis*. Environmental differences among individuals can also lead to phenotypic differences between them. Behavioral genetic research offers some of the best evidence for the importance of environmental influences on development. The environmental component of variance can be separated into *shared environmental influences,* which are any environmental influences that contribute to phenotypic similarity among family members, and *nonshared environment,* which is defined as any environmental influence that makes family members different from one another. A major development in behavioral genetics over the past two decades is the testing of explicit models rather than the simple examination of correlations. Model-fitting techniques are especially useful when combination designs, yielding many different familial correlations, are employed. Although model-fitting techniques are somewhat complex, they are overviewed here briefly because much of the current research is reported in terms of model-fitting analyses.

   Behavioral genetic model-fitting techniques are based on path analysis, a method first described by Wright in 1921. The path diagram in Fig. 3.1 represents the basic

(presence or absence of disease) do not usually present estimates of heritability. Such results are usually presented in a descriptive manner, indicating whether identical twins are more concordant for a characteristic than are fraternal twins. In general, presentation of results in the present chapter follows the original researchers' method of presentation.

proposition that phenotypic variance can be due to genetic and environmental variance. Thus, variability in genotypes (G) and environments (E) cause variability in the phenotype (P). That is, $P = G + E$, and G and E are assumed to be uncorrelated. The path labeled h is the square root of heritability (h^2), and is defined as the proportion of the standard deviation of the phenotype (e.g., a health characteristic of interest) that is caused by variation in the genotype. The path e similarly represents the environmentally induced phenotypic variation.

Figure 3.2 represents a simple path diagram for twins or siblings. For twins, $P1$ represents the score of one member of the twin pair on the health characteristic of interest, and $P2$ refers to the score of the other twin. G and Es refer to genotypic and shared environmental variables, respectively. The model assumes that r_g (the genetic correlation) is 1.0 for identical or monozygotic (MZ) twins and 0.5 for fraternal or dizygotic (DZ) twins if the genetic influences operate in an additive manner, and 1.0 for MZ and 0.25 for DZ twins if the genetic influences operate in a

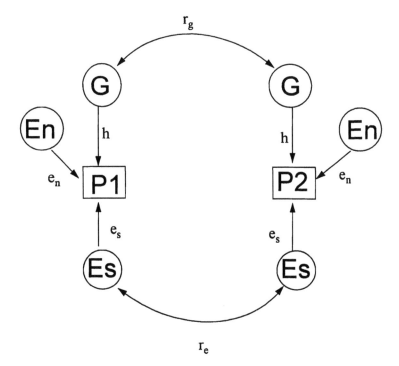

FIG. 3.2.   A path diagram representing the resemblance between members of a twin or sibling pair. $P1$ is the trait of interest in one member of the pair and $P2$ is the corresponding value for the other member of the pair. G is the genotypic value; Es represents the influence of shared environment; En reflects the nonshared environmental influences that make family members different from one another (including error of measurement); rg is the genetic correlation and re is the environmental correlation.

nonadditive way (i.e., via dominance or epistasis). r_e (the environmental correlation) is specified as 1.0 if the twins are reared together (T), and 0.0 if the twins are reared apart (A). This does not mean that the actual correlation for a particular trait is 1.0 for either genetic or environmental reasons; the model merely indicates that identical twins reared together (MZT) share all genetic effects that influence the trait of interest, and they share all environmental effects on the trait that occur as a result of living together. The parameter labeled *En* represents nonshared environmental influences that do not contribute to twin similarity. In other words, *En* represents the environmental factors that contribute to differences between twins (or other family members), including error of measurement.

To illustrate, the intraclass twin correlations for height (in twins over the age of 70 in the Swedish Adoption/Twin Study of Aging [SATSA]) are as follows: $rMZA = .64$; $rMZT = .84$; $rDZA = .23$ and $rDZT = .42$. The pattern of correlations indicates genetic influence because on average the MZ twin correlations (.74) are higher than the average DZ twin correlations (.33). The correlations also suggest some influence of shared rearing environment, because twins reared together on average (.63) are more similar than twins reared apart (.44). Quantitative genetic model-fitting analyses provide a powerful tool for assessing genetic and environmental influences on behavior because they estimate the parameters simultaneously, and provide both standard errors for the parameter estimates and a chi-square goodness-of-fit index (Loehlin, 1987). Results of model-fitting analyses for height using LISREL indicate that 53% of the variance is due to additive genetic influences, 17% to shared rearing environment, and the remaining balance (30%) to nonshared environmental factors.

Developmental behavioral genetics merges developmental questions with behavioral theories and methodologies. One of the most basic developmental questions is whether the relative importance of genetic variance (heritability) differs with age. The "differential heritability" is most often assessed cross-sectionally by comparing individuals of different ages in studies or by comparing results across studies that focus on different age groups. Reviews of behavioral genetic research indicate differences in the results of behavioral genetic analyses in infancy, childhood, adolescence, adulthood, and old age. Because most of this work to date is cross-sectional, however, it only addresses the question of whether the relative contribution of genetic and environmental influences differ in various age groups. Thus, cross-sectional research can provide information about *age differences*, but not about *age changes*, in heritability. As a result, the comparison of individuals in different age groups might reflect cohort differences rather than the developmental processes that occur as individuals age. For example, characteristics associated with specific cohorts (e.g., epidemics) or factors related to historical change (e.g., development of antibiotics) can contribute to different estimates of genetic and environmental influence on health. This occurs because heritability is a population-specific parameter, and quantitative genetic parameter estimates change when genetic and environmental sources of variation change.

In summary, quantitative behavioral genetic methodologies serve as tools for estimating the degree to which complex health traits or characteristics are influenced by genetic and environmental factors. Identical and fraternal twins, pairs of family members, and adopted siblings differ in genetic relatedness. In addition, these family members might have been reared together or apart (i.e., adopted apart), providing groups of individuals that differ in environmental similarity as well. Such methods allow for the exploration of questions such as the extent to which health characteristics are influenced by genetic factors, environmental factors, or both. The next section of this chapter reviews research relevant to this type of question. Health characteristics reviewed in this chapter include disorders that have been examined at different points in the life span such as obesity, cardiovascular (CV) disease, juvenile- and adult-onset diabetes mellitus (DM), as well as longevity, a more global index of health.

BEHAVIORAL GENETIC RESEARCH
ON HEALTH ACROSS THE LIFE SPAN

Obesity

Obesity has been linked with numerous health problems, such as increased risk for heart disease, diabetes, certain cancers, and psychological problems. As a result, understanding the etiology of weight in both the normal and extreme range is crucial to a broad understanding of individual differences in health. Obesity is also one of the few health-related characteristics that has been studied across the life span using behavioral genetic methodology—albeit most studies are cross-sectional, and as such are limited by the issues previously discussed.

Reviews of weight and obesity (Foch & McClearn, 1980; Grilo & Pogue-Geile, 1991; Maes, Neale, & Eaves, 1997) indicate that body weight and obesity are substantially influenced by heredity. Although several forms of obesity can be attributed to single-gene disorders, such as Bardet-Biedle, Laurence-Moon, and Alstrom syndromes, fewer than 5% of cases of obesity can be attributed to such single-gene effects. It is also conceivable that some cases of obesity may be attributed to an overriding environmental factor, such as an overwhelmingly stressful life event. Most incidences of obesity, however, are probably due to the cumulative effects of many genetic loci and environmental factors. In addition, the extent to which genes and environment influence obesity might differ at different points in the life course. Family, twin, and adoption studies using samples of various ages have enabled us to examine the relative influences of heredity, shared environmental, and nonshared environmental influences across the life span.

The Louisville Twin Study has supplied longitudinal information about the heritability of physical characteristics during infancy and early childhood (Wilson, 1976). At birth, MZ and DZ correlations for weight are essentially equivalent (r_{MZ}

$= .62$ and $r_{DZ} = .66$), suggesting that shared environmental effects, such as prenatal conditions, account for the majority of the variation in newborn body weight. By 6 months of age, however, heritability was estimated to be 34% ($r_{MZ} = .78$ and $r_{DZ} = .61$), and from 12 months to 6 years, heritabilities stabilized at around 60%, which is closer to estimates found in adult samples (Grilo & Pogue-Geile, 1991).

Unfortunately, obesity has been defined and assessed in various ways, and depending on how obesity is measured, estimates of the relative influence of genetic and environmental factors differ. In one study, using a composite measure of subscapular and triceps skinfolds as an index of fatness, researchers reported heritability estimates that were different for children compared to adolescents and adults (Brook, Huntley, & Slack, 1975). When twin pairs were divided into groups of under or over 10 years of age, heritability was greater for older twins ($h^2 = .98$) than in younger twins ($h^2 = .52$). High heritability estimates were also obtained from a longitudinal study of adult twins aged 20 and 45 (Stunkard, Foch, & Hrubec, 1986). Using the Body Mass Index (BMI) as a measure of obesity (weight [kg] / height $[m]^2$), Stunkard and colleagues estimated heritability to be about 80% for both adult age groups.

Obesity has also been measured as a categorical variable. The co-twin concordance rate for individuals who were 25% overweight at age 20 was 47% for identical twins and 28% for fraternal twin pairs; for those overweight at age 45, concordance rates were 54% and 26%, respectively (Stunkard et al., 1986). Similar concordance rates were found in another sample of adult twins with a larger age range (Medlund, Cederlöf, Floderus-Myrhed, Friberg, & Sörensen, 1976). Interestingly, five times as many individuals were obese at age 45, compared to age 20, but the pattern of concordance rates was fairly similar over time (slight increase in heritability). That is, although the incidence of obesity increased with age, the pattern of twin similarity remained constant. It is also important to note that these results indicate that the high extreme of the normal weight distribution occurs for reasons that are similar to those that affect the rest of the population.

In addition to studies using twins, several studies have used the sibling-adoption design to examine genetic and environmental influence on obesity. The sibling-adoption design is especially useful for directly testing the importance of shared rearing environment because adopted siblings who live in the same household do not share any hereditary influences. Thus, any resemblance between biologically unrelated pairs of individuals indicates the influence of shared environment. Biron, Mongeau, and Bertrand (1977) reported nonsignificant adoptive sibling correlations for weight (age of siblings: 1 to 21 years). Likewise, Bouchard, Savard, Depres, Tremblay, and Leblanc (1985) reported nonsignificant adoptive sibling correlations on measures of tricep and subscapular skinfold indices (age of siblings: 8 to 26 years). Together, these results suggest no effect of shared family experience for weight or fatness. One study contradicts findings from Biron et al. (1977) and Bouchard et al. (1985): Garn, Cole, and Bailey (1979) found that unrelated siblings aged 0 to 18 were significantly correlated ($r = .31$). However, Garn et al.'s (1979) study differs from the other two in that the sample included stepsiblings. To the extent that assortative mating occurs, that is, couples remarry on the basis of similar characteristics, and bring with them their children who are biologically related to themselves, correlations would be artificially inflated. In other words, shared environmental factors are confounded with assortative mating effects.

If the data are available, the adoption design can also permit examination of resemblance between biological parents and their adopted-away offspring. The Colorado Adoption Project (Plomin & DeFries, 1985) is one such longitudinal project to provide information of this type. Model-fitting analyses of BMI from birth to age 9 yielded nonsignificant heritability estimates from birth to 3, but significant heritabilities from ages 3 to 9 (year-to-year heritability estimates ranged from .37 to .57; Cardon, 1994). Thus, even though biological parents and their adopted-away children do not share living conditions, and they differ substantially in age, results again support the general finding that body mass is heritable and estimates indicate that heritability increases with development, at least from infancy to middle childhood.

Finally, identical twins who are reared apart (MZA) provide us with unique data to examine genetic and environmental influences because MZA twin resemblance is attributable only to their shared genes, not environmental experiences (assuming no selective placement). Five major studies of weight in MZA twins have been published (see Grilo & Pogue-Guile, 1991, for a review). Of particular relevance is the recent large study reported by Stunkard, Harris, Pedersen, and McClearn (1990) from the SATSA (average age = 59). Overall, across ages and gender, MZA correlations average .72 for weight and .62 for BMI. When correlations are compared to those of MZ twins reared together (.80 for weight and .74 for BMI), the similarity is striking, again suggesting little additional effect of shared rearing environment over that of shared genes.

Despite different designs and methodologies for assessing obesity, behavioral genetic studies converge on the finding that heritability appears to increase in influence on body weight and obesity from infancy through adulthood. In addition, there is little evidence that *shared* family environment contributes to obesity during adulthood. These results do not imply that obesity (or lack thereof) is inevitable because, nonshared environmental effects, or those factors that make twins different are important throughout the life span. In terms of prevention strategies, interventions could be targeted toward children and adults who are at genetic risk for becoming obese. For example, using an animal model, Stern and Johnson (1977) found that simply increasing physical activity prevented the development of obesity in 50% of yellow mice that had been bred for obesity and limited the extent of obesity among the other 50%.

Cardiovascular Disease

One area of health that is related to obesity (especially in adulthood) is CV disease. Atherosclerosis is a disease of the large arteries and is the major cause of heart disease and stroke in middle age and later life (Lusis, Rotter & Sparks, 1992). Research indicates that it is a complex disorder that is determined by numerous genetic as well as environmental factors. Behavioral genetic studies of coronary heart disease have recently been reviewed; for more a more detailed overview see deFaire and Pedersen's work (1994). The discussion here briefly reviews studies of genetic and environmental influences on risk factors for heart disease (especially in children and young adults) as well as the etiology of CV disease more broadly.

Although CV disease is not a widespread problem in children, several studies have examined CV risk factors (e.g., high blood pressure) in younger populations. Resemblance between newborns (aged 48 to 96 hours) and their mothers was significant for diastolic blood pressure (DBP) and was in the same direction, but not significant for systolic blood pressure (SBP; Lee, Rosner, Gould, Lowe, & Kass, 1976). Likewise, sibling–sibling (aged 2 to 14) and mother–child similarity, based on regression coefficients, were .34 and .16 for SBP and .32 and .17 for DBP, respectively (Zinner, Levy, & Kass, 1971). Greater sibling–sibling than parent–child resemblance might reflect a cohort or age effect. It is important to remember, however, that estimates based on family resemblance cannot be used to disentangle genetic and environmental effects.

Rice, Vogler, Pérusse, Bouchard, and Rao (1989) used both twins and adoptive families to examine resemblance in SBP, DBP, and mean arterial blood pressure (MBP) in a sample of French Canadians aged 8 to 25. Heritability estimates were lower for models using parent–offspring data (e.g., heritabilities ranged from 10% to 15%) than for models using twin or adoptive sibling data (40% to 50%), which again suggests a possible cohort or age effect. Shared environment estimates were substantial for SBP and MBP for both generations (30% to 40%) but were higher in parents (43%) than in offspring (21%) for DBP.

Interestingly, sibling correlations examining gender effects for SBP and MBP suggest that female sibling pairs are more similar than male siblings, with the opposite pattern for DBP. Although Rice et al. (1989) found no evidence to support specific gender effects in parent–offspring resemblance, a Belgian study (Joossens, 1980) found that the parent–offspring group with greatest resemblance for blood pressure (BP) was for father–son pairs, and the group with the lowest degree of similarity was for father–daughter dyads. However, other studies have not found such gender differences in parent–offspring resemblance (e.g., Havlik et al., 1979). Clearly, more research is required in the area of age and gender effects for familial resemblence in BP.

It is important to keep in mind that BP is often correlated with other characteristics (e.g., obesity). Thus far, one behavioral genetic study on children has examined whether such associations between BMI and BP were genetically mediated. Multivariate genetic analyses indicated that there are significant genetic paths that are shared between BMI and SBP, and between SBP and DBP, but not between BMI and DBP (Schieken, 1993). These results suggest that there may be some overlap in genetic etiologies for markers of BP and BMI.

The study of hypertension in children, which is defined somewhat differently than in adults, might yield different etiological results compared to the examination of normal-range BP. Although it is somewhat of an arbitrary cutoff, children whose BP is in the upper 95th percentile for age, gender, and race, are generally classified as *hypertensive* (Mongeau, 1987). In the examination of the percentage of children with hypertension when one or both parents were hypertensive, there was some support for genetic effects. Depending on the geographical location of the sample, the incidence of hypertension in children varies from 15.9% to 56.8% if one parent is hypertensive and from 44% to 73.3% if both parents are hypertensive (Miyao & Furusho, 1978). Although results suggest increased genetic risk when both parents are hypertensive, effects due to shared environment cannot be ruled out from such family designs. In addition, results from a study by Lauer, Burns, and Clarke (1985) suggest that childhood hypertension may have different developmental trajectories. They found that one group of children, who were in the 95th percentile for their age, gender, and race, continued to remain hypertensive as they developed, whereas another group had BP readings around the 50th percentile early in life, but with time, readings increased to abnormally high values (Lauer et al., 1985). Such results suggests that there may be multiple ways in which hypertension develops. A cautionary note is warranted, however; the results are based on a single study and more behavioral genetic work is needed on hypertension in childhood.

In adulthood, the risk of death from myocardial infarction (heart attack) is 1.5 to 2 times greater in a man whose male sibling died at an early age (less than 50 years of age). This type of premature coronary heart disease is a single-gene defect, affecting lipoprotein metabolism, that accounts for about 5% of coronary disease in the population (Schumaker & Lembertas, 1992). The abnormality is related to hypercholesterolemia via apolipoprotein B (Ose & Tolleshaug, 1989; Rajput-Williams et al., 1988), and the gene (located on Chromosome 19) is associated with obesity, high blood cholesterol levels, and increased risk of coronary heart disease.

Because CV disease is a multidimensional disorder, attributes related to coronary artery disease, such as blood pressure, cholesterol levels, and glucose intolerance have been studied in adults. Heritability estimates of .44 for SBP and .34 for DBP were reported in a study using data from the SATSA (Hong, deFaire, Heller, McClearn, & Pedersen, 1994). In addition, depending on the model being tested (total sample; separated by age group or by gender), shared family environment accounted for up to 27% of the variance. Model-fitting analyses also indicated significant age differences in heritability for serum lipid (e.g., cholesterol) and apolipoproteins (Heller, deFaire, Pedersen, Dahlén, & McClearn, 1993). In the young cohort (age < 65) the heritability estimate for total cholesterol was 63%, whereas in the older group (age ≥ 65) the heritability was 26%. Although there is clearly an indication of the importance of hereditary factors, genetic influences appear to be more important at younger ages. Shared rearing environment was also important for individual differences in total cholesterol levels, especially in the older cohort, accounting for 16% and 36% of the variance in the young and old cohorts, respectively.

A report from the National Heart, Lung, and Blood Institute (NHLBI; Feinleib et al., 1977) focused on CV disease risk factors in middle-aged men. The patterns of twin similarity suggest that the familial aggregation of CV disease results from a genetic influence on BP (h^2 = .60 for SBP and .61 for DBP), hematocrit (h^2 = .25), uric acid (h^2 = .53), triglyceride levels probably resulting in obesity (h^2 = .56), and glucose intolerance (h^2 = .88). In addition to shared environment, genetic influences accounted for 14% to 31% (corrected for a variance difference in DZ vs. MZ twins) of individual differences in cholesterol levels in these twins. In a 16-year follow-up of this sample, an inverse relation between plasma high density lipoprotein cholesterol and the risk for the complication for arteriosclerosis (h^2 = .56) was found (Christian et al., 1990).

Although multiple studies have assessed vascular disease (primarily CV), few studies have looked at the etiology of cerebrovascular accidents, more commonly referred to as stroke. Using male twins from the National Academy of Sciences–National Research Council (NAS–NRC) Twin Registry, researchers reported concordance rates of 17.7% for MZ and 3.6% for DZ twins (Brass, Isaacsohn, Merikangas, & Robinette, 1992). Although there were too few pairs of twins with stroke to reliably estimate the magnitude of heritability, these results indicate a nearly fivefold increase in the co-occurrence of stroke in MZ twins compared to DZ twins. This finding suggests that genetic factors may be important contributors to the etiology of stroke. Additional research is needed, however, to verify these conclusions.

In summary, behavioral genetic studies on vascular and CV disease suggest the importance of both genetic and environmental influences. Moreover, when potential indicators of CV disease such as BP are examined for different age groups, estimates of genetic and environmental influences appear to be roughly equivalent. However, similarities between parents and offspring are typically lower than resemblance between siblings within a family, suggesting that cohort or age is important to consider. Gender may also be a factor, however, studies do not always converge on whether genetic and environmental effects differ according to gender. And given that many studies, especially on adults, control for possible gender effects by including only males in their sample, we may be missing some important information regarding the role that gender plays in genetic and environmental etiologies of CV disease and its physiological markers.

Diabetes Mellitus

Diabetes mellitus applies to a number of disorders that involve inappropriate hyperglycemia and absolute or relative insulin deficiency. In the past few decades, advances have been made in understanding the nature of familial predisposition to diabetes. Among these advances are two diabetic classifications—insulin-dependent

DM (Type I) and non-insulin-dependent DM (Type II)—that appear to have distinct etiologies. For example, in terms of familial risk, close relatives of patients with DM have increased risk of developing the disease, but the risk is almost exclusively for the same form of the disorder (insulin- or non-insulin-dependent DM) as is present in the proband (MacDonald, 1974).

The age at which onset occurs is often—but not always—related to the type of DM. Insulin-dependent DM generally has an onset before age 45 and patients are typically of normal weight. Non-insulin-dependent diabetes, on the other hand, usually occurs after age 40, and affected patients are often obese. Insulin therapy may be necessary to prevent symptomatic hyperglycemia in some non-insulin-dependent DM patients, but caloric restriction or oral medication is frequently sufficient. Because of the age-related differences in onset of the insulin and non-insulin-dependent forms of DM, some have referred to· the former as "juvenile" diabetes and the latter as "adult-onset" diabetes, although insulin dependence, rather than age, is a better criterion for distinguishing the two types (Craighead, 1978). To avoid confusion, we use the terms *Type I DM* to indicate juvenile or insulin-dependent DM and *Type II DM* to represent adult-onset or non-insulin-dependent DM.

Evidence for genetic distinction between Type I and Type II DM generally comes from twin studies. Although twin studies often differ in their reported concordance rates for MZ versus DZ twins, studies that have compared concordance rates for Type I versus Type II diabetes have reached similar conclusions: Heritability appears stronger for Type II diabetes than for Type I diabetes. For example, concordance rates in MZ pairs for Type I diabetes range from 10% to 50%, whereas those for Type II diabetes range from 70% to 100% (see Friedman & Fialkow, 1980, for a review).

In addition to probable distinct etiologies for Type I and Type II DM, there may be different mechanisms by which the two forms of DM develop. In other words, within each type of DM, heterogeneity exists (Friedman & Fialkow, 1980). Pyke and Nelson (1976) observed that an MZ twin who does not develop DM within 3 years of his or her Type I diabetic co-twin probably never will have the disease (based on follow-ups of more than 10 years), which suggests that environmental factors might play a role in its development or expression. Several environmental factors have been suggested. For example, dietary agents such as certain proteins found in cow's milk (Coleman, Kuzava, & Leiter, 1990) and preservatives used in curing mutton (Helgason, Ewen, Ross, & Stowers, 1982) have been implicated in several studies of Type I DM. Some studies have also suggested that exposure to viruses at a young age might be linked to triggering immune problems that then leads to Type I diabetes (Gamble, 1977). It is also possible that such environmental factors negatively influence only those individuals who are genetically susceptible to the disease (Blom & Dahlquist, 1985; Leslie & Elliott, 1994). In addition, Leslie and Elliott suggested that Type I diabetes may be initiated by single or multiple exposures of an environmental factor during a critical period in early childhood.

Thus, genetic and environmental factors might interact to make certain individuals more susceptible than others in developing Type I DM.

In the case of Type II DM, there is evidence for a mutation in the gene for the insulin receptor and in enzymes of sugar metabolism (Shimada et al., 1990.) In addition, there is at least one monogenic type of DM, called maturity-onset diabetes of young people, that appears to be the result of an autosomal dominant allele (Fajans et al., 1976). However, other forms of Type II DM may have a more complex etiology. For example, twin studies of Type II DM have indicated that the concordance rates for MZ twins range from 55% to 100%, but only 4% to 46% for DZ twins indicating substantial genetic influence (Friedman & Fialkow, 1980; Shohat, Raffel, Vadhaim, & Rotter, 1992). Perhaps the strongest evidence for genetic influence on Type II DM comes from a study on glucose intolerance. For example, data from the NHLBI study described earlier indicate that the heritability for glucose intolerance was .88 (Feinleib et al., 1977). However, Friedman and Fialkow (1980) suggested that environmental agents (e.g., diet) may be important in determining the severity of glucose intolerance in genetically predisposed people.

In summary, Type I and Type II DM appear to have distinct etiologies, with Type II being under more genetic control than Type I; however both conditions appear to involve complex processes. In addition, the types and timing of exposure to certain environmental factors might be critical in disease onset or severity.

Longevity

Perhaps one of the most viable indicators of overall health status is longevity. The notion that longevity has a familial component has been around for a long time. In fact, more than a century ago Oliver Wendell Holmes presented the following advice: "those wishing long lives should advertise for a couple of parents, both belonging to long-lived families" (Cohen, 1964, p.133). Genealogical studies (e.g., Pearl & Pearl, 1934), have consistently established a significant, but modest, familial component to human longevity. Because familial resemblance includes both genetic and environmental influences, however, family studies alone do not provide conclusive evidence for a genetic component to longevity. Results from studies using twin and adoption designs also provide support for the conclusion that genetic factors play a role in how long people live. The most extensive work of this type comes from the Danish Twin Registry (Hougaard, Harvald, & Holm, 1992a, 1992b; McGue, Vaupel, Holm, & Harvald, 1993; Vaupel, Harvald, Holm, Yashin, & Xiu, 1992). Results from one study, for example, indicated a moderate heritability ($h^2 = .22$) for life span (McGue, Vaupel, et al., 1993). Interestingly, most of the variance was environmental, but was of the nonshared type. That is, the environmental influences that are important determinants of longevity contribute to twin differences, rather than to twin similarity.

One reason suggested to explain why the relation between parents and offspring for longevity is modest is that what children inherit from their parents is not longevity per se, but rather frailty. That is, children inherit susceptibility to disease or other risk factors that contribute toward their chances of death at different ages (Vaupel, 1988; Vaupel, Manton, & Stallard, 1979). Results from a Danish adoption study, indicating that the premature death of a biological parent related to a twofold increase in mortality of the adoptee, supported this hypothesis (Sorensen, Nielsen, Andersen, & Teasdale, 1988). Similar results were found in the NAS–NRC (Hrubec & Neel, 1981). In this sample, genetic differences for liability to death from disease accounted for 54% of the individual differences for this trait, indicating that familial resemblance for disease mortality is primarily due to genetic influences.

IMPLICATIONS FOR THEORY AND RESEARCH
ON HEALTH ACROSS THE LIFE SPAN

Two general hypotheses have been posited to describe potential change in the relative influences of genetic and environmental factors. First, developmental behavioral geneticists have suggested that when heritability changes with development, it increases (Plomin, 1986; Plomin & Thompson, 1988). Supporting this hypothesis are results from longitudinal studies of infant and childhood obesity, coupled with results from studies on adult obesity, that indicate that heritability estimates are higher once children exit the infant and toddler period. Such a pattern suggests that early environments, which are less under the control of the infant (e.g., prenatal environment and limited control in food selection postnatally), might override genetic propensities for body weight. Indeed, Scarr and McCartney (1983) proposed that as individuals become older, they gain increasing control over their environment and in essence, "niche-pick." That is, older individuals may be become more active in selecting environments that support or even promote their genetic tendencies. In the obesity example, individuals with a genetic propensity for being overweight may create an environment through their lifestyle (e.g., poor diet, lack of exercise) that correlates with, and even promotes, their genetic predispositions.

Proponents of an alternative hypothesis about the relative influences of nature and nurture across the life span suggest that as individuals have a greater number of life experiences, the impact of the environment plays an increasingly important role in determining the course of human development (Baltes, Reese, & Lipsett, 1980). As a result, it is speculated that heritability will decrease with age. There is generally little evidence for a decrease in heritability across the life span, although there is some indication that the heritability for self-reported physical health might be lower in older age groups than in younger ones (Harris, Pedersen, McClearn, Plomin, & Nesselroade, 1992). The environmental influences on development, which are primarily of the nonshared type, provides some support for the second hypothesis.

At this point, however, empirical support for either of these hypotheses is lacking because the majority of the research in this area is based on cross-sectional analyses. The results of cross-sectional studies of genetic and environmental influences on health have indicated that there may be some important etiological differences at various points in the life span. Heritability and environmentality are considered static estimates because they are based on findings from a certain population at a given point in time; different estimates of heritability (and environmentality) can be obtained from samples of study participants who have vastly different experiences due to their cohort, socioeconomic status, culture, or other factors that contribute to differential experience.

Apparent differences in heritability across the life span could also be due to selection effects on longevity or functional capacity (Boomsma, 1993). For example, genetic influences might appear to be more important for health characteristics in middle adulthood, because characteristics that are highly heritable might result in the death of one or both of the twins; an example of this is CV disease (Bergeman, 1997). The effect of the loss of these participants from the sample (or potential sample) is an artificially lower heritability estimate for the later age groups.

Even if estimates of heritability do not change with age, levels of heritability can be the same at two ages for different genetic reasons. That is, the genes that affect the trait at one age could be different from the genes that affect the trait at another age, but the overall magnitude of genetic effects (heritability) could be the same at the two ages. Traditionally, the variance due to age is statistically controlled for in behavioral genetic analyses or removed by selecting participants from narrow age bands because age effects cannot be assigned to either a genetic or an environmental component of variance (see McGue & Bouchard, 1984, for details). Thus, caution should be exercised when generalizing the results beyond the age or cohort of the samples used, because without a longitudinal design, there is no way to disentangle effects due to age (age change) versus experience (age differences). Thus, longitudinal designs are crucial in the study of stability or change in genetic and environmental effects.

There are several longitudinal behavioral genetic studies on health-related issues across age groups (e.g., Louisville Twin Study, Colorado Adoption Project, SATSA). Valuable data are also available from twin registries that have been established in many Scandinavian countries. Unfortunately, most of these data are limited to short segments of the life span (e.g., infancy to adolescence). For this reason, these studies provide little information about the etiology of health across the entire life span, and comparisons have to be made across different studies, using different measures and study participant populations. For example, studies differ in their definition of the disease (e.g., obesity; hypertension) or the samples differ (e.g., many studies of heart disease have focused only on men). Perhaps because different health issues are more salient in some age groups (e.g., CV disease), longitudinal studies may seem less relevant to other age groups. However, as a more comprehensive understanding of the biological processes involved prior to disease onset is gained, the utility of conducting longitudinal behavioral genetic twin studies of seemingly age-specific diseases should become more apparent.

To date, much of behavioral genetic research on health-related issues focus on the extent to which certain health characteristics are influenced by genetic, shared environmental, and nonshared environmental factors. These results have important implications for understanding health issues all across the life span. For example, it is important to avoid the mistaken notion that even when measures of health show substantial heritability—as in the case of obesity—this does not mean that the problems are inevitable. Changes in the environment can alter the extent to which a genetic characteristic is phenotypically expressed. For example, phenylketonuria, which results in mental retardation if left untreated, is completely heritable (i.e., it is a recessive, single-gene disease). If the amount of phenylalanine in the diet is restricted until the early school years, however, the manifestation of the disorder is circumvented. Thus, although the genetic defect results in the inability to produce phenylalanine hydroxylase (an enzyme that converts phenylalanine to tyrosine), a completely environmental intervention strategy can change the expression of the underlying problem.

Behavioral genetic research can guide health professionals toward appropriate intervention strategies by elucidating the etiology of the health problem of interest. Because the health problems discussed in this chapter are complex, it is unlikely that a single intervention will be appropriate. Given the results of behavioral genetic research to date, it may prove fruitful to examine the ways in which combinations of genotypes and environments work; an example of this is coronary heart disease. Research has indicated that even individuals who eat essentially the same diet show large individual differences in coronary heart disease, probably due to genetic differences (Lusis et al., 1992). In fact, research has indicated that a high blood cholesterol level appears to be a prerequisite for the deleterious effect of other secondary factors, such as hypertension, diabetes, autoimmune disorders and coagulation factor levels. Thus, if an individual is not genetically predisposed to high levels of low-density lipoprotein cholesterol, then the other risk factors such as smoking or high blood pressure may not be as important.

In summary, theory and research in genetic (nature) and environmental (nurture) influences are beginning to converge on a common ground model of active organism–environment interaction in which nature and nurture play a "duet" rather than one directing the performance of the other (Plomin, 1995). It seems clear that some of the most interesting questions for genetic research on health behaviors involve the environment, and some of the more interesting questions for environmental research involve heredity.

REFERENCES

Baltes, P. B., Reese, H. W., & Lipsitt, L. P. (1980). Life-span developmental psychology. *Annual Review of Psychology, 31,* 65–110.

Bergeman, C. S. (1997). *Aging: Genetic and environmental influences.* Thousand Oaks, CA: Sage.

Biron, P., Mongeau, J. G., & Bertrand, D. (1977). Familial resemblance of body weight and weight/height in 374 homes with adopted children. *Journal of Pediatrics, 91,* 555–558.

Blom, L., & Dahlquist, G. (1985). Epidemiological aspects of the natural history of childhood diabetes. *Acata Pediatrica Scandinavia, Suppl. 320,* 20–25.

Boomsma, D. I. (1993). Current status and future prospects in twin studies of the development of cognitive abilities: Infancy to old age. In T. J. Bouchard & P. Propping (Eds.), *Twins as a tool of behavioral genetics* (pp. 69–82). New York: Wiley.

Bouchard, C., Savard, R., Despres, J-P., Tremblay, A., & Leblanc, C. (1985). Body composition in adopted and biological siblings. *Human Biology, 57,* 61–75.

Brass, L. M., Isaacsohn, J. L., Merikangas, K. R., & Robinette, C. D. (1992). A study of twins and stroke. *Stroke, 23,* 221–223.

Brook, C. G. D., Huntley, R. M. C., & Slack, J. (1975). Influence of heredity and environment in determination of skinfold thickness in children. *British Medical Journal, 2,* 719–721.

Cardon, L. (1994). Height, weight, and obesity. In J. C. DeFries, R. Plomin, and D. W. Fulker (Eds.), *Nature and nurture during middle childhood* (pp. 165–172). Cambridge, MA: Blackwell.

Christian, J. C., Carmelli, D., Castelli, W. P., Fabsitz, R., Grim, C. E., Meany, F. J., Norton, J. A.; Reed, T., Williams, C. J., & Wood, P. (1990). High density lipoprotein cholesterol: A 16-year longitudinal study in aging male twins. *Arteriosclerosis, 10,* 1020–1025.

Cohen, B. H. (1964). Family patterns of mortality and life span. *Quarterly Review of Biology, 39,* 130–181.

Coleman, D. L., Kuzava, J. E., & Leiter, E. H. (1990). Effect of diet on incidence of diabetes in nonobese diabetic mice. *Diabetes, 39,* 432–436.

Craighead, J. E. (1978). Current views on the etiology of insulin-dependent diabetes mellitus. *New England Journal of Medicine, 299,* 1439–1445.

deFaire, U., & Pedersen, N. L. (1994). Studies of twins and adoptees in coronary heart disease. In U. Goldbourt, U. deFaire, & K. Berg (Eds.), *Genetic factors in coronary heart disease* (pp. 55–68). Dordrecht: Kluwer.

Fajans, S. S., Floyd, J. C., Tattersall, R. B., Williamson, J. R., Pek, S., & Taylor, C. I. (1976). The various faces of diabetes in the young. *Archives of Internal Medicine, 136,* 194–202.

Feinleib, M., Garrison, R. J., Fabsitz, R. R., Christian, J. C., Hrubec, Z., Borhani, N. O., Kannel, W. B., Rosenman, R., Schwartz, J. T., & Wagner, J. O. (1977). The NHLBI Twin Study of cardiovascular disease risk factors: Methodology and summary of results. *American Journal of Epidemiology, 106,* 284–295.

Foch, T. T., & McClearn, G. E. (1980). Genetics, body weight, and obesity. In A. J. Stunkard (Ed.), *Obesity* (pp. 48–71). Philadelphia: Saunders.

Friedman, J. M., & Fialkow, P. J. (1980). The genetics of diabetes mellitus. In A. Steinberg, A. Bearn, A. Motulski, and B. Childs (Eds.), *Progress in medical genetics: Vol. 4. Genetics of gastrointestinal disease* (pp. 199–232). Philadelphia: Saunders.

Gamble, D. R. (1977). Viruses and diabetes: An overview with special reference to epidemiological studies. In J. S. Bajaj (Ed.), *Proceedings of IXth Congress of the International Diabetes Federation* (pp. 285–293). Amsterdam: Oxford.

Garn, S. M., Cole, P. E., & Bailey, S. M. (1979). Living together as a factor in family-line resemblances. *Human Biology, 51,* 565–587.

Grilo, C. M., & Pogue-Geile, M. F. (1991). The nature of environmental influences on weight and obesity: A behavior genetic analysis. *Psychological Bulletin, 110,* 520–537.

Harris, J. R., Pedersen, N. L., McClearn, G. E., Plomin, R., & Nesselroade, J. R. (1992). Age differences in genetic and environmental influences for health from the Swedish Adoption/Twin Study of Aging. *Journal of Gerontology: Psychological Sciences, 47*, 213–220.

Havlik, R. J., Garrison, R. J., Feinleib, M., Kannel, W. B., Castelli, W. P., & McNamara, P. M. (1979). Blood pressure aggregation in families. *American Journal of Epidemiology, 110*, 304–312.

Helgason, T., Ewen, S. W. B., Ross, J. S., & Stowers, J. M. (1982). Diabetes produced in mice by smoked/cured mutton. *Lancet II*, 1017–1022.

Heller, D. A., deFaire, U., Pedersen, N. L., Dahlén, G., & McClearn, G. E. (1993). Genetic and environmental influences on serum lipid levels in twins. *New England Journal of Medicine, 328*, 1150–1156.

Hong, Y., deFaire, U., Heller, D. A., McClearn, G. E., & Pedersen, N. L. (1994). Genetic and environmental influence on blood pressure in elderly twins. *Hypertension, 24*, 663–670.

Hougaard, P., Harvald, B., & Holm, N. V. (1992a). Assessment of dependence in the lifetimes of twins. In J. P. Klein & P. K. Goel (Eds.), *Survival analysis: State of the art* (pp. 77–97). Dordrecht: Kluwer.

Hougaard, P., Harvald, B., & Holm, N. V. (1992b). Measuring similarities between the lifetimes of adult Danish twins born between 1881–1930. *Journal of American Statistical Association, 87*, 17–24.

Hrubec, Z., & Neel, J. V. (1981). Familial factors in early deaths: Twins followed 30 years to ages 51–61 in 1978. *Human Genetics, 59*, 39–46.

Joosens, J. V. (1980). Stroke, stomach cancer, and salt: A possible clue to the prevention of hypertension. In J. Kesteloot & J. V. Joossens (Eds.), *Epidemiology of arterial blood pressure* (pp. 489–506). The Hague: Martinus Nijhoff.

Lauer, R. M., Burns, T. L., & Clarke, W. R. (1985). Assessing children's blood pressure—considerations of age and body size: The Muscatine Study. *Pediatrics, 75*, 1081–1090.

Lee, Y. H., Rosner, B., Gould, J. B., Lowe, E. W., & Kass, E. H. (1976). Familial aggregation of blood pressures of newborn infants and their mother. *Pediatrics, 58*, 722–729.

Leslie, R. D. G., & Elliott, R. B. (1994). Early environmental events as a cause of IDDM: Evidence and implications. *Diabetes, 43*, 843–850.

Loehlin, J. C. (1987). *Latent variable models: An introduction to factor, path, and structural analysis.* Hillsdale, NJ: Lawrence Erlbaum Associates.

Lusis, A. J., Rotter, J. I., & Sparkes, R. S. (Eds.). (1992). *Molecular genetics of coronary artery disease.* New York: Karger.

MacDonald, M. J. (1974). Equal incidence of adult-onset diabetes among ancestor juvenile diabetics and nondiabetics. *Diabetologia, 10*, 767–773.

Maes, H. H. M., Neale, M. C., & Eaves, L. J. (1997). Genetic and environmental factors in relative body weight and human adiposity. *Behavior Genetics, 27*, 325–351.

Medlund, P., Cederlöf, R., Flodérus-Myrhed, B., Friberg, L, & Sörensen, S. A. (1976). A new Swedish Twin Registry. *Acta Medica Scandinavia [Suppl.], 600*, 1–111.

McGue, M., & Bouchard, T. J. (1984). Adjustment of twin data for the effects of age and sex. *Behavior Genetics, 14*, 325–343.

McGue, M., Vaupel, J. W., Holm, W., & Harvald, L. S. (1993). Longevity is moderately heritable in a sample of Danish twins born 1870–1880. *Journal of Gerontology, 48*, B237-B224.

Miyao, S., & Furusho, T. (1978). Genetic study of essential hypertension. *Japanese Circulation Journal, 42*, 1161–1186.

Mongeau, J. G. (1987). Heredity and blood pressure in humans: An overview. *Pediatric Nephrology, 1*, 69–75.

Ose, L., & Tolleshaug, H. (1988). International symposium on familial hypercholesterolemia, *Arteriosclerosis, 9 (Suppl)*, I1–I186.

Pearl, R., & Pearl, R. D. (1934). *The ancestry of the long-lived.* Baltimore: Johns Hopkins University Press.

Plomin, R. (1986). *Development, genetics and psychology.* Hillsdale, NJ: Lawrence Erlbaum Associates.

Plomin, R. (1995). Genetics, environmental risks and protective factors. In J. R. Turner, L. R. Cardon, & J. K. Hewitt (Eds.), *Behavior genetic approaches in behavioral medicine* (pp. 217–235). New York: Plenum.

Plomin, R., & DeFries, J. C. (1985). *Origins of individual differences in infancy: The Colorado Adoption Project.* Orlando, FL: Academic Press.

Plomin, R., & Thompson, L. (1988). Life-span developmental behavioral genetics. In P. B. Baltes, D. L. Featherman, & R. M. Lerner (Eds.) *Life-span development and behavior: Vol. 8* (pp. 1–31). Hillsdale, NJ: Lawrence Erlbaum Associates.

Pyke, D. A., & Nelson, P. G. (1976). Diabetes mellitus in identical twins. In W. Creutzfeldt, J. Kobberling, & J. V. Neel (Eds.), *The genetics of diabetes mellitus* (pp. 194–202). New York: Springer-Verlag.

Rajput-Williams, J., Wallis, S. C., Yarnell, J., Bell, G. I., Knott, T. J., Sweetnam, P., Cox, N., Miller, N. E., & Scott, J. (1988). Variation in the apolipoprotein-B gene is associated with obesity, high blood cholesterol levels, and increased risk or coronary heart disease. *Lancet II,* 1442–1445.

Rice, T., Vogler, G. P., Pérusse, L., Bouchard, C., & Rao, D. C. (1989). Cardiovascular risk factors in a French Canadian population: Resolution of genetic and familial environmental effects of blood pressure using twins, adoptees, and extensive information on environmental correlates. *Genetic Epidemiology, 6,* 571–588.

Scarr, S., & McCartney, K. (1983). How people make their own environments: A theory of genotype → environment effects. *Child Development, 54,* 424–435.

Schieken, R. M. (1993). Genetic factors that predispose the child to develop hypertension. *Pediatric Clinic of North America, 40,* 1–11.

Schumaker, V., & Lembertas, A. (1992). Lipoprotein metabolism: Chylomicrons, very-low-density lipoproteins and low-density lipoproteins. In A. J. Lusis, J. I. Rotter, & R. S. Sparkes (Eds.), *Molecular genetics of coronary artery disease.* New York: Karger.

Shimada, F., Taira, M., Suzuki, Y., Hashimoto, N., Nozaki, O., Tatibana, M., Ebina, Y., Tawata, M., Onaya, T., Makino, H., & Yoshida, S. (1990). Insulin-resistant diabetes associated with partial deletion of insulin-receptor gene. *Lancet, 335,* 1179–1181.

Shohat, T., Raffel, L. F., Vadhaim, C. M., & Rotter, J. (1992). Diabetes Mellitus and coronary heart disease genetics. In A. J. Lusis, H. I. Rotter, & R. S. Sparks (Eds.), *Molecular genetics of coronary artery disease* (pp. 272–310). New York: Karger.

Sorensen, T., Nielsen, G., Andersen, P., & Teasdale, T. (1988). Genetic and environmental influences on premature death in adult adoptees. *New England Journal of Medicine, 318,* 727–732.

Stern, J. S., & Johnson, P. R. (1977). Spontaneous activity and adipose cellularity in the genetically abese Zucker rat. *Metabolism, 26,* 371–380.

Stunkard, A. J., Foch, T. T., & Hrubec, Z. (1986). A twin study of human obesity. *The Journal of the American Medical Association, 256,* 51–54.

Stunkard, A. J., Harris, J. R., Pedersen, N. L., & McClearn, G. E. (1990). The body-mass index of twins who have been reared apart. *The New England Journal of Medicine, 322,* 1483–1487.

Vaupel, J. W. (1988). Inherited frailty and longevity. *Demography, 25,* 277–287.

Vaupel, J. W., Harvald, B., Holm, W., Yashim, A., & Xiu, L. (1992). Survival analysis in genetics: Danish twin data applied to a gerontological question. In J. P. Klein & P. K. Goel (Eds.), *Survival analysis: State of the art* (pp. 121–138). Dordrecht, Netherlands: Kluwer.

Vaupel, J. W., Manton, K. G., & Stallard, E. (1979). The impact of heterogeneity in individual frailty on the dynamics of mortality. *Demography, 16,* 439–454.

Wilson, R. S. (1976). Concordance in physical growth for monozygotic and dizygotic twins. *Annals of Human Biology, 3,* 1–10.

Wright, S. (1921). Correlation and causation. *Journal of Agricultural Research, 20,* 557–585.

Zinner, S. H., Levy, P. S., & Kass, E. H. (1971). Familial aggregation of blood pressure in childhood. *The New England Journal of Medicine, 284,* 401–404.

4

Poverty and Health
Across the Life Span

Erika E. Bolig
John Borkowski
Jay Brandenberger
University of Notre Dame

ALTHOUGH the United States is the richest nation in the world, millions of adults and children live in poverty. In 1995, 36.4 million people were reported to be living below the poverty threshold, which then was $15,569 for a family of four (Weinberg, 1996). Alarmingly, 40% of those in poverty are children. This rate is the highest for any age group, with one in five children living below the poverty level. The poverty rate is significantly greater for minorities than for nonminorities and for female-headed households than for male- or two-parent-headed households (Sabol, 1991; Weinberg, 1996). In addition, the risk of being poor during older adulthood is significantly greater for women than for men (Hardy & Hazelrigg, 1993).

Many factors contribute to the fact that there is a large number of children and adults living in poverty, among them are high levels of unemployment among the unskilled and undereducated, particularly for African American males; lower wages for women; and the growing number of female-headed households (Hardy & Hazelrigg, 1993; Sabol, 1991). In addition, jobs that pay minimum wages generally do not generate enough income to lift a wage earner above the poverty threshold, and rarely provide benefits such as health insurance and child care (Tarnowski & Rohrbeck, 1993). Another contributing factor is the failure to complete high school, a phenomenon that is more common among adolescents from low-income families; dropping out of high school not only increases adolescents' chances of living in poverty during adulthood but also decreases their chances of escaping poverty for many years after they drop out (Schorr, 1989). Among older people, particularly women, greater longevity results in higher health costs, and a lack of adequate personal assets or governmental assistance place hundreds of thousands

TABLE 4.1
Threats to Health and Well-Being Across the Life Span

Prenatal Development and Infancy	Childhood	Adolescence	Adulthood
Inadequate prenatal care	AIDS	Substance abuse	Mental health problems
Congenital syphilis	Asthma	Pregnancy	AIDS
Perinatally contracted AIDS	Bacterial meningitis	Sexually transmitted diseases	Substance abuse
Prenatal drug or alcohol exposure	Rheumatic fever	AIDS	Domestic violence
Low birthweight	Diabetic ketoacidosis	Mental health problems	Hypertension
Neonatal and postneonatal mortality	Impaired vision	Suicide	Heart disease
Sudden infant death syndrome	Ear infections	Homicide	Diabetes
Stunted growth	Exposure to toxic chemicals	Gang violence	Cancer
Malnutrition or undernutrition	Gastrointestinal disorders		Tuberculosis
Anemia	Poor dental health		Sexually transmitted diseases
Lead poisoning	Allergies		Cumulative effects of inadequate medical care
Failure to thrive	Respiratory problems		Lack of resources for care
	Diseases and bites from rodents		
	Accidents		
	Poisoning		
	Abuse, neglect and/or maltreatment		

of individuals at greater risk for living in poverty during old age (Hardy & Hazelrigg, 1993).

In addition to its financial consequences, poverty also affects in profound ways the cognitive, emotional, social, and physical well-being of individuals. For example, poor children are twice as likely as other children to be born with low birthweight, three times as likely to receive necessary immunizations off schedule, and three to four times as likely to die of childhood diseases (Oberg, Bryant, & Bach, 1995). At the behavioral level, undernourished and malnourished children are three times as likely to experience concentration problems and irritability (which affects their learning, verbal skills, and motor skills), four times as likely to experience fatigue, and 12 times as likely to experience periods of dizziness. It is often difficult for children to overcome these adverse effects of early poverty because they affect so many aspects of their lives.

This chapter focuses on significant health problems across the life span that can be traced directly to poverty and discusses the implications of providing effective, adequately funded programs for those living in poverty. For the purposes of this discussion, the life span is divided into four age groups: prenatal development and infancy, childhood, adolescence, and adulthood. For each age group, critical health problems and their major risk factors are highlighted. The scope of this chapter is demonstrated in Table 4.1, which details the major health problems associated with poverty during the four developmental periods. The chapter concludes with a discussion of intervention programs designed to improve the health and well-being of the poor across key points in the life span and overviews plans for future programs and actions at the federal, state, and community levels.

POVERTY AND HEALTH IN INFANCY AND CHILDHOOD

Prenatal Development and Infancy

Children living in poverty are not only more likely to experience a greater number of health problems than other children but they also experience more severe problems (McGauhey & Starfield, 1993). Health problems among the poor begin even before birth (Sherman, 1994). During the prenatal and infancy periods, poor children are at increased risk for little or no prenatal care (Tarnowski & Rohrbeck, 1993), congenital syphilis (Klerman, 1996), perinatally contracted AIDS (Zuckerman, 1993), prenatal drug and/or alcohol exposure (Abel, 1995; Coles et al., 1991; Hawley & Disney, 1992), low birthweight (Children's Defense Fund, 1993), neonatal and postneonatal mortality (Garbarino, 1992; Oberg et al., 1995), sudden infant death syndrome (Sherman, 1994), stunted growth (Tarnowski & Rohrbeck, 1993), malnutrition or undernutrition (Brown & Pollitt, 1996), iron deficiency anemia (Oberg et al., 1995; Pollitt, 1994), lead poisoning, and failure to thrive (Black & Dubowitz, 1991).

Although these health threats are serious and often life threatening in their own right, they are also associated with—and sometimes cause—additional health or developmental problems. For example, low birthweight, which can be caused by inadequate prenatal care, smoking, alcohol use, or drug use during pregnancy (Coles, Platzman, Smith, James, & Falek, 1992; Tarnowski & Rohrbeck, 1993), has been linked to infant mortality (Oberg et al., 1995; Sherman, 1994), neurodevelopmental problems, birth defects, learning problems, and cognitive delays (Korenman, Miller, & Sjaastad, 1995). Sherman (1994) highlighted the reciprocal and adverse relations that link infant health problems and poverty: "A disadvantaged background often makes children more vulnerable to the effects of low birthweight. And, as in other interactions, the reverse is necessarily true as well: low birthweight makes children more vulnerable to the effects of poverty" (p. 56).

Malnutrition during the prenatal or infancy periods is another early health threat that has lifelong implications for the children's development. In the absence of intervention, early malnutrition has lingering effects that negatively affect a child's later cognitive, social, and behavioral development (Grantham-McGregor, Powell, Walker, Chang, & Fletcher, 1994; Morgane et al., 1993; Stein & Susser, 1985; Zeskind & Ramey, 1981). These findings, along with evaluation research documenting the cost-effectiveness of intervention programs such as the Women, Infants, and Children's program (WIC) (Schramm, 1985), underscore the importance of providing nutritional assistance during pregnancy and good prenatal care for successful development in infancy and childhood.

Childhood

The disadvantaged child not only might experience the lingering consequences of health problems from the prenatal and infancy periods, but also new threats can emerge that further jeopardize development. Growth retardation, anemia, poor nutrition, and lead poisoning often persist as problems (Klerman, 1996; Tarnowski & Rohrbeck, 1993). Added to these threats are childhood AIDS (Rosenbaum, 1992; Sabol, 1991), asthma, bacterial meningitis, rheumatic fever, diabetic ketoacidosis, impaired vision (Oberg et al., 1995), frequent ear infections, illness from exposure to toxic chemicals (Sherman, 1994), gastrointestinal disorders, and poor dental health (Rosenbaum, 1992). Numerous children living in poverty also contract diseases that could have been prevented by timely immunizations (Klerman, 1996; Liu & Rosenbaum, 1992; Oberg et al., 1995; Rosenbaum, 1992). Homelessness or long-term poverty further increase health, mental health, and developmental risks (Grant, 1990; Masten, 1992; Molnar & Rath, 1990; Wright, 1991; Ziesemer, Marcoux, & Marwell, 1994).

A child's safety can also be compromised by growing up in poverty. As a result of living in unsafe environments, disadvantaged children are at increased risk for accidents, including fatal accidents, and poisoning (Klerman, 1996; Oberg et al., 1995). In addition, parents trapped in poverty are less likely to engage in prevention behaviors such as learning the poison control phone number and ensuring that their water temperature is such that it would not cause scalding (Klerman, 1996), and installing latches on cabinets to prevent children from access to household cleaners, poisons, and medicines (Sherman, 1994). They are also less likely to use car seats and seat belts for their children (Tarnowski & Rohrbeck, 1993) and to have smoke detectors in their homes (Sherman, 1994).

Children's health and safety also can be greatly compromised by child abuse, neglect, and maltreatment. Although mistreatment of children occurs in all socioeconomic classes, it seems to occur more frequently in families living below the poverty line (Dore, 1993; Sherman, 1994; Williams, 1983); this is true particularly for severe and very severe cases of violence (Gelles, 1992). Other correlates of child mistreatment include single parenthood (particularly in low-income, female-headed families), limited parental education, and minority status (Dore, 1993).

Early Health Risks. Many factors contribute to increased risk for health problems during poor children's prenatal, infancy, and childhood periods. One of these factors is health insurance. From conception, children living in poverty face obstacles in receiving needed medical services. Lack of health insurance, inadequate coverage, and coverage that is not accepted by many doctors (e.g., Medicaid) are among the major reasons why poor women do not receive adequate prenatal care (Oberg et al., 1995; St. Clair, Smeriglio, Alexander, & Celentano, 1989). Low-income adolescents, unwed mothers, and African-American women are less likely than other groups to receive adequate prenatal care (Covington, Churchill, & Wright, 1994).

Each year, the number of uninsured children increases (Teitelbaum, 1994), a phenomenon that prompted Congressional action in 1997. For poor children, the lack of insurance often means little or no health care because available financial resources are needed for food and shelter. Thus, children may not receive the immunizations needed to guard against childhood diseases; in addition, many illnesses go untreated (Oberg et al., 1995). The consequences of this lack of preventative care and prompt treatment can be significant for a child's current and future development (e.g., polio, tetanus, and diphtheria as a result of not receiving immunizations; hearing loss and language disorders as a result of untreated ear infections).

Many features in the environment also contribute to poor children's heightened risk for health problems. Exposure to excessive amounts of crime and violence can lead to injury, death, and posttraumatic stress syndrome (Garbarino, 1995). Unsafe and crowded environments, as well as limited supervision, increase the disadvantaged child's risk for accidents and poisoning (Klerman, 1996; Oberg et al., 1995; Sherman, 1994). Living in crowded housing conditions also can cause children to experience more stress, get less sleep, and have greater susceptibility to illnesses. Low-income neighborhoods place children at greater risk for exposure to toxic chemicals, lead paint, and pollution (Kozol, 1995; Sherman, 1994), which can lead to cancer, lung damage, brain damage, and cognitive deficits (Needleman, 1994; Sherman, 1994). Other aspects of poverty can make the effects of exposure to toxic chemicals even graver. For example, the lack of proper nutrition can lead to iron deficiency which, in turn, can magnify the effect of lead in the bloodstream. More specifically, due to a lack of iron, blood cells absorb more lead, causing higher levels of lead in the child's bloodstream and, thus, more severe levels of lead poisoning.

Insufficient heat and damp housing conditions, common in low-income housing, can contribute to health problems in childhood such as allergies, asthma, and respiratory problems (Sherman, 1994). In addition, health problems can be caused by cockroaches, rats, and mice, which are more common in low-income housing (Moeller, 1992; Sherman, 1994). Rats and mice also place children at greater risk for injury due to bites and diseases.

POVERTY AND HEALTH:
ADOLESCENCE AND ADULTHOOD

During adolescence and adulthood, disadvantaged individuals experience new threats to their health and well-being, as well as continue to experience the lasting effects of earlier health problems caused or exacerbated by poverty.

Adolescence

For low-income youth, adolescence "stands in marked contrast to the mainstream adolescent experience, characterized by prolonged dependence, lack of adult responsibilities, and economic uselessness" (Crockett, 1997, p. 40). It can also be a time when the accumulation of chronic multiple stressors associated with poverty leads to school dropout, delinquency, mental health problems, suicide, drug or alcohol abuse, and violence (Rosella & Albrecht, 1993). The incidence of fatal and nonfatal violence is particularly high for low-income African Americans; for example, homicide has been reported to be the leading cause of death for African Americans between the ages of 15 and 34 (Hammond & Yung, 1991).

Other developmentally related problems that surface during adolescence include teen pregnancy (Merrick, 1995), sexually transmitted diseases (Koniak-Griffin, Nyamathi, Vasquez, & Russo, 1994), and AIDS (Rosenbaum, 1992), each of which occurs at higher rates in disadvantaged adolescents than their middle- and upper class counterparts. Although teenage pregnancy is associated with health problems for the mother (Scholl, Hediger, & Belsky, 1994), the health and developmental risks for the child are sometimes more extensive and debilitating (Furstenberg, Brooks-Gunn, & Morgan, 1987; Ketterlinus, Henderson, & Lamb, 1990), particularly when the young mother receives little or no prenatal care.

Risk Factors During Adolescence. Long-term exposure to poverty significantly affects the beliefs, attitudes, and cognitions that adolescents have about
themselves, others, and their futures. In turn, these attitudes and cognitions influence health-related behaviors. For instance, a lack of positive future orientation is
often displayed in the form of rage and disrespect for human life (Garbarino,
1995). As a result, youths might turn to gang life, which not only encourages and
provides an outlet for their rage but also provides a sense of belongingness, self-
worth, and security that low-income adolescents often lack (Garbarino, 1995;
Koniak-Griffin et al., 1994). Surrounded by increasing violence, many low-income
adolescents plan for their funerals rather than their futures; parents take out murder insurance policies rather than dreaming of their children's graduation cere-
monies (Rucker & Greene, 1995). Depression, suicide, drug and alcohol abuse,
school dropout, and delinquency are also common responses to a sense of hopelessness due to limited current and future opportunities (Dillihay, 1989; Rosella &
Albrecht, 1993).

Another response by adolescents faced with the realities of poverty is teenage
pregnancy. Whereas for middle-class teenagers pregnancy is often considered non-
normative, for low-income teenagers it is more typical. For low-income adolescents, having a child can provide a source of self-esteem and elevated income
(Merrick, 1995). The choice to become pregnant during adolescence also might
reflect the expectation of shorter life spans—and hence condensed life-event
timetables—for low-income individuals due to poor living conditions, inadequate medical care, and poor nutrition (Burton, 1990). Although teenage pregnancy can be an "adaptive" response to the conditions of poverty, it often has negative consequences for both the child and mother.

Low-income adolescents are also at increased risk for contracting AIDS (Koniak-
Griffin et al., 1994). Overwhelmed with the daily, constant stressors associated with
poverty, adolescents might not project their thoughts into the future and, thus, fail
to protect themselves from a disease whose effects might not be felt for several
years. As a result, low-income adolescents are more likely to engage in sexual risk-
taking than individuals not overwhelmed by the stressors of poverty, putting
themselves at increased risk for AIDS and other sexually transmitted diseases.

Adulthood

Poverty continues to tax a person's health during adulthood, as previous health
problems again continue to take their toll and new problems emerge. Adults in
poverty, particularly women and minorities, are at increased risk for mental health
problems, such as depression (Belle, 1990; Bennett, 1988; Dore, 1993). They also
experience greater numbers of stressful events, and these stressors often last for
long periods of time (Parker, Greer, & Zuckerman, 1988). The mental health problems and stresses associated with poverty not only affect an individual's functioning but also affect parenting behaviors and subsequent child outcomes (Mc-

Loyd & Wilson, 1991). For instance, low levels of social support, which are more commonly reported by disadvantaged families, negatively influence the quality of parent–child interactions, which, in turn, hinder children's development (Parker et al., 1988). Similarly, other health problems during adulthood have intergenerational consequences, including AIDS (Zuckerman, 1993), substance abuse, and domestic violence (Richie & Kanuha, 1993; Sullivan & Rumptz, 1994).

Common adult health problems influencing the quality of life of the poor are hypertension (Gilligan, 1996), heart disease (Ward, 1993), diabetes, cancer, tuberculosis, and sexually transmitted diseases. Not surprisingly, adults living in poverty tend to have shorter life expectancies than those not living in poverty (Pappas, Queen, Hadden, & Fisher, 1993), with the life expectancy for African Americans being shorter than that for Euro-Americans (Mechanic, 1986). As a result of shorter life expectancies, health problems encountered by those in poverty during the latter part of their life span have not been researched as much as problems encountered earlier in the life cycle.

Risk Factors During Adulthood. Many factors contribute to health problems in economically disadvantaged adults; many of these are structural. For example, unemployment (Bartley, 1994) and homelessness (Wright, 1990) place individuals at greater risk for acute and chronic health problems. Those in poverty also often do not have the ability or desire to engage in health-promoting or health-maintaining behaviors (Clark, 1996). More extensively documented than these factors, however, are the economic barriers to health care and their subsequent effect on health.

Millions of poor adults and children do not have health insurance. Thus, gaining access to the health care they need is very difficult because the poor cannot afford the care or doctors refuse to treat them because they do not have insurance (Liu & Rosenbaum, 1992; Teitelbaum, 1994). Even those with government-supported Medicaid coverage often find access to health care difficult to obtain. For example, many doctors refuse to treat Medicaid patients due to low reimbursement (Aday, 1993). In addition, individuals with low incomes often have difficulty paying for expenses (e.g., deductible, co-pay) not covered by Medicare (Davis & Schoen, 1978). Sexism and racism are additional barriers to health care for the poor (Kahn et al., 1993; Richie & Kanuha, 1993). Furthermore, disadvantaged patients tend to receive poorer quality care than do patients who are not disadvantaged (Kahn et al., 1993), and are less likely to receive needed long-term care (Hall, 1993). Those health care facilities that are designed specifically for low-income individuals face other barriers including lack of sufficient funding and resources (Aday, 1993; Liu & Rosenbaum, 1992). In addition, there is often a failure to coordinate different services for the poor, making it difficult for the poor to receive the kind of integrated care needed (Rivera, Regan, & Rosenbaum, 1995).

Thus, poor people are at greater risk for health problems, and also face numerous barriers to receiving adequate health care. This lack of attention to the health needs of the poor and the message it sends to the disadvantaged provide their own commentary on the value our society places on the lives of disadvantaged people. This message is sent not only through the health care sector but also through the quality of schools (Kozol, 1991), the conditions of the neighborhoods (Kozol, 1995), and the shortage of well-designed, adequately funded, comprehensive programs designed to help disadvantaged people overcome the vicious cycle of poverty. This lack of investment in disadvantaged people not only affects their lives but also affects all citizens in diverse ways, such as increased violence and crime, wasted human potential, and the significantly elevated costs of failing to invest adequately in early prevention programs (Edelman, 1992; Parker et al., 1988).

RESILIENCY, PREVENTION, AND INTERVENTION

Resiliency

In addition to the examination of the negative outcomes associated with poverty during infancy, childhood, adolescence, and adulthood, considerable attention has been given to identifying protective factors that lead to resiliency among the poor (Engeland, Carlson, & Sroufe, 1993; Nettles & Pleck, 1993; Werner, 1986, 1993). Both internal factors (e.g., the ability to elicit positive responses from others, easy temperament, and perceptions of personal control over life outcomes) and external factors (e.g., a strong social support network beyond the family, positive academic experiences, and good role models) have been identified as protective factors. Furthermore, it has been suggested that intervention programs should be the "means whereby protective mechanisms are provided or set in motion" (Nettles & Pleck, 1993, p. 13). Werner (1986) argued that

> the identification and assessment of risk factors in young children "makes sense" *only* if it plugs into practical intervention programs, and that there is a periodic follow-up to determine the efficacy of education, rehabilitation or treatment. Such efforts are ultimately based on the faith that the odds *can* be changed, if not for every vulnerable child, at least for many; if not all the time, at least some of the time; if not everywhere, at least in some places. (p. 19)

Given the extensive available knowledge on risk and protective factors that has been gained through longitudinal research (e.g., Werner, 1986, 1993), greater attention should be paid to the lessons derived from this knowledge through the implementation and adequate funding of intervention programs designed to help "provide or set in motion" critical protective factors.

General Qualities of Successful Programs for the Poor

Successful programs for the poor should be multigenerational, multidimensional, flexible, contextual, and respectful (Lerner, Ostrom, & Freel, 1997; Schorr, 1989,

1993). In addition, they should be outcome-based and preventive in orientation. Because poverty influences all aspects of an individual's life, programs designed to help the poor should coordinate services in multiple domains (Schorr, 1993). Programs focusing only on one domain (such as health) often fail to address factors that originally led to problems in the targeted domain or could cause future problems in the targeted domain as well as other domains. Programs should also be flexible, working to meet the unique needs of each family and should take into consideration the context in which the family and individual are functioning and ways that the contextual developmental system might be changed to maximize successful outcomes following intervention.

Respect for the individual and the family is also essential in programs for the poor, as is building trusting relationships. Without respect and trust, poor people might not be invested in the program, or the program facilitator may not be truly invested in helping the individual. Another attribute of successful programs is that they focus on the quality and outcome of their services rather than on how many people are served. Finally, programs for the poor should focus on prevention and addressing potential problems early, which is "when it is most effective and economical to intervene" (Schorr, 1993, p. 47).

To be most effective, prevention programs should be longitudinal and consistent rather than providing a short-term intervention based on the hope that the initial impact will be maintained for years. Fade-out effects are often the result of interventions that are not long enough in duration and of returning individuals to high risk environments without continued services to maintain the intervention effectiveness (cf. Lee & Loeb, 1995) and/or without services designed to alter key features of negative environments. Additional attributes of successful programs specific to each of the age groups discussed previously are presented in the following sections.

Prenatal and Infancy Interventions

In recognizing the significance of the prenatal and infancy periods for satisfactory life-span development, many community-based, family-oriented programs have pursued the goal of enhancing poor children's growth and development through educating parents on topics such as the types of care needed by infants prior to and after birth, child development, beneficial parent–child interactions, and positive discipline methods. In some programs, a family outreach worker is paired with a pregnant adolescent or woman and works with the mother (visiting her at home weekly and later monthly) prior to the birth and for the first few years of the child's life (Allen, Brown, & Finlay, 1994; Schorr, 1989). In less intensive programs, parents "drop in" to a family and parent center and attend workshops or parenting support groups.

One exemplar early intervention program is The Family Place in Washington, DC (Allen et al., 1995). The mission of The Family Place is to help pregnant women and women with children younger than 3 years of age to receive necessary prenatal care throughout their pregnancy, educate mothers on their role in fostering child development, and ensure that young children receive adequate health care. Classes are offered on topics such as prenatal nutrition and exercise, breast feeding, and infant and child development. In 1990, the average birthweight of the babies born to women who had worked with The Family Place was more than 7 pounds, and only one baby was born prematurely.

The Family Place works in conjunction with other agencies such as Planned Parenthood, The Red Cross, and The Handicapped Infant Intervention Project to provide additional coordinated services to the women. When needed, The Family Place provides money for transportation to health clinics and shelters (e.g., for battered women). In addition, the program offers life skill courses in areas such as English as a second language and literacy, which help to prepare the mothers for employment. The programs are sensitive to the culture and values of the neighborhood (one Family Place is located in a predominantly Spanish-speaking neighborhood in the city, another in a predominantly African American neighborhood). Thus, the programs provided by The Family Place are multigenerational, multidimensional, preventive, and ethnically sensitive.

Childhood Interventions

Like intervention and prevention programs during the prenatal and infancy years, quality programs during childhood are aimed at helping both the child and the parent. The most widely known of these is Head Start, a federally funded, comprehensive preschool program for low-income children. Created in 1965 as part of the War on Poverty, Head Start was designed to meet the needs of the whole child, including his or her educational, social, nutritional, physical health, and mental health needs. Parents are strongly encouraged to become involved in the program and their child's education by volunteering in the child's classroom, serving on the policy council, or working for Head Start. Services are also provided to help the parents (e.g., high school equivalency [GED] courses). In addition, a family service worker is assigned to each child's family, and works with the family to identify resources in the community which may help the family meet its specific needs.

Although there have been disagreements regarding the long-term effectiveness of Head Start, when appropriate measures are used (e.g., measures of social competence rather than IQ), the efficacy of Head Start has been supported. Head Start children appear to benefit socially, emotionally, physically, and cognitively both while enrolled in the program and later when they begin school. Sleeper effects due to the intervention have also been documented, including decreased risk for school dropout, teen pregnancy, and juvenile delinquency (Schweinhart & Weikart, 1986; Zigler, 1973, 1994). It has been estimated that for every $1 spent on Head Start, at least $4.75 is saved in educational and societal costs during adolescence and adulthood (Edelman, 1992; Parker et al., 1988). However, despite its reported success, only about 30% of children who are eligible for Head Start actually attend a local program due to funding limitations (Gomby, Larner, Stevenson, Lewit, & Behrman, 1995).

Adolescence Interventions

During adolescence, the goals of prevention and intervention efforts not only should be to affect the knowledge and cognitions of the individual but also should be to direct important behavioral decisions; all too often programs designed only to increase the knowledge of the adolescent do not also result in changes in behavior (Rodrigue, Tercyak, & Lescano, 1997). To change behavior, it has also been argued that the individual must be motivated to engage in the new behaviors. For this reason, intervention programs should consider including a carefully targeted motivation component. Furthermore, intervention and prevention programs for adolescents should provide opportunities for individuals to learn and to practice new behaviors. Activities designed to enhance self-efficacy are also important for adolescents to help teens believe that they are capable of engaging in the new behaviors and believe in the effectiveness of those behaviors. Finally, programs for adolescents should also be culturally sensitive, developmentally appropriate, longitudinal, and delivered through a variety of communication modes such as the media and peer groups (Rodrigue et al., 1997).

An interesting example of an adolescent intervention program is the Life Skills Training approach to drug abuse and violence prevention that is being examined with inner-city minority adolescents (Botvin & Scheier, 1997). This school-based intervention consists of seventeen 45-minute activities that focus on personal skills, social skills, drug abuse, and violence. In addition, there is a parent intervention component that uses videotapes, written materials (e.g., a manual on drug abuse and violence, newsletters), homework assignments, and workshops. Although data on the effectiveness of the program with this population are not yet available, research using the Life Skills Training approach with other populations has indicated that the approach successfully reduces high-risk behaviors (e.g., drug and alcohol use); the beneficial effects of the approach has been documented up to 2 and 3 years after intervention (Botvin, 1996; Botvin & Scheier, 1997).

Adulthood Interventions

Research suggests that during adulthood and old age there are multiple barriers that prevent low-income individuals from engaging in health-promoting behaviors, such as exercise (e.g., Clark, 1996). For example, although walking tends to be the preferred type of exercise activity for older adults, for low-income older adults, unsafe, and crowded neighborhoods make engaging in this activity difficult or undesirable. In addition, low-income adults tend to have lower efficacy and outcome expectations relating to exercise, which contribute to their decreased likelihood of engaging in exercise as a health promoting behavior. Another barrier to fitness is financial limitations which often prevent the elderly from joining a fitness club, taking exercise classes, or purchasing exercise equipment.

Information from a focus group conducted by Clark (1996) with poor, inner-city minority women between the ages of 55 and 70 suggests that programs designed to increase the efficacy and outcome expectations relating to exercise for older low-income adults could increase the likelihood of their engaging in exercise as a health promoting behavior. In addition, it was suggested that intervention programs for low-income older adults be conducted in the home rather than at centers. The in-home approach allows greater access to the programs for those who could benefit most from the intervention—those with deteriorating health, less activity, or no transportation to a center-based program. In addition, engaging in exercise in one's own home might be safer than walking in unsafe and crowded neighborhoods. However, it is also important to note that peer support can play a very important role in an elder person's willingness to engage in exercise and commitment to continued exercising. In this sense, group-based, in-home programs could be very beneficial for older, low-income adults because of increased social contact and peer-based motivation.

PROPOSED ACTIONS TO MAKE HEALTH CARE MORE ACCESSIBLE TO THE POOR

In response to the growing number of uninsured children in the United States, bills to provide health insurance coverage for children who do not have health insurance and whose families are not Medicaid eligible have been introduced in Congress. For such programs to be successful, however, local doctors and hospitals must be willing to accept the insurance. In addition, there is a need for the access to necessary health care to continue during the child's adolescent and adulthood years. Treatment during the childhood years, although reducing health threats during this period, does not necessarily inoculate against later threats to the individual's health and well-being during subsequent developmental periods.

At the state level, bills have also been proposed to make health insurance more accessible to the poor. One program in Michigan would allow low-income families who have gotten off welfare to purchase managed care health insurance for 2 years after their year-long Medicaid coverage has expired (Putnam, 1997); the current policy provides transitional Medicaid coverage for 1 year after the family leaves welfare. Insurance premium costs would be shared with the state, with the family paying 25% more of the cost every 6 months. The program would not only allow a greater number of children and adults to continue receiving health care after going off welfare, but would also help prevent families from returning to welfare. With the current policy, many families are not able to afford insurance after the transitional year and, thus, either are uninsured after this point or return to welfare to receive health insurance coverage. As with the proposed federal insurance programs, the success of this type of state program in part depends on the willingness of doctors and hospitals to provide health care for those covered by this insurance.

Although the proposed health insurance actions are very important and necessary, it should be acknowledged that these actions alone will not eliminate threats to the health of disadvantaged individuals. For example, health insurance coverage does not reduce the violence or improve poor housing conditions that many low-income individuals face and that pose significant threats to their health and well-being. Although health insurance might allow disadvantaged individuals to have access to health care once problems have already developed, programs and actions are also needed to prevent the problems from developing in the first place.

CONCLUSIONS

Throughout the life span, individuals living in poverty not only are at greater risk for developing health problems, but also have decreased opportunities to access needed health care services. As a result, health problems worsen, problems develop in other areas of functioning, future problems become more likely, and life expectancy is shortened. This chain of events results not only in "rotten outcomes" for individuals in poverty (Schorr, 1989, 1993), but also for society as a whole in terms of wasted human potential and increased violence and crime (Hammond & Yung, 1991). Given the knowledge we have about the consequences of poverty and the ways to prevent these predictable negative consequences, clear and forceful steps need to be taken. Comprehensive, coordinated, multidimensional planning is required at all levels of government, and in the private sector, to root out poverty and to foster human health and development across the entire life span.

REFERENCES

Abel, E. L. (1995). An update on incidence of FAS: FAS is not an equal opportunity birth defect. *Neurotoxicology and Teratology, 17,* 437–443.

Aday, L. A. (1993). *At risk in America: The health and health care needs of vulnerable populations in the United States.* San Francisco: Jossey-Bass.

Allen, M. A., Brown, P., & Finlay, B. (1994). *Helping children by strengthening families: A look at family support programs.* Washington, DC: Children's Defense Fund.

Bartley, M. (1994). Unemployment and ill health: Understanding the relationship. *Journal of Epidemiology and Community Health, 48,* 333–337.

Belle, D. (1990). Poverty and women's mental health. *American Psychologist, 45,* 385–389.

Bennett, M. B. H. (1988). Afro-American women, poverty and mental health: A social essay. *Women & Health, 12,* 213–228.

Black, M., & Dubowitz, H. (1991). Failure-to-thrive: Lessons from animal models and developing countries. *Journal of Developmental and Behavioral Pediatrics, 12,* 259–267.

Botvin, G. J. (1996). Substance abuse prevention through Life Skills Training. In R. DeV. Peters & R. J.

McMahon (Eds.), *Preventing childhood disorders, substance abuse, and delinquency* (pp. 215–240). Thousand Oaks, CA: Sage.

Botvin, G. J., & Scheier, L. M. (1997). Preventing drug abuse and violence. In D. K. Wilson, J. R. Rodrigue, & W. C. Taylor (Eds.), *Health- promoting and health-compromising behaviors among minority adolescents* (pp. 55–86). Washington, DC: American Psychological Association.

Brown, J. L., & Pollitt, E. (1996). Malnutrition, poverty and intellectual development. *Scientific American, 274*, 38–43.

Burton, L. M. (1990). Teenage childbearing as an alternative life- course strategy in multigeneration Black families. *Human Nature, 1*, 123–143.

Children's Defense Fund. (1993). *Decade of indifference: Maternal and child health trends 1980–1990.* Washington, DC: Author.

Clark, D. O. (1996). Age, socioeconomic status, and exercise self-efficacy. *The Gerontologist, 36*, 157–164.

Coles, C. D., Brown, R. T., Smith, I. E., Platzman, K. A., Erickson, S., & Falek, A. (1991). Effects of prenatal alcohol exposure at school age. I. Physical and cognitive development. *Neurotoxicology and Teratology, 13*, 357–367.

Coles, C. D., Platzman, K. A., Smith, I., James, M. E., & Falek, A. (1992). Effects of cocaine and alcohol use in pregnancy on neonatal growth and neurobehavioral status. *Neurotoxicology and Teratology, 14*, 23–33.

Covington, D. L., Churchill, M. P., & Wright, B. D. (1994). Factors affecting number of prenatal car visits during second pregnancy among adolescents having rapid repeat births. *Journal of Adolescent Health, 15*, 536- 542.

Crockett, L. J. (1997). Cultural, historical, and subcultural contexts of adolescence: Implications for health and development. In J. Schulenberg, J. L. Maggs, & K. Hurrelmann (Eds.), *Health risks and developmental transitions during adolescence* (pp. 23–53). New York: Cambridge University Press.

Davis, K., & Schoen, C. (1978). *Health and the war on poverty: A ten-year appraisal.* Washington, DC: Brookings Institution.

Dillihay, T. C. (1989). Suicide in Black children. *The Psychiatric Forum, 15*, 24–27.

Dore, M. M. (1993). Family preservation and poor families: When "homebuilding" is not enough. *Families in Society: The Journal of Contemporary Human Services, 74*, 545–556.

Edelman, M. W. (1992). *The measure of our success: A letter to my children and yours.* New York: HarperCollins.

Engeland, B., Carlson, E., & Sroufe, L. A. (1993). Resilience as a process. *Development and Psychopathology, 5*, 517–528.

Furstenberg, F. F., Brooks-Gunn, J., & Morgan, S. P. (1987). *Adolescent mothers in later life.* New York: Cambridge University Press.

Garbarino, J. (1992). The meaning of poverty in the world of children. *American Behavioral Scientist, 35*, 220–237.

Garbarino, J. (1995). The American war zone: What children can tell us about living with violence. *Developmental and Behavioral Pediatrics, 16*, 431–435.

Gelles, R. J. (1992). Poverty and violence toward children. *American Behavioral Scientist, 35*, 258–274.

Gilligan, J. (1996). *Violence: Our deadly epidemic and its causes.* New York: Putnam.

Gomby, D. S., Larner, M., Stevenson, C., Lewit, E., & Behrman, R. (1995). Long term outcomes of early childhood programs: Analysis and recommendations. *The Future of Children, 5*(3), 6–24.

Grant, R. (1990). The special needs of homeless children: Early intervention at a welfare hotel. *Topics in Early Childhood Special Education, 10*, 76–91.

Grantham-McGregor, S., Powell, C., Walker, S., Chang, S., & Fletcher, P. (1994). The long-term follow-up of severely malnourished children who participated in an intervention program. *Child Development, 65*, 428–439.

Hall, C. (1993). Long-term care and the minority elderly. *Pride Institute Journal of Long Term Home Health Care, 12*(4), 3–8.

Hammond, W. R., & Yung, B. R. (1991). Preventing violence in at- risk African-American youth. *Journal of Health Care for the Poor and Underserved, 2*, 359–373.

Hardy, M. A., & Hazelrigg, L. E. (1993). The gender of poverty in an aging population. *Research on Aging, 15*, 243–278.

Hawley, T. L., & Disney, E. R. (1992). Crack's children: The consequences of maternal cocaine abuse. *Social Policy Report: Society for Research in Child Development* (Vol. VI, No. 4). Ann Arbor: Society for Research in Child Development.

Kahn, K. L., Pearson, M. L., Harrison, E. R., Rogers, W. H., Brook, R. H., Desmond, K., & Keeler, E. B. (1993). *Analysis of quality of care for patients who are Black or poor in rural and urban settings.* Santa Monica, CA: RAND/UCLA/Harvard Center for Health Care Financing Policy Research.

Ketterlinus, R. D., Henderson, S. H., & Lamb, M. E. (1990). Maternal age, sociodemographics, prenatal health and behavior: Influences on neonatal risk status. *Journal of Adolescent Health Care, 11*, 423–431.

Klerman, L. V. (1996). Child health: What public polices can improve it? In E. Zigler, S. L. Kagan, & N. W. Hall (Eds.), *Children, families and government: Preparing for the 21st century* (2nd ed, pp. 188–206). New York: Cambridge University Press.

Koniak-Griffin, D., Nyamathi, A., Vasquez, R., & Russo, A. A. (1994). Risk-taking behaviors and AIDS knowledge: Experiences and beliefs of minority adolescent mothers. *Health Education Research, 9*, 449–463.

Korenman, S., Miller, J. E., & Sjaastad, J. E. (1995). Long-term poverty and child development in the United States: Results from the NLSY. *Children and Youth Services Review, 17*, 127–155.

Kozol, J. (1991). *Savage inequalities: Children in America's schools.* New York: HarperPerennial.

Kozol, J. (1995). *Amazing grace.* New York: Crown.

Lee, V. E., & Loeb, S. (1995). Where do Head Start attendees end up? One reason why preschool effects fade out. *Educational Evaluation and Policy Analysis, 17*, 62–82.

Lerner, R. M., Ostrom, C. W., & Freel, M. A. (1997). Preventing health-compromising behaviors among youth and promoting their positive development: A developmental contextual perspective. In J. Schulenberg, J. L. Maggs, & K. Hurrelmann (Eds.), *Health risks and developmental transitions during adolescence* (pp. 498–521). New York: Cambridge University Press.

Liu, J. T-Y., & Rosenbaum, S. (1992). *Medicaid and childhood immunizations: A national study.* Washington, DC: Children's Defense Fund.

Masten, A. S. (1992). Homeless children in the United States: Mark of a nation at risk. *Current Directions in Psychological Science, 1*, 41–44.

McGauhey, P. J., & Starfield, B. (1993). Child health and the social environment of White and Black children. *Social Science & Medicine, 36*, 867–874.

McLoyd, V. C., & Wilson, L. (1991). The strain of living poor: Parenting, social support, and child mental health. In A. C. Huston (Ed.), *Children in poverty: Child development and public policy* (pp. 105–135). New York: Cambridge University Press.

Mechanic, D. (1986). Health care for the poor: Some policy alternatives. *Journal of Family Practice, 22*, 283–289.

Merrick, E. N. (1995). Adolescent childbearing as career "choice:" Perspective from an ecological context. *Journal of Counseling & Development, 73*, 288–295.

Moeller, D. W. (1992). *Environmental health.* Cambridge, MA: Harvard University Press.

Molnar, J. M., & Rath, W. R. (1990). Constantly compromised: The impact of homelessness on children. *Journal of Social Issues, 46*(4), 109–124.

Morgane, P. J., Austin-LaFrance, R., Bronzino, J., Tonkiss, J., Diaz-Cintra, S., Cintra, L., Kemper, T., & Galler, J. R. (1993). Prenatal malnutrition and development of the brain. *Neuroscience and Biobehavioral Reviews, 17*, 91–128.

Needleman, H. L. (1994). Preventing childhood lead poisoning. *Preventive Medicine, 23*, 634–637.

Nettles, S. M., & Pleck, J. H. (1993). *Risk, resilience, and development: The multiple ecologies of Black adolescents* (Rep. No. 44). Baltimore, MD: Johns Hopkins University, Center for Research on Effective Schooling for Disadvantaged Students.

Oberg, C. N., Bryant, N. A., & Bach, M. L. (1995). A portrait of America's children: The impact of poverty and a call to action. *Journal of Social Distress and the Homeless, 4,* 43–56.

Pappas, G., Queen, S., Hadden, W., & Fisher, G. (1993). The increasing disparity in mortality between socioeconomic groups in the United States. *New England Journal of Medicine, 329,* 103–109.

Parker, S., Greer, S., & Zuckerman, B. (1988). Double jeopardy: The impact of poverty on early child development. *Pediatric Clinics of North America, 35,* 1227–1240.

Pollitt, E. (1994). Poverty and child development: Relevance of research in developing countries to the United States. *Child Development, 65,* 283–295.

Putnam, J. (1997, May 12). Plan provides insurance for working poor. *The Ann Arbor News,* p. C5.

Richie, B. E., & Kanuha, V. (1993). Battered women of color in public health care systems: Racism, sexism, and violence. In B. Bair & S. E. Cayleff (Eds.), *Wings of gauze: Women of color and the experience of health and illness* (pp. 288–299). Detroit, MI: Wayne State University Press.

Rivera, L., Regan, C., & Rosenbaum, S. (1995). *Managed care and children's health: An analysis of Early and Periodic Screening, Diagnosis, and Treatment services under state Medicaid managed care contracts.* Washington DC: Children's Defense Fund.

Rodrigue, J. R., Tercyak, K. P., & Lescano, C. M. (1997). Health promotion in minority adolescents: Emphasis on sexually transmitted diseases and the human immunodeficiency virus. In D. K. Wilson, J. R. Rodrigue, & W. C. Taylor (Eds.), *Health-promoting and health-compromising behaviors among minority adolescents* (pp. 87–105). Washington, DC: American Psychological Association.

Rosella, J. D., & Albrecht, S. A. (1993). Toward an understanding of the health status of Black adolescents: An application of the stress-coping framework. *Issues in Comprehensive Pediatric Nursing, 16,* 193–205.

Rosenbaum, S. (1992). Child health and poor children. *American Behavioral Scientist, 35,* 275–289.

Rucker, N., & Greene, V. (1995). The myth of the invulnerable self of adolescence. *The American Journal of Psychoanalysis, 55,* 369–379.

Sabol, B. J. (1991). The urban child. *Journal of Health Care for the Poor and Underserved, 2,* 59–73.

Scholl, T. O., Hediger, M. L., & Belsky, D. H. (1994). Prenatal care and maternal health during adolescent pregnancy: A review and meta-analysis. *Journal of Adolescent Health, 15,* 444–456.

Schorr, L. B. (1989). *Within our reach: Breaking the cycle of disadvantage.* New York: Anchor Books.

Schorr, L. B. (1993). What works: Applying what we already know about successful social policy. *American Prospect, 13,* 43–54.

Schramm, W. F. (1985). WIC prenatal participation and its relationship to newborn medicaid costs in Missouri: A cost/benefit analysis. *American Journal of Public Health, 75,* 851–857.

Schweinhart, L. J., & Weikart, D. P. (1986). What do we know so far? A review of the Head Start Synthesis Project. *Young Children, 41,* 49–55.

Sherman, A. (1994). *Wasting America's future: The Children's Defense Fund report on the costs of child poverty.* Boston: Beacon Press.

St. Clair, P. A., Smeriglio, V. L., Alexander, C. S., & Celentano, D. D. (1989). Social network structure and prenatal care utilization. *Medical Care, 27,* 823–832.

Stein, Z., & Susser, M. (1985). Effects of early nutrition on neurological and mental competence in human beings. *Psychological Medicine, 15,* 717–726.

Sullivan, C. M., & Rumptz, M. H. (1994). Adjustment and needs of African-American women who utilized a domestic violence shelter. *Violence and Victims, 9,* 275–286.

Tarnowski, K. J., & Rohrbeck, C. A. (1993). Disadvantaged children and families. In T. H. Ollendick & R. J. Prinz (Eds.), *Advances in clinical child psychology* (Vol. 15, pp. 41–79). New York: Plenum Press.

Teitelbaum, M. A. (1994, March). *The health insurance crisis for America's children.* Washington, DC: Children's Defense Fund.

Ward, M. C. (1993). A different disease: HIV/AIDS and health care for women in poverty. *Culture, Medicine, and Psychiatry, 17,* 413–430.

Weinberg, D. H. (1996). *Press briefing on 1995 income, poverty, and health insurance estimates.* U.S. Bu-

84 BOLIG, BORKOWSKI, BRANDENBERGER

reau of the Census [Online]. Available: http://www.census.gov/ftp/pub/hhes/income/income95/ prs96asc.

Werner, E. (1986). The concept of risk from a developmental perspective. *Advances in Special Education, 5*, 1–23.

Werner, E. (1993). Risk, resilience, and recovery: Perspectives from the Kauai Longitudinal Study. *Development and Psychopathology, 5*, 503–515.

Williams, G. J. R. (1983). Child abuse reconsidered: The urgency of authentic prevention. *Journal of Clinical Child Psychology, 12*, 312–319.

Wright, J. D. (1990). Poor people, poor health: The health status of the homeless. *Journal of Social Issues, 46*, 49–64.

Wright, J. D. (1991). Poverty, homelessness, health, nutrition, and children. In J. H. Kryder-Coe, L. M. Salamon, & J. M. Molnar (Eds.), *Homeless children and youth: A new American dilemma* (pp. 71–103). New Brunswick, NJ: Transaction.

Zeskind, P. S., & Ramey, C. T. (1981). Preventing intellectual and interactional sequelae of fetal malnutrition: A longitudinal, transactional, and synergistic approach to development. *Child Development, 52*, 213–218.

Ziesemer, C., Marcoux, L., & Marwell, B. E. (1994). Homeless children: Are they different from other low-income children? *Social Work, 39*, 658–668.

Zigler, E. (1973). Success or failure? *Learning, 1*, 43–47.

Zigler, E. (1994). Reshaping early childhood intervention to be a more effective weapon against poverty. *American Journal of Community Psychology, 22*, 37–47.

Zuckerman, B. (1993). Developmental considerations for drug- and AIDS-affected infants. In R. P. Barth, J. Pietrzak, & M. Ramler (Eds.), *Families living with drugs and HIV: Intervention and treatment strategies* (pp. 37–58). New York: Guilford.

PART II

Children, Family, and Health

5

Environmental Influences on Prenatal Development and Health

Kathleen J. Sipes Kolberg
University of Notre Dame

DESPITE ITS apparently isolated containment, the developing individual is affected by the rich, diverse environment of the womb. The mother's body sends hormonal signals to the fetus that fluctuate with diurnal rhythms and maternal effects, such as stress. Stimuli experienced by the mother are transmitted to the fetus with varied degrees of filtration. For example, small molecules (e.g., alcohol, simple sugars) tend to pass easily through maternal circulation to the child, but larger ones (e.g., larger proteins) do not. External sounds are dampened in varied degrees, depending on the frequency of the sound, whereas internal sounds are transmitted well. Light is almost completely blocked. Environmental inputs might be damaging (e.g., alcohol, viruses) or supportive (e.g., nutrients, movement, voice, etc.). The developing embryo and fetus is susceptible to damage by environmental factors in two major ways: direct insult to fragile, immature tissues and perturbations of the developing system that alter the trajectory of development (e.g., damage to cells at the tip of the limb bud can stop development of the limb). From a positive perspective, the sensory and hormonal environment of the uterus supports embryonic and fetal development, especially the development of nervous system function.

One indicator of the sensitivity of the developing conceptus is the rate of anomalies seen in miscarriages, stillbirths, and live births. Major structural anomalies are estimated to occur in 20% or more of all conceptions. Most of the concepti with these anomalies spontaneously abort, but 2% to 4% of children are born with significant malformations. Deviations in the genotype are known to cause 20% to 25% of these malformations (Brent & Beckman, 1990), whereas known environmental causes, such as maternal illness (e.g., diabetes or hypertension), infection, mechanical obstruction or constriction, chemicals, drugs, radiation, and temperature extremes account for 10% of congenital anomalies. The etiology of two thirds of all birth defects remains unknown. Brent proposed that these defects are derived from polygenic defects, multifactoral interactions (genetic sensitivity combined with environmental influences), unknown environmental agents, combinations of agents in synergism (i.e., agents that are safe separately but harmful in combination), and accidents of development (e.g., additional sites of gastrulation on a single embryonic disc leading to conjoined twins). The specific environmental causes of birth defects in humans are difficult to ascertain due to the wide variety of agents, such as industrial, consumer, medical, and agricultural chemicals to which the mother is exposed, the variety of combinations of agents, and the poor documentation of such exposures.

Less attention has been paid in the empirical literature to environmental inputs that facilitate normal embryonic and fetal development and behavior. Many traits previously believed to be innate (traits that do not require learning) are now seen as developing through the interaction of the fetus and the its environment. For example, the approach behavior of the gull chick to the parent's call was considered innate or hardwired because it was present at birth in all chicks observed. However, this behavior has now been shown to be a function of environmental inputs, specifically the exposure of the egg to parental calls (Impekoven & Gold, 1973).

This chapter discusses the environmental context in which prenatal development occurs, the ramifications of negative environmental influences, the role of environmental inputs in normal development, and the implications of this knowledge for fetal, prenatal, and infant medicine.

PRENATAL DEVELOPMENT

Stages of Development

The effects of the uterine environment on the developing individual greatly depend on the stage of development during which environmental exposure occurs. The developmental period from conception to birth is far from homogeneous. The different characteristics of the stages of development before birth affect the nature and extent of environmental influence. Prenatal life is commonly divided into three main stages: early events (from conception to gastrulation), embryogenesis, and fetal stages. The early events, which take place during the first 2 weeks, involve rapid cell division, partitioning of the cells into the inner cell mass (forming the embryo and amnion, or the sac immediately surrounding the embryo) and the trophoblast outer layer (forming the chorion, or the embryonic contribution to the placenta), followed by implantation, and gastrulation. On Day 6 the trophoblast layer interacts with the uterine lining to perform implantation, typically in the upper portion of the uterus. Gastrulation begins at the end of Week 2 and involves the division of the embryo into the three germ layers that provide the foundation for the formation of the organs. Multiple sites of gastrulation result in twinning (conjoined or complete, depending on the space between the sites). These important early processes seem to be driven internally but require an environment that is physically and chemically supportive. Developmentally, the early stage is a risky period, during which approximately 50% of conceptuses are spontaneously aborted, because mistakes at these stages tend to be lethal (Hertig, 1967; Robert & Lowe, 1975).

The embryonic stage follows the early period and runs from Week 2 to the beginning of Week 9. During this stage organs take shape and become functional at different times and to varying degrees. For example, the heart becomes functional very early in the embryonic stage, but the lungs do not mature until late in the fetal period. Organogenesis, the formation of organs, is the result of many interactions. Embryology texts provide numerous examples of how organs form from the interaction of two or more layers of germ layer primordia. These interactions are sensitive to environmental perturbations that induce errors (e.g., failure of facial processes to attach and fuse, leaving clefts) that often have effects on gross morphology. The degree of specialization that occurs during organogenesis creates a diversity of receptors and compartmentalization that lead to more restricted action of some environmental agents. Because of this compartmentalization, damage to the embryo is often specialized, as opposed to general. The embryonic period is the realm of classic teratology, and primarily drugs that cause structural malformations act during this period. Although embryonic death can occur during this stage, this outcome is less common than it is during the earlier stage.

The fetal period runs from Week 9 until birth and involves histogenesis (i.e., tissue formation and cellular differentiation), acquisition of function, and growth. The fetal period makes up the bulk of the prenatal period and is the period during which important functions appear. It is less well defined than the embryonic period and not as extensively cataloged. The fetus gradually becomes capable of accepting sensory stimulation and responding to it peripherally as well as centrally. Inputs affecting the fetus might be chemical, physical, or stimulatory in nature. The sensory systems become functional in a predictable sequence among vertebrate species, with touch and vestibular systems emerging first, followed by the chemosensory functions of smell and taste, then the auditory and finally the visual system. Sensory function emerges with initial differentiation of the terminal sensory organ, and the subsequent innervation and connection of the peripheral sensors to central processing at spinal, brainstem, ganglionic, and cortical levels. Some sensory function can occur at lower levels prior to its connection to the cortex. Important processes, such as neuronal pruning and proliferation of neuronal connections, are initiated during the fetal stage and continue during the perinatal and infancy periods. Research on the fetal period has contributed significantly to our knowledge regarding environmental influences on development.

Damage to developing systems during the fetal stage generally leads to functional deficits, such as blindness, deafness, and mental retardation. Although the fetal period appears to be less sensitive to environmental insult than previous periods, a number of common teratogens, such as alcohol and tobacco, lead to functional deficits. Fetal and neonatal death is a possible outcome of negative events during this period but is less common than in the earlier stages.

The Prenatal Environment

While the conceptus is developing, the environment in which it resides also changes. During the early stages, as the conceptus is swept down the uterine tube toward the uterus, the environmental influences occur via the secretions of the uterine tube and the uterus and movement along the uterine tube. One critical environmental aspect of this early phase is the ability of the mother's reproductive tract to carry the conceptus down the uterine tube to the upper portion of the uterus before the trophoblast portion of the conceptus is ready for implantation. If travel is too slow, the conceptus can implant in the uterine tube (a tubal ectopic pregnancy). In order for the conceptus to implant properly, the endometrial lining of the uterus must be adequately mature and supportive of the implantation and the muscles of the uterus must be calm. These processes are influenced by estrogen and progesterone levels. After implantation, the placenta, a joint organ of the maternal lining and the trophoblast or chorion (specifically, chorion frondosum) of the conceptus, forms.

The placenta is the exchange interface between maternal and infant circulations, as well as a physical point of attachment. Passage of nutrients, hormone and waste products occur through the placenta by diffusion, facilitated diffusion, and active transport. During fetal development the placenta thins and becomes more permeable. Up to Week 18, the placenta allows passage of viruses, lipid soluble substances, and chemicals up to 500 molecular weight (mw; as a point of reference, glucose has a molecular weight of 180), whereas past Week 18 bacteria and chemicals up to 1000 mw can pass through.

In terms of physical space, the embryo or fetus is enclosed in the chorion and the amnion and surrounded by amniotic fluid, which is derived from several sources. Early in the pregnancy, amniotic fluid is mainly produced by the placenta and amnion. Later it is secreted by fetal tissues; for example, amniotic fluid is swallowed by the fetus, passes through the circulation, and is recirculated as fetal urine. Amniotic fluid contains waste products, immunological factors, as well as diffused chemicals from the circulations (including odor cues). This fluid filled environment is important for several developmental functions. It facilitates fetal movement through most of the pregnancy because its liquid produces a lower resistance and a reduced gravity effect. However, just prior to birth the amniotic sac and uterus become virtually filled with the fetus, thus providing little room for gross motor movement. When the 35-week and older fetus makes large movements, it does so against the resistance of the uterine wall. Amniotic fluid also provides a reservoir of hydraulic pressure for amniotic breathing. As the fetus "breathes," amniotic fluid is pulled into the mouth and pharynx, allowing the lungs, which are filled with secreted lung fluid, to expand. Amniotic fluid also provides surface lubrication, helping to prevent skin adhesions. Early large ruptures of the amnion pose risks related to the interference with functions such as those just described as well as increased risk of infection from exposure to the external environment.

The uterine environment provides a rich sensory environment for the fetus. Touch and vestibular stimulation are provided through containment of the uterus and maternal movement. Fetal movement and uterine contractions add to this stimulation. Chemosensory stimulation (olfactory and gustatory) is provided by dissolved chemicals in the amniotic fluid. Auditory inputs are also available, predominately through maternal voice, digestive sounds, and circulatory sounds. External airborne sounds are dampened and skewed to the lower frequencies (Abrams, Gerhardt, & Peters, 1995). The fetus has little visual input because at least 98% of ambient light is blocked by the mother's body. Stimulation to the visual cortex before birth seems to be internally driven by the fetus and is thought to occur in conjunction with rapid-eye movement sleep.

Thus, the interaction of the conceptus and the prenatal environment changes over the course of the pregnancy, the conceptus changes with respect to its ability to interact with the environment and its ability to resist damage from that environment. In the next section, the negative influences of specific environmental agents on the developmental processes are discussed.

THE UTERINE ENVIRONMENT AS A SOURCE OF RISK

The biological fields of teratology and developmental toxicology involve the study of environmental agents that impair the health and development of embryos and fetuses. Whereas teratology is concerned with agents that alter developmental trajectory, developmental toxicology is more inclusive, examining any negative effects due to environmental exposures. A teratogen is an environmental agent that adversely affects embryonic and fetal developmental processes. In routine use, teratogens are generally considered synonymous with developmental toxins. Teratogens can be chemical, physical or mechanical, or infectious agents or maternal conditions that alter the uterine environment. Chemical agents include lifestyle drugs (e.g., alcohol), pharmaceuticals (e.g., tetracycline, lithium, isotretinoin [Accutane], and thalidomide), and workplace or environmental chemicals (e.g., methylmercury, acetone, and lead). Physical–mechanical agents include radiation (e.g., x-ray), pressure (e.g., amniotic bands), and maternal fever. Infectious agents include viruses (e.g., rubella and cytomegalovirus), bacteria (e.g., syphilis), and parasites (e.g., toxoplasmosis). Maternal conditions affecting the developing fetus include insulin-dependent diabetes and other endocrine disorders.

Gregg's 1941 study of the rubella epidemic in Australia and the relation of this disease to congenital anomalies and miscarriage brought teratology to the attention of the medical community. In the early 1960s, public interest in teratology increased as the effects of thalidomide became known. This drug, used from 1959 to 1961 as a mild sedative by pregnant women, produced a previously rare malformation of the limbs in more than 10,000 children, primarily in Europe. Although the Food and Drug Administration (FDA) had not approved thalidomide for use in the United States, this tragedy helped to lay the groundwork for more stringent testing requirements for drugs used by pregnant women.

Establishing the teratogenicity of an agent requires more than the association between its use and an adverse pregnancy outcome. Five basic rules for determining the developmental toxicity of environmental agents are outlined by Brent and Beckman (1990). These rules require an understanding of stage sensitivity, dose response relations, threshold levels, genetic variation in susceptibility, and cases that call for exceptions to the first four rules.

Stage sensitivity refers to the stage of development during which a teratogen can induce damage or adversely affect development. The period during which a specific type of damage can be induced is called the *sensitive period, vulnerable period*, or *window of susceptibility*. The end of the sensitive period, after which a defect cannot be induced, is the *teratogenic termination point*. This stage specificity only holds for true cases of malformation and not for disruption or deformation of previously well-formed organs. Most teratogens have a narrow window in which they can negatively affect development. Thus, what is teratogenic on a given day may not be so a week later. Periods of sensitivity have been determined for specific organs. For example, phocomelia, a defect caused by thalidomide in which the long bones of the limb are absent or deficient, is specific to the time frame of 39 to 44 days postconception (Lenz & Kapp, 1962). Anencephaly, a failure of the neural tube to close in the anterior region, preventing formation of the cerebral hemispheres, occurs prior to the 26th day after conception. The fetal stage is receiving more attention as we become more interested in functional deficits such as mental retardation and behavioral anomalies. For example, the effects of alcohol on mental function are thought to be related to exposure during the fetal periods.

Whether a certain agent will act as a teratogen also depends on the amount delivered to the conceptus. If increasing dosage levels of an agent are associated with increasing incidence and severity of adverse effects, a dosage response effect is evident. A dose-response relation is important in establishing causality between the teratogenic agent and the adverse effects. Calculation of the dose-response relation is difficult in the prenatal environment because of the imperfect correlation between maternal and embryonic or fetal exposure. This variability of the dosage might be due to several factors, such as permeability of the placenta, the immaturity of fetal metabolism, and the specific distribution and storage of agents in fetal tissues. These variability factors also change over the course of the pregnancy.

As mentioned earlier, the placenta is an exchange organ, designed to be highly permeable to nutrients, hormones, and waste products. Depending on the stage of development, this permeable barrier allows a wide range of other agents to cross thereby exposing the embryo or fetus. For example, ethyl alcohol is a smaller molecule than simple sugars, and there is no mechanism for selectively blocking its passage, whereas larger, non-fat-soluble proteins might not be able to cross the placenta from the maternal circulation, precluding any exposure to the embryo or fetus. Because of adult–fetal metabolic differences, the immature fetal metabolism also affects the extent of the effect of a teratogenic agent in embryonic or fetal tissues. A short-term exposure to a potential teratogenic agent by the mother might be a long-term exposure to the fetus. A drug such as caffeine, which is half cleared from adult systems within 7 hours, takes 40 to 231 hours to fall the same amount in newborns (Aranda, Hales, & Rieder, 1992). The distribution of a potential agent in the body is also often different between adult and developing systems. For example the blood–brain barrier, which ultimately will prevent many blood-borne agents from entering neural tissue, does not develop its full protective capabilities until well after birth. Thus, the exposures to potential teratogenic agents for the developing embryo or fetus might be greater in both dosage and time as compared to those for adults.

Fetal or embryonic susceptibility to a potential teratogen also depends on the threshold dose. The *threshold dose* is the lowest dose for which toxicity can be detected above the background level. Below the threshold dose, the agent is considered safe. Knowledge of the threshold dose is useful in defining safety guidelines for pharmaceuticals and work place chemicals. Many teratogens have a threshold dose for developmental toxicity below that for adult toxicity; that is, a dosage may be in the safe range for the mother but toxic to the developing system in her. For example, the clinically prescribed dose of thalidomide was well below the threshold dose for toxicity to the mother but above the threshold dose for developmental toxicity to the embryo within the mother.

Genetic variability also alters susceptibility to potential teratogens by creating differences in absorption, metabolism, placental transport, and distribution of an agent, as well as the ability of the agent to bind to proteins or receptors. This variability is thought to be important in multifactoral defects that have some correlation to inheritance, such as neural tube defects.

Finally, secondary disruptive forces, infections, and deficiency-induced malformations do not conform to these tenets of stage sensitivity, dosage effect, and threshold dose. Secondary disruptive forces, which damage previously well-formed organs, do not exhibit stage sensitivity, although they are more common in the latter stages of pregnancy. For example, hydranencephaly, the replacement of brain tissue with fluid, is a disruption that occurs after the brain is formed and can be caused by viral infections (Kitano, Ohzono, Yasuda, & Shimizu, 1996) or vascular accidents. Infectious agents may not exhibit a dose response or a threshold dose. Infections are generally described in terms that do not lend themselves to dosage response curves. Certain malformations have been linked to deficiencies of certain substances, such as the role of folic acid deficiency in neural tube defects, and these deficiency malformations follow the guidelines of other deficiency diseases.

DEVELOPMENTAL TOXINS

In this section, some of the diverse types of agents that can act as developmental toxins are briefly discussed. These examples include ethanol, tobacco, rubella, external pressure, radiation, and maternal stress.

Ethanol

The effects of ethanol on the embryo have been categorized by Jones and Smith (1973) and Streissguth, Bookstein, Sampson, and Barr (1993). Fetal alcohol syndrome (FAS) describes a cluster of defects seen in the newborn babies of approximately one third of alcoholic mothers, including facial anomalies, growth retardation with small head size, and mental retardation. Children with a prenatal history of ethanol exposure who manifest outcomes in two of the three categories are described as manifesting fetal alcohol effect (FAE). The window of vulnerability for damage from prenatal alcohol exposure extends throughout the pregnancy, with different types of damage at different stages. The facial defects are induced during the embryonic period, growth retardation is introduced mainly in the third trimester, and mental retardation results from exposure throughout the fetal period (Coles, 1994). Facial anomalies include short palpebral fissures (eye openings), underdeveloped midface with slow nose growth, and smooth philtrum (paired ridges from the upper lip to the nose). These facial anomalies become less distinctive as the children age. In addition to mental retardation, early and late behavioral problems associated with FAS include irritability in infancy, distractibility, high level of activity, communication skill deficits, impulsivity, difficulty with abstract concepts, and problem-solving difficulties (Streissguth, 1986; Streissguth et al., 1991). FAS and FAE are the most common preventable causes of mental retardation and most common preventable cause of birth defects. The high numbers of affected children are largely due to the prevalence of alcohol use and the extended period of sensitivity. The threshold dose for alcohol-induced prenatal damage is not firmly established but is estimated from standard procedures to be 0.35 ounces of alcohol per week. Using standard risk to benefit assessment, the recommended dosage is zero (Jacobson & Jacobson, 1994). For a general discussion of the effect of prenatal alcohol exposure on the lives of the children, the reader is referred to *The Broken Chord* (Dorris, 1989).

Tobacco

Approximately 30% of women of childbearing age smoke and 14.6% continue to smoke during their pregnancy (Guyer, Strobino, Ventura, MacDorman, & Martin,

1996). Although tobacco use has not been shown conclusively to be associated with congenital malformations, it is linked with other negative pregnancy outcomes. Smoking is the leading risk factor associated with low birthweight and early death, including sudden infant death syndrome (SIDS). Smoking has also been linked with respiratory difficulty after birth. Because tobacco smoke contains a large number of chemicals, mechanisms of damage are difficult to ascertain. However, smoking increases the level of carbon monoxide in maternal blood, thereby reducing oxygen availability to the fetus. Nicotine is readily passed to the embryo or fetus and has direct cytotoxic and central depressive effects, particularly in regard to amniotic breathing.

Rubella

Prenatal rubella exposure has been linked to embryonic or fetal death, congenital blindness, deafness, heart defects, and low birthweight. Maternal rubella during pregnancy produces a one in six chance of birth defects. The degree of risk changes depending on the timing of the infection. Birth defect rates of 47% for infants exposed in the first month, 22% in the second month, and 7% in the third month have been reported. The viral transmission rate from mother to embryo or fetus is higher, however, than the rate of actual birth defects (Miller, Cradock-Watson, & Pollock, 1982). Rubella creates embryonic or fetal damage through cell death, inhibition of cell division, decreased blood supply to tissue, and increased formation of scar tissue.

External Pressure

A variety of conditions can exert excess pressure on the body of the developing embryo or fetus. These conditions include uterine anomalies (small uterus, divided uterus), amniotic bands (constriction of the amnion), umbilical cord bands, or oligohydramnios (less than normal amount of amniotic fluid). Depending on the location and extent of pressure, embryonic or fetal structures can be distorted, stunted, cut off from circulation or amputated. Most commonly, pressure causes a distortion of the limb bones and joints. Pressure might also inhibit closure of clefts of the face and neck and closure of the abdominal cavity. For example, amniotic banding across the face might result in malposition of the eyes, specifically because the direct pressure of the band impedes the migration of the eye from the lateral to frontal position.

Radiation

Radiation, the particles or waves emitted from atomic or nuclear decay, have been shown to cause birth defects. Epidemics of birth defects were found among the infants of Marshall Islands and Japanese women after atomic blasts. X-rays, artificially produced gamma rays, are the most common source of radiation exposure.

They have been linked to miscarriage, congenital deformities, and childhood leukemia.

Maternal Stress

Maternal stress response to social environments can be classified as a developmental toxin if it negatively affects the health of the embryo or fetus or alters the fetal and infant developmental trajectory. The stress response affects maternal levels of hormones (cortisol, gonadotropins, estrogen, and progesterone), nutrient and oxygen availability to the embryo or fetus, blood flow, and alcohol, tobacco, and illicit drug use; all of which are potentially damaging to the embryo or fetus.

Maternal stress has been shown to provoke fetal stress response, intrauterine growth deficits (Field, Sandberg, Quetel, Garcia, & Rosario, 1985; Lederman, Lederman, Work & McCann, 1981), premature birth (Hedegaard, Henriksen, Secher, Hatch, & Sabroe, 1996), spontaneous abortion (Fenster et al., 1995), as well as pregnancy-induced maternal hypertension (Landbergis & Hatch, 1996; Klonoff-Cohen, Cross, & Pieper, 1996). In Klonoff-Cohen et al.'s case-control study (1996), the link between work stress and preeclampsia (hypertension, proteinurea, and edema) was found, even when other correlated factors such as age, smoking, alcohol, family history, and socioeconomic status were controlled. Chisholm found that the temperament differences in Navajo, Aboriginal, and Euro-American infants were partly attributable to differences in maternal blood pressure and stress, with stressed mothers having children with more sensitive (lower threshold for stimulation) temperaments (Chisolm, 1989). Other effects of stress on the embryo or fetus are suggested by animal studies including altered social behavior, premature birth, altered neurochemistry (e.g., opiates and catecholamines), and cognitive problems (Clark, Soto, Bergholz, & Schneider, 1996; Insel, Kinsley, Mann, & Bridges, 1990; Peters 1990; Weinstock, Fride, & Herzberg, 1988,).

One reason so little is known about the effects of prenatal stress is that stress research is difficult to perform. The lack of a universally agreed on tool to measure the "dosage" of stress is an important barrier. Life event scales, daily hassles indices, and other self-report measures show low correlation to biological indices of stress, such as endocrine levels, cardiovascular response, and rates of illness (for a review of measurement issues see Workman, 1997). Coping factors, such as social support, also alter the biological response of an individual to stressors.

THE UTERINE ENVIRONMENT
AS A DEVELOPMENTAL STIMULUS

The fetus needs certain types of environmental inputs to proceed through normal development. The supportive role of the uterus in development is well accepted in regard to the provision of nutrients, waste removal, temperature regulation, and physiological function, but the role of the uterus as a rich and varied environment that facilitates fetal sensory and behavioral development is only beginning to be understood. Development of the nervous system has been strongly linked to reciprocal interactions between the nervous tissue, the rest of the body, and the environment (Purves, 1988). Environmental factors have been shown to play important stimulatory and disruptive roles in cell proliferation, location, form (differentiation), connectivity, and survival.

Research into the positive prenatal inputs required for development is particularly important for safeguarding and improving fetal environments and as well as improving the environments of premature infants. Studies in this area have been facilitated by both improved prenatal imaging technology and observation of the capabilities of premature infants. Many questions confront researchers in developmental psychobiology, for example, which developmental events require environmental inputs to proceed normally? What role does the environment play in fetal sensory, motor, and cognitive development? What are the environmental requirements for tactile, kinesthetic, olfactory, gustatory, auditory, and visual development? Does prenatal exposure to speech affect speech development?

The fetus becomes capable of reacting to uterine sensory stimuli in fetal period, showing both short- and long-term evidence of the effects of these interactions. Touch and vestibular senses, which mature very early in the fetal period, are stimulated frequently through maternal movement, position changes, maternal speech vibration, as well as fetal movement and position changes. Touch and vestibular stimulation in animals and human preterms and neonates are related to basic physiologic processes, such as growth and respiration (Anderson, 1995; Evoniuk, Kuhn, & Schanberg, 1979). Patterns of common maternal and fetal movement and fetal position in the field of movement might be linked to neonatal postural preferences and postnatal preferences such as handedness (Michel, 1987; Previc, 1991).

The sensation of odor can be traced to the liquid environment of the uterus and the development of the vomeronasal and main olfactory systems. Animal research has demonstrated the ability of fetuses and neonates to respond to and recall unusual odors injected into the amniotic fluid. These unusual odor cues affected the feeding preference of newborn animals (preferring a nipple swabbed with the unusual scent experienced before birth). In utero exposure to unusual chemicals also cause physiological responses, such as alteration in the heart rate (Schaal & Orgeur, 1992). Moreover, full-term human infants show a preference for their mother's scent (Porter & Schaal, 1995).

Fetuses can respond physiologically to sounds, with the extent of the response related to the frequency and intensity of the sound, the developmental stage of the fetus, and behavioral state of the fetus (sleep and wake states). Typical responses to sound include movements, sucking responses, and changes in fetal breathing and heart rate. Fetuses and preterm infants show a physiologic response to sound by 26 to 27 weeks of gestation, in the form of changes in heart rate, respiration rate, and blood oxygen. By 32 weeks of gestation, connections to the auditory cortex become increasingly complete and infants can habituate to sounds. The number of trials needed to habituate to a vibration stimulus in utero was altered by exposure to cigarette smoke, barbiturates, or alcohol (Leader, 1995). The stimulation from the mother's voice provides a rich sensory experience for the fetus, with kinesthetic and tactile experience accompanying the sound.

Newborn infants respond differently to sounds encountered before birth, such as voices or certain stories or songs, from the way they respond to novel sounds. Bates (1994) made a compelling case that voice exposure during the fetal period and early infancy is important for the development of language capabilities. Seelback, Intrator, Lieberman, and Cooper (1994) demonstrated that a neural network computer program could produce categories of speech from inputs designed to model speech as heard by the fetus. Finally, prosody, the emotional aspect of speech, might play a role in emotional development before and after birth (Bates, 1994; Fifer & Moon, 1988).

Sensory experience inside the womb takes on additional significance when the effects of such stimulation on neural development are examined. Multiple lines of evidence show that prenatal experience (or early postnatal in immature newborn animals such as kittens and mice) plays an important role in shaping the nervous system. Animal models suggest an organizing role of the sequence of sensory stimulation (the order in which they come online and function). If function in one mode is prematurely activated out of sequence, other modalities might be affected adversely (intersensory interference). In most studies, visual stimulation prior to encoding of auditory information prevented the full function of auditory identification of mother and species members (for a review see Lickliter, 1995).

One of the most striking lines of evidence regarding the critical supportive role of prenatal stimulation comes from research examining the effect of sensory stimulation on programmed cell death and cellular differentiation in the sensory tracts. Sensory stimulation effects on the neural tissues continue from the fetal period into infancy. Early work with newborn animals, such as kittens, provided some of the first lines of evidence in the area of vision, which in turn catalyzed research on other modalities. The development of the pathway from the retina to the cortex is very sensitive to stimulation. Ocular dominance and distinct layering of the lateral geniculate nucleus (a relay station from the optic tract to the visual cortex) only occur with electrical stimulation of the system. Stimulation has been shown to alter the physiology of the neurons in the optic pathway, the amount of branching, and the organization of the neurons into lateral layers and horizontal columns (Shatz & Stryker, 1988; Stryker & Harris, 1986). Connection of elements in the visual system fail to form when the eyes of kittens are sutured shut at birth (Callaway & Katz, 1990). Suturing one eye (monocular deprivation) in the cat or monkey causes the animal to be essentially blind in the sutured eye due to weaker cortical connections and degenerative effects in the lateral geniculate (LeVay, Wiesel, & Hubel, 1980). Dark rearing or binocular suturing in cats and rats reduces the numbers of dendritic spines and the size of the dendritic field.

Another sensory modality examined is a specialized tactile pathway in rodents. The development of a specialized multistep neuronal pathway from rodent vibrissae (whiskers) through the brain stem and thalamus to an area of the sensory cortex seems to be dependent on sensory stimulation. The upper levels of this pathway, in the sensory cortex and thalamus, develop after birth and are dependent on the stimulation of the vibrissae. The development of these upper levels can be prevented by removal of the vibrissae soon after birth (Woolsey, Durham, Harris, Simons, & Valentino, 1981).

As interesting as both the visual and tactile stimulation data are, the question remained whether prenatal stimulation plays a similar role. The vibrissae of rodents provide a model for prenatal stimulation through the lower levels of the pathway in the brain stem and trigeminal nuclei, which are developed by birth. However, it was important to determine whether these lower levels of the system require prenatal stimulation to develop. The deprivation of stimulation was problematic until Li, Erzurumlu, Chen, Jhaveri, and Tonegawa (1991) developed a mouse strain in which postsynaptic transmission was prevented. The specialized whisker-specific arrangements in the trigeminal nuclei fail to develop in this strain, presumably due to the prevention of neural stimulation up the pathway. These results show that the pattern seen in early postnatal stimulation was also occurring in processes involving prenatal stimulation.

Attention has also been given to other types of stimulation that might affect the development of the embryo or fetus, such as circadian rhythms. Many stimuli delivered by the mother have diurnal rhythms. For example, maternal movement and hormones, such as catecholamines and melatonin, follow the day–night cycle. Rat and primate fetuses have circadian clock function, which has been shown to respond (entrain) to maternal circadian cues, such as melatonin. Newborn primates respond to light by a shift in their circadian cycle. If this circadian stimulation is important in development of the fetus, it may alter the way in which newborns are cared for in the newborn intensive care units (NICU). There is some preliminary evidence that this stimulation may be valuable to preterm infants in the NICU. For example, premature infants who received day–night cycling of light showed better outcomes than infants in constant light (Miller, White, Whitman, O'Callaghan, & Maxwell, 1995). For a review of the circadian literature as it pertains to the fetal and perinatal period, the reader is referred to Rivkees (1997).

The motor neurons also rely on prenatal function to develop normally. Practice of movement continues to affect connections at the cerebellar levels into adulthood. Prenatal motor and sensory experience is important in the development of the components of the motor system (particularly muscles, bones, and joints). Prenatal immobilization leads to joint abnormalities, contractions, and muscle wastage.

One important process in motor neurons, affected by prenatal experience, is programmed cell death. Motor neurons that do not connect to appropriate target cells in a firing sequence do not survive. The connection to the target cell and sensory inputs in the firing sequence provide trophic factors, chemicals that stimulate the neuron and protect it from cell death. Unlike the sensory tracts, the number of motor neurons is not increased with increasing activity of the tract. Increasing the mass or growth of the target region leads to an increase in the number of surviving motor neurons, but increased firing actually decreases the number of surviving neurons. The firing seems to lead to competition among the neurons for the trophic factors, with the firing of one neuron's inhibiting activity in nearby neurons, but the exact nature of this competition is not well understood. Immobilizing a limb in chick embryos leads to decreased motor neurons, whereas chemically produced paralysis in the embryo increases the number of surviving neurons. The difference in the outcomes could be due to muscle wastage, decreasing target tissue inputs. Self-generated movement plays a role in coordination of movement, with basic movements becoming more complex and organized. Although evidence for the importance of prenatal motor experience accumulates, the mechanisms of development of this system and the full ramifications of this experience on development are still largely unknown.

IMPLICATIONS FOR TREATMENT, CARE, AND RESEARCH

The newborn infant is the product of the interpenetration of a genetic program and numerous environmental interactions. The uterine environment typically provides for the physiological needs of the conceptus and the sensory stimulation of the fetus. However, the environment also can contain risks capable of altering developmental trajectories. For example, environmental agents can poison or damage tissues, interfere with growth, alter neurological function, trigger premature birth, or even cause death of the conceptus. Although proven teratogens are responsible for only 10% of congenital defects, this fraction still includes a large number of infants born every year with preventable birth defects. Known teratogenic damage is responsible for more than 5,000 children per year affected with mental retardation through FAS and is the one of the most important determinants of SIDS risk via smoking. Effective management of these risks would greatly affect child health and development. Further research into the unknown causes of birth defects could also lead to better management of risk.

Research regarding the supportive aspects of the uterine environment has provided considerable information about the impact of the uterine environment and the way it shapes fetal neonatal development and health. Research documenting the importance of touch and vestibular stimulation in fetal development has influenced care practices for preterm infants. As information on the importance of maternal voice, odor and gustatory cues, and circadian rhythmicity in the fetal period becomes clearer, further changes in the NICU environment, as well as changes in specific treatment practices, might result.

The information on the risks of the uterine experience has considerable implications for safety regulation and clinical management of pregnancy and premature infants. Safety regulatory agencies, such as the FDA and the Occupational Safety and Health Administration (OSHA), consider known teratogenic risks when setting standards of safety for medical treatments and workplace environments. Moreover, adding protective agents, such as folic acid, to foods to reduce neural tube defects, is now recommended. Obstetrical practice also manages teratogenic risks by assessing immunity to teratogenic pathogens, treatment of maternal illnesses, prudent use of pharmaceuticals, dietary supplementation to avoid deficiency malformations and complications, and counseling on lifestyle drugs that affect the developing embryo or fetus.

Despite these safeguards and attempts at protection, risks persist, as demonstrated by the number of children born each year with FAS. Researchers are attempting to formulate more effective methods of intervention to reduce the presence of lifestyle drugs in the uterine environment (Hankin, 1994). Neonatologists face complicated challenges connected with this field of knowledge. They must develop suitable environments that provide for the physiological stability and developmental trajectory of an infant who is fetal by age, but not by environment (i.e., airbreathing, cold, loud, and motionless). Teams that provide care to the premature infant must help the infant adapt to an environment for which they are not developmentally ready. As more is discovered about the types of stimulation that promote or impair the development of the fetus, the clinical application of that information might be adapted for the preterm infant. Conversely, neonatology provides information about the capabilities of the preterm infants that can provide direction to fetal research. In combination, the cooperation of laboratory research, medicine, and environmental regulation can continue to improve pregnancy outcomes and provide infants with their best chance of thriving on their continued developmental path.

REFERENCES

Abrams, R. M., Gerhardt, K. J., & Peters, A. (1995). Transmission of sound and vibration to the fetus. In J. Lecanuet, W. Fifer, N. Krasnegor, & W. Smotherman (Eds.), *Fetal development: A psychobiological perspective* (pp. 315–330). Hillsdale, NJ: Lawrence Erlbaum Associates.

Anderson, G. (1995). Touch and the kangaroo care method. In T. Field (Ed.), *Touch in early development* (pp. 35–51). Mahwah, NJ: Lawrence Erlbaum Associates.

Aranda, J., Hales, B., & Rieder, M. (1992). Developmental Pharmacology. In A. A. Fanaroff & R. J. Martin (Eds.) *Neonatal-perinatal medicine: Diseases of the fetus and infant.* (pp. 123–146). Chicago: Mosby.

Bates, E. (1994). Modularity, domain specificity and the development of language. *Discussion in Neuroscience, 10,* 136–149.

Brendt, R. L., [sic] & Beckman, D. A. (1990). Teratology. In R. Eden & F. Boehm (Eds.), *Assessment and care of the fetus* (pp. 223–244). Norwalk, CT: Appleton and Lange.

Callaway, E. M., & Katz, L. C. (1991). Effects of binocular deprivation on the development of clustered horizontal connections in cat striate cortex. *Proceedings of the National Academy of Science USA, 88,* 745–749.

Clark, A. S., Soto, A., Bergholz, T., & Schneider, M. L. (1996). Maternal gestational stress alters adaptive and social behavior in adolescent rhesus monkey offspring. *Infant Behavior and Development, 19*(4), 451–462

Chisolm, J. S. (1989). Biology, culture and the development of temperament: A Navajo example. In J. K. Nugent, B. M. Lester, & T. B. Brazelton (Eds.), *The cultural context of infancy: Vol. 1* (pp. 341–364). Norwood, NJ: Ablex.

Coles, C. (1994). Critical periods for prenatal alcohol exposure: Evidence from animal and human studies. *Alcohol Health and Research World, 18*(1), 22–29.

Dorris, M. (1989). *The broken cord.* New York: Harper and Row.

Evoniuk, G. E., Kuhn, C. M., & Schanberg, S. M. (1979). The effect of tactile stimulation on serum growth hormone and tissue ornithine decarboxylase activity during maternal deprivation in rat pups. *Communications in Psychopharmacology, 3,* 363–370.

Fenster, L., Schaefer, C., Mathur, A., Hiatt, R., Pieper, C., Hubbard, A., Von Behren. J., Swan, S. (1995). Psychologic stress in the workplace and spontaneous abortion. *American Journal of Epidemiology, 142,* 1176–1183.

Field, T., Sandberg, D., Quetel, T., Garcia, R., & Rosario, M. (1985). Effects of ultrasound feedback on pregnancy anxiety, fetal activity and neonatal outcome. *Obstetrics and Gynecology, 66,* 525–528.

Fifer, W. P., & Moon, C. (1988). Auditory experience in the fetus. In W. P. Smotherman & S. R. Robinson (Eds.), *Behavior of the fetus* (pp. 175–188). Caldwell, NJ: Telford Press.

Gregg, N. (1941). Congenital cataract following German measles in the mother. *Transactions of the Ophthalmological Society of Australia, 3,* 35–46.

Guyer, B., Strobino, D. M., Ventura, S. J., MacDorman, M., & Martin, J. A. (1996). Annual summary of vital statistics 1995. *Pediatrics, 98,* 1007–1019.

Hankin, J. (1994). FAS prevention strategies: Passive and active measures. *Alcohol Health and Research World, 18*(1), 62–66.

Hedegaard, M., Henriksen, T., Secher, N., Hatch, M., & Sabroe, S. (1996). Do stressful life events affect duration of gestation and risk of preterm delivery? *Epidemiology, 7*(4), 339–345.

Hertig, A. T. (1967). The overall problem in man. In K. Bernischke (Ed.), *Comparative aspects of reproductive failure* (pp. 11–41). Berlin: Springer-Verlag.

Impekoven, M., & Gold, P. (1973). Prenatal origins of parent-young interactions in birds: A naturalistic approach. In G. Gottlieb (Ed.) *Behavioral embryology: Vol. 1. Studies on the development of behavior and the nervous system* (pp. 325–356). New York: Academic Press.

Insel, T., Kinsley, C., Mann, P., & Bridges, R. (1990). Prenatal stress has long term effects on brain opiate receptors. *Brain Research, 511,* 93–97.

Jacobson, J., & Jacobson, S. (1994). Prenatal alcohol exposure and neurobehavioral development: Where is the threshold? *Alcohol Health and Research World, 18*(1), 30–36.

Jones, K., & Smith, D. (1973). Recognition of fetal alcohol syndrome in early infancy. *Lancet II* (7836), 999–1001.

Kitano, Y., Ohzono, H., Yasuda, N., & Shimizu, T. (1996). Hydranencephaly, cerebellar hypoplasia, and myopathy in chick embryos infected with the aino virus. *Veterinary Pathology, 33,* 672–681.

Klonoff-Cohen, H. S., Cross, J. L., & Pieper, C. F. (1996). Job stress and preeclampsia. *Epidemiology, 7*(3), 245–249.

Landbergis, P., & Hatch, M. (1996). Psychosocial work stress and pregnancy-induced hypertension. *Epidemiology, 7,* 346–351.

Leader, L. (1995). The potential value of habituation in the prenate. In J. Lecanuet, W. Fifer, N. Krasnegor, & W. Smotherman (Eds.), *Fetal development: A psychobiological perspective* (pp. 383–405). Hillsdale NJ: Lawrence Erlbaum Associates.

Lederman, R., Lederman, E., Work, B., & McCann, D. (1981). Maternal psychological and physiological correlates of fetal-newborn health status. *American Journal of Obstetrics and Gynecolgy, 139,* 956–958.

Lenz, W., & Kapp, K. (1962). Thalidomide embryopathy. *Archives of Environmental Health, 5,* 100–105.

LeVay, S., Wiesel, T., & Hubel, D. (1980). The development of ocular dominance columns in normal and visually deprived monkeys. *Journal of Comparative Neurology, 191*(1), 1–51.

Li, Y., Erzurumlu, R. S., Chen, C., Jhaveri, S., & Tonegawa, S. (1994). Whisker-related neuronal patterns fail to develop in the trigeminal brainstem nuclei of NMDAR1 knockout mice. *Cell, 76,* 427–437.

Lickliter, R. (1995). Embryonic sensory experience and intersensory development in precocial birds. In J. Lecanuet, W. Fifer, N. Krasnegor, & W. Smotherman (Eds.), *Fetal development: A psychobiological perspective* (pp. 281–294). Hillsdale NJ: Lawrence Erlbaum Associates.

Michel, G. (1987). Self-generated experience and the development of lateralized neurobehavioral organization in infants. *Advances in the Study of Behavior, 17,* 61–83.

Miller, E., Cradock-Watson, J. E., & Pollock T. M. (1982). Consequences of confirmed maternal rubella at successive stages of pregnancy. *Lancet II* (8302), 781–784.

Miller, C., White, R., Whitman, T., O'Callaghan, M., & Maxwell, S. (1995). The effects of cycled versus noncycled lighting on growth and development in preterm infants. *Infant Behavior and Development, 18,* 87–95.

Peters, D. (1990). Maternal stress increases fetal brain and neonatal cerebral cortex 5-hydroxytrypamine synthesis in rats: A possible mechanism by which stress influences brain development. *Pharmacology, Biochemistry and Behavior, 17,* 721–725.

Porter, R. H., & Schaal, B. (1995). Olfaction and development of social preferences in neonatal organisms. In R. L. Doty (Ed.), *Handbook of clinical olfaction and gestation* (pp. 299–321). New York: Marcel Dekker.

Previc, F. (1991). A general theory concerning the prenatal origins of cerebral lateralization in humans. *Psychological Review, 98,* 299–334.

Purves, D. (1988). *Body and brain: A trophic theory of neural connections.* Cambridge, MA: Harvard University Press.

Rivkees, S. (1997). Developing circadian rhythmicity. Basic clinical aspects. *Pediatric Clinics of North Amermica, 44*(2), 467–487.

Robert, C. J., & Lowe, C. R. (1975). Where have all the conceptions gone? *Lancet I* (7906), 498–499.

Schaal, B., & Orgeur, P. (1992). Olfaction in utero: Can the rodent model be generalized? *Quarterly Journal of Experimental Psychology, 44B,* 245–278.

Seelback, B. S., Intrator, N., Lieberman, P., & Cooper, L. N. (1994). A model of prenatal acquisition of speech parameters. *Proceedings of the National Academy of Science USA, 91,* 7473–7476.

Shatz, C., & Stryker, M. (1988). Prenatal tetrodotoxin infusion blocks segregation of retinogeniculate afferents. *Science, 242,* 87–89.

Streissguth, A. (1986). The behavioral teratology of alcohol: Performance, behavioral, and intellectual deficits in prenatally exposed children. In J. West (Ed.), *Alcohol and brain development* (pp. 3–44). New York: Oxford University Press.

Streissguth, A., Aase, J., Clarren, S., Randels, S., LaDue, R., & Smith, D. (1991). Fetal Alcohol Syndrome in adolescents and adults. *Journal of the American Medical Association, 265*(15), 1961–1967.

Streissguth, A., Bookstein, F., Sampson, P., & Barr, H. (1993). *The enduring effects of prenatal alcohol exposure on child development: Birth through seven years, a partial least squares solution.* Ann Arbor: University of Michigan Press.

Stryker, M., & Harris, W. (1986). Binocular impulse blockade prevents formation of ocular dominance columns in cat visual cortex. *Journal of Neuroscience, 6,* 2117–2133.

Weinstock, M, Fride, E., & Hertzberg, R. (1988). Prenatal stress effects on functional development in the offspring. *Progress in Brain Research, 73,* 319–331.

Woolsey, T., Durham, D., Harris, R., Simons, D., & Valentino, K. (1981). Somatosensory development. In R. Aslin, J. Alberts and M. Peterson (Eds.), *Development of perception: Vol. 1. Audition, somatic perception and the chemical senses* (pp. 259–292). New York: Academic Press.

Workman, E. (1997). The measurement of stress and its effects. In J. Hubbard & E. Workman (Eds.), *Handbook of stress medicine: An organ systems approach* (pp. 295–308). New York: CRC Press.

6

Environmental Aspects
of Infant Health and Illness

Thomas L. Whitman
Robert D. White
Kathleen M. O'Mara
Marcie C. Goeke-Morey
University of Notre Dame

INFANCY IS a period of rapid change along biological and psychological continua. Infants' major tasks are to grow and learn, which they accomplish at a rate unmatched at any other time in the life span. Infants typically double their length and quadruple their birthweight by 2 years of age. Although most of the neurons of the infant brain have been generated prior to birth, the arborization process through which the brain becomes interconnected is only beginning. Many of the infants' early interactions with their environments are structured by reflexes that control vital functions, including their approach to food and avoidance of aversive stimuli. The infants' motor responses, initially dominated by underlying reflexes, gradually come under intentional control. Gross uncoordinated action is slowly replaced by fine coordinated action. Infants' sleep patterns change, with both alert states and deep sleep states gradually emerging, sleep periods increasing in length and rhythmicity, and the amount of daily sleep decreasing. The sensory systems, already functioning to varying extents before birth, continue to develop after birth, with the auditory and particularly visual systems maturing last. With increasing periods of alertness, infants quickly become active information processors, with learning occurring at breakneck speed. Although the basic structure of the infant's temperament is in place early, the development of the emotional system and attachment responses awaits the emergence of the cognitive system. As motor, sensory, cognitive, and emotional development proceeds, infants progress toward becoming active, self-regulatory, and social beings.

Although amazingly well adapted for survival, infants are biologically vulnerable. Their ability to adapt to life outside the womb can be disrupted easily if they are born too soon, have congenital biological problems, or are placed in stressful environments that make demands that exceed infant resources. Infancy, as a developmental period, is unique in the degree to which the immediate environment plays a role in determining health outcomes. Because of their immature status, infants rely almost entirely on their social environment to satisfy their basic needs for nurturing and stimulation. The way this environment is structured can have profound effects on their survival, health and general development. When properly arranged, the infants' social environment can facilitate growth, even under biologically challenging conditions.

This chapter examines the factors that place infants at risk for illness and protect them from health problems. Although biological causes of infant illness are discussed briefly in the next section, this chapter emphasizes examining how the physical and social environments in which infants live affect their health. Prevention and intervention strategies for improving infant health are identified. Finally, research questions in need of investigation are discussed.

EARLY BIOLOGICAL INFLUENCES ON INFANT HEALTH

In the past decade, concern about children's health in the United States has been widely registered. According to statistics released by the Children's Defense Fund, about 25% of American babies are born to mothers who do not receive early prenatal care (Children's Defense Fund, 1994). The United States ranked higher than at least 20 other nations in infant mortality and infants born with low birthweight. The overall infant mortality in the United States in 1995 was 7.5 per 1,000 live births. For Black infants, the mortality rate was almost twice as high, 14.9 deaths per 1,000 births. Black infant mortality in the United States was higher than for infants in countries such as Cuba, Chile, Lithuania, and Jamaica. Seven percent of U.S. babies were of low birthweight (less than 5.5 pounds). Infants surviving birth are at risk for a myriad of health problems, including congenital defects (e.g., neural tube defects such as spina bifida), complications of prematurity (including chronic lung disease and intraventricular hemorrhage), viral and bacterial infections, physical injuries, failure to thrive, and sudden infant death syndrome (SIDS).

Estimates of birth defects in babies born in the United States range from 3% to 5%. Although the exact etiology of many of these anomalies are unknown, their causes are primarily genetic or teratogenic in nature. More than 7,000 chromosomal and single-gene defects have been identified, and more are discovered every year (McKusick, 1994). Well-known single-gene disorders include galatosemia, phenylketonuria, cystic fibrosis, Tay-Sach, and sickle cell anemia. Common chromosomal syndromes include Down, Turner, Edward, and Fragile X. The majority of infants born with genetic and chromosomal disorders also have health-related problems (see Batshaw & Perret, 1992). For example, infants with Down syndrome commonly have respiratory and cardiac problems. Although the environment certainly can affect the course of infants with genetic defects, through both medical and social interventions, their developmental trajectory is influenced to a considerable extent by their defects.

Maturational factors also influence infant health. Like many birth defects, the normative schedule of infant maturation has a strong genetic basis, although it is environmentally influenced to some extent. Health problems can develop when infants confront an environment for which they are not maturationally prepared. This maturational mismatch is most clearly seen in preterm births. Preterm infants, particularly those born before 28 weeks, are at risk for bronchopulmonary problems because their lungs are immature and not fully capable of respiratory function. They are also subject to intraventricular brain bleeds because their vascular walls are thin and regulation of cerebral blood flow is immature. As is discussed later, the incidence of these types of problems can be reduced with proper medical technological and environmental supports. Full-term infants are also vulnerable due to their maturational status. For example, at birth the infant's immunological system is only beginning to develop, although the infant's defenses against disease can be reinforced through breast-feeding and inoculations. (See chapters 2 and 5, this volume, for further discussion of early biological risk factors.)

ENVIRONMENTAL INFLUENCES
ON INFANT HEALTH

As indicated earlier, the focus of this chapter is on examining the relation between environment and infant health. The environmental influences on infant health are many and diverse, operating prenatally and postnatally. Environmental influences include any biological or chemical agents introduced into the infant's body, medical interventions (including the use of drugs and surgery), physical and social arrangements surrounding the delivery of medical treatments, and social factors that operate in living settings, such as the family. Ultimately, all of these environmental influences exert their effects on health through biological channels. Because a considerable amount has been written about the prenatal and perinatal periods (see chapter 5, this volume), this section emphasizes the postnatal period of development. Special attention is devoted to the discussion of environmental prevention and intervention programs.

Prenatal Influences

A range of substances, commonly referred to as *teratogens,* can produce prenatal and congenital health problems. Teratogens are biological agents, introduced from the environment through the mother into the developing embryo and fetus, that cause physical malformations. The effect of a teratogen depends on its biological action and on the specific stage of embryological or fetal development in which exposure to the teratogen occurs. Teratogenic effects are also related to the size of the teratogen, the permeability of the placenta, and to the dosage level of the teratogen. Early exposure to teratogens during the embryological period might cause severe damage, resulting in spontaneous abortion. Some teratogens, including alcohol, can exert their adverse effects throughout fetal development, whereas other agents, such as the rubella virus or syphilis, are most likely to cause damage during specific periods of prenatal development.

Agents that might act as teratogens include drugs (e.g., alcohol, cocaine, and thalidomide), chemical substances (e.g., lead and mercury), radiation, maternal infections (such as syphilis, toxoplasmosis, rubella, and cytomegalovirus), and maternal metabolic disorders (e.g., diabetes). The range of impact of such teratogens is extremely diverse, potentially affecting each of the organ systems of the body. Some of the more frequently occurring congenital defects that are produced by teratogens include fetal alcohol syndrome, microcephaly, hydrocephaly, neural tube disorders (e.g., spina bifida), growth retardation, and mental retardation (Batshaw & Perret, 1992). Many of these problems can be prevented through education and prenatal medical care programs (see chapter 5, this volume, and Batshaw & Perret, 1992, for more extensive discussions of prenatal influences on fetal development).

Perinatal Influences

A range of events surrounding the baby's delivery, to some extent controllable through medical or environmental interventions, can affect the health and physical status of the child. For example, precipitous or delayed deliveries can result in anoxic brain damage. Drugs used to reduce maternal discomfort, such as tranquilizers, sedatives, and analgesics, have been the subject of controversy; the short- and long-term effects of these drugs on the infant seem to vary with type of drug and infant characteristics. The impact on infant development of Cesarean deliveries, which significantly alters the baby's birth experience, has also been the subject of empirical study and debate.

In recent decades, a variety of childbirth strategies have been advocated including standard delivery (which employs liberal use of analgesics), natural child birth, and the LeBoyer method. Current childbirth practices tend to be more flexible than those of a generation ago, with more emphasis on maternal and family choices, cognitive preparation, and the use of techniques such as relaxation and controlled breathing. Increasingly, there have also been efforts to create more homelike environments in hospitals, which allow fuller family participation.

As interest in natural childbirth has increased, so too has the assistance with delivery of midwives and doulas, woman who provide physical care and emotional support to the mother before, during, and after the birth of her infant. In a meta-analytic review, Klaus (1995) found that the presence of a doula was associated with reduction in cesarean section (50%), length of labor (25%), oxytocin use (40%), pain medication (30%), need for forceps (40%), and requests for epidurals (50%). Klaus suggested that doulas, by supporting mothers during and after birth, help teach them how to mother their babies. He observed that women who received support from a doula were more likely to breast-feed, feed on demand, be satisfied with their babies and husbands, and perhaps, most important, spend more time with their babies. Unfortunately, data concerning the infants was not available. However, if the mother generally is more pain free, secure, and satisfied, it seems likely that the infant would also derive health benefits.

For a more complete discussion of perinatal influences on health, the reader is referred to chapter 5 (this volume), Batshaw & Perret (1992), and Santrock (1996).

Postnatal Influences: The Hospital Environment

In the past several decades, concern has grown about how the physical aspects and social caretaking arrangements in hospital environments influence infant health. For example, it has been suggested that preterm infants in hospitals might be deprived and need more stimulation to grow and mature appropriately. In contrast, it has also been argued that preterm infants are often overstimulated in hospitals, with environmental inputs serving as stressors that tax the infant's biological and behavioral coping resources, thus producing medical problems and intefering with growth. Proponents of a stimulus deprivation hypothesis have sought to supplement the infant's environment by providing enriching auditory, visual, kinesthetic, and propreceptive inputs, whereas advocates of the overstimulation hypothesis have emphasized reducing input from the environment, especially light, noise, and painful procedures.

This debate sometimes oversimplifies a much more complex issue. As Brazelton and Field (1990) pointed out, there is a tremendous range of stimulation, from excessive to optimal to a state of deprivation, which they refer to as *violation*. Violation occurs when the lack of stimulation results in the disorganization of the infant. Depending on the circumstances, stimulation either might facilitate or inhibit the development of biological structures (Hunt, 1961; Schanberg, 1995). A developmental perspective emphasizes that infants are not static entities but rather are dynamic organisms made up of different subsystems (e.g., respiratory, cardiovascular, sensory, motor, and attentional) that evolve at different rates. The empirical questions that needs to be addressed concern the types and levels of stimulation that are appropriate for infants at different developmental stages. As this section details, this type of question is only beginning to be addressed by researchers.

Physical Aspects of Hospital Environments. Since the 1960s, medical care for infants has changed significantly. For example, technological advances have occurred that have allowed for the successful treatment of many medical complications associated with premature birth and full-term infants in distress at birth. Through creating special environments and providing specific aids, these technologies have replaced or assisted bodily functions. These technologies include special beds and incubators, respiratory aids (e.g., endotracheal tubes and mechanical ventilation), and nutritive procedures (e.g., gavage feeding and intravenous assistance). In addition, an array of special monitoring devices (e.g., to monitor respiratory, cardiac, and oxygenation functions) have been developed to evaluate infant medical status. Whereas, in the 1970s, the survival rate for prematurely born infants weighing 1500 grams was about 50%, in the 1990s this same advantage was experienced by infants weighing 750 grams. To a great extent, this improved survival is due to the development of new technologies as well as medications such as surfactant, which is used for preterm infants with immature lung development. However, as mortality rates for infants have improved, morbidity concerns have increased.

As White (1996) pointed out, until recently it was felt that premature infants were oblivious to their surroundings, seeming to tolerate the new technological environments created in the neonatal intensive care unit (NICU), along with routine aspects of this setting, such as bright lights, noise, frequent handling, and painful medical procedures. In the past decade, however, clinical researchers have suggested that the hospital environments created to accommodate the special needs of preterm infants might have adverse side effects on infant health. For example, there is now concern that the underdeveloped nervous system of the premature infant can be overwhelmed through sensory bombardment produced by new technologies and as a consequence of this overstimulation, be at greater risk for physical problems, such as apnea, bronchopulmonary dysplasia, seizures, bradycardia, intraventricular hemorrhages, and retinopathy of prematurity.

Concern has been especially focused on the high noise levels and bright continuous lighting conditions in NICU settings. The 1970s brought the sounds of ventilators, including intravenous pumps and monitors, to the NICU often designed as a single room holding 40 or more babies. Noise levels were significantly higher in NICUs than in normal nurseries, comparable to levels associated with street traffic, as well as of a quality different from noise in the average home. Some empirical studies suggest that these noise levels interfere with sleep and result in increases in heart rates and peripheral vasoconstriction. Other research indicates an association between environmental noise levels and apneic episodes, oxygen desaturation, and increased intracranial pressure (see Miller, White, Whitman, O'Callaghan, & Maxwell, 1995).

A variety of research has also raised serious concerns about the effect of bright and continuous lighting conditions in hospitals. Continuous bright lighting has been linked to numerous problems in both animals and humans, including retinal pathology, disruption of circadian rhythms, reduced melatonin secretion, insomnia, fatigue, affective disorders, and performance problems. In contrast, lower level and cyclical lighting has been postulated to be a more appropriate type of sensory stimulation, preventing many of the problems associated with continuous bright lighting (Miller et al., 1995).

Until recently, little has been known about the effects of ambient lighting on infant growth and development. Although some studies suggest that cycled lighting would be beneficial to infants in NICUs, the effects of such lighting arrangements on infants in the long term has not been examined. This issue was addressed by Miller et al. (1995). Preterm infants in structurally identical critical care units were provided either cycled or noncycled lighting during a lengthy hospital stay. Lighting conditions were looked at in relation to multiple aspects of infant development and staff behavior. Compared to infants in the noncycled lighting condition, infants assigned to the cycled lighting condition had a greater rate of weight gain, were able to be fed orally sooner, spent fewer days on the ventilator and on phototherapy, and displayed enhanced motor coordination. There was no evidence in this study that lighting conditions affected staff behavior or that staff mediated the effect of lighting on infant outcomes. In the past decade, in part catalyzed by research such as that previously cited, changes are beginning to be initiated in NICUs. The guideline of 100-foot-candles illumination, widely accepted in the 1980s, is now used in only a minority of NICUs. Because of improved monitoring systems, the need for continuous bright lights has diminished. The psychological benefits of windows and natural lighting increasingly have been emphasized.

As indicated earlier, a number of clinical researchers have suggested that intensive care nurseries for preterm infants may also be a source of sensory deprivation and that supplemental stimulation needs to be provided. Some investigators have argued that this stimulation should approximate the experiences of the intrauterine fetus, whereas other researchers have emphasized the biological differences of the preterm infant from the fetus and suggest the needs for other kinds of stimulation. In a literature review, Field (1980) summarized the results of studies that provided preterm infants supplemental stimulation, ranging from a recorded mother's voice, nonnutritive sucking, to rocking, stroking, handling, oscillating waterbeds, rocking beds, and heartbeat recordings, to sensorimotor exercises. Although the studies varied considerably in their choice of type of preterm subjects (and parameters such as age, weight, and presence of medical complications), their dependent variables, their experimental designs, and the nature of the supplemental stimulation, Field (1980) pointed out that as a group they indicated the benefits of supplemental enriching stimulation for infants, including better weight gain, greater milk intake, fewer medical complications, shorter hospital stays, improved motor and sensory functioning, increased activity, less crying, and more quiet sleep. However, comparisons between specific studies also revealed inconsistent results and considerable individual differences in response.

Against this backdrop, more controlled studies are starting to be conducted that examine the benefits of adding certain sounds back into the hospital environment. For example, a recent study by Kawakami, Takai-Kawakami, Kurihara, Shimizu, and Yanaihara (1996) found that infants, presented with either white noise or recorded heartbeats during a heelstick procedure, were less stressed than infants presented no supplemental sounds. Increased consideration is also being given to the creation of microenvironments for infants, similar to incubators, that can regulate lighting levels and cycles, noise, tactile, and proprioceptive inputs along with temperature and oxygenation level (White, 1996). The ideal environment is likely not to be static but adjustable, accommodating to the emerging behavioral and sensory competencies of the infant. In designing these new types of environments, the unique and sometimes conflicting needs of the child, family, and medical staff must be considered.

Nursing Care. In addition to specific physical arrangements in hospital settings, the structure of nursing care routines have been scrutinized (Mouradian & Als, 1994). Concern has been expressed regarding the nature of stimulation that occurs during interactions between medical caregivers and infants, interactions that have been characterized variously as exclusively medical, too frequent, aversive, and noncontingent. Clinicians have suggested that infant physiological status, growth and development could be improved through changing nursing practices, for example, by reducing the number of medical interventions, clustering interventions and timing interventions so that their application is not associated with high infant arousal.

Consistent with these suggestions, Als (1994) introduced the concept of individualized care for preterm infants. She noted that preterm infants exhibit a number of observable behaviors (e.g., autonomic and visceral responses, movements, postures, and state levels) that provide information concerning their level of stress. To optimize infant physiological and behavioral status, she suggested that if staff, as they apply medical interventions, were trained to recognize these biological and behavioral signals, infant stress might be reduced and infant development and growth facilitated.

Als (1994) incorporated this idea into her study of individualized care for very low birthweight preterm infants. Thirty-eight infants with no known congenital abnormalities were assigned to an experimental or a control group. All infants weighed less than 1250 grams, were less than 30 weeks gestational age at birth, and were mechanically ventilated in 3 hours of delivery. Infants in the experimental intervention group received individualized care from a group of trained nurses and their parents. This specialized care consisted of placing the infant in a flexed position to encourage restfulness, holding infants after stressful medical procedures, creating sleep and feeding schedules that conformed to the infant's own individual sleep and feeding cycles, and reducing lighting and noise levels. The control groups were given primary care nursing, their incubators were covered with blanket covers, and a 24-hour visiting policy for the parents was available. Comparisons with the control group revealed that infants in the experimental group developed significantly fewer intraventricular hemorrhages, better motor and autonomic integration, and self-regulatory competencies. Overall, these results suggested that individualized care provided by staff and parents improved the physical and behavioral development of the preterm infant.

Recently, Als and Gilkerson (1995) proposed specific guidelines for what they described as developmentally supportive care in hospital settings. They suggested that the infant should be an active collaborator in his or her own care, specifically because the infant provides the best information from which to design a care program. Developmentally supportive care emphasizes caretakers' learning to observe and interpret infant behavior before developing an individualized care plan, the provision of consistent and collaborative caregiving by a team that includes parents and hospital personnel, structuring care on a 24-hour basis to provide the infant sufficient rest and support growth, and pacing caregiving so the infant will be less stressed. Other components of developmental care include providing the infant feeding support, positioning support, opportunities for skin-to-skin contact, and a quiet soothing environment.

Family-Centered Care. Als and Gilkerson (1995) emphasized that individualized caregiving is appropriate not only for hospital staff but also for parents. Increasingly, hospitals are encouraging families of preterm infants to assume primary caregiver responsibilities before their children are discharged. Family-centered care acknowledges the significant impact that parents and other family members can have on an infant's health and encourages dialogue and cooperation between family and staff in planning and implementing caretaking for the infant. This type of care emphasizes the importance of human contact and distinctly contrasts with traditional medical care, which has been characterized as pragmatic, often involving painful encounters and lacking in tender-loving attention. Family-centered care is sometimes conjoined with a rooming-in program. Most rooming-in programs provide family members with a separate sleeping and living area near the NICU, where the infant can spend periods of time being cared for by its family under the supervision of staff members (Johnson, 1995). The combination of new medical technologies with rooming-in results in a holistic program that provides comprehensive medical care without sacrificing human contact with the infant. Rooming-in and family care programs are also viewed as promoting the family's bond with the infant.

Several hospitals have emerged as leaders in redesigning and reestablishing the concept of rooming-in in the NICU. One such hospital is the Transitional Care Center (TCC) at Rainbow Babies and Children's Hospital in Cleveland, Ohio. Since 1992, the TCC has sought to create a family-centered environment in which parents serve as individualized caregivers, with the welfare of the infant being closely aligned with the state of the parent–child relationship (Forsythe, 1995). This program also furnishes the infant with environmental supports to promote the neurobehavioral organization of the infant. As a result of these practices, Rainbow Hospital has noted improved medical outcomes in its NICU patients and reduced duration of hospital stays (Johnson, 1995).

Feeding on demand, a component of individualized care, is also a major feature of most family-centered programs. Individualized feeding is most easily executed in a rooming-in situation because the mother and the rest of the family are constantly available to monitor the infant's behaviors and to respond to its signals of hunger. Rooming-in at night seems particularly appropriate if a mother is breast-feeding, given that prolactin (the hormone that stimulates lactation and maternal behavior) is secreted at a higher level at night than during the day (see Anderson, 1989).

A number of researchers have suggested that family-centered and rooming-in programs benefit both parents and infants. Anderson (1989) reported that preterm infants who roomed with their mothers had significantly lower blood pressures than control infants. This research also indicated that preterm infants, who were gently held by a foster caregiver during the first 4 hours after birth, cried an average of 2 minutes, in contrast to control infants who cried an average of 38 minutes. Premature infants are especially vulnerable to the harmful effects of crying, which can lead to their respiratory complications and increase the threat of later intracranial hemorrhages.

The Importance of Touch.   The findings just mentioned, described by Anderson (1989), suggest that one of the most important components of family-centered, individualized care and rooming-in programs, is the involvement of caretakers in the active handling and touching of their infants. A study by Field et al. (1986) provides evidence for the effectiveness of a tactile and kinesthetic stimulation intervention with 20 preterm neonates. This intervention consisted of body stroking and passive movement of limbs for three 15-minute periods per day for 10 days. In comparison with a control group, infants receiving the intervention showed substantially greater weight gain per day (47%), a greater percentage of time in active and alert states, more mature habituation, orientation, motor and range of state behaviors on the Brazelton Neonatal Behavior Assessment Scale, and shorter hospital stays. A variety of other research has also suggested the beneficial effects of touch on the development of the autonomic, immune, neurological, and attachment systems (see reviews by Field, 1980, 1995a, 1995b).

A biological basis for the beneficial effects of touch is suggested in a study by Schanberg (1995), who examined the effects of maternal separation on the development of rat pups. The results of this study indicate that when rat pups were separated from their mother, levels of growth-promoting hormones (prolactin, growth hormone, and insulin) decreased. When pups were returned to an accepting female, however, the levels of growth-promoting hormones returned to normal. Schanberg (1995) speculated that the licking and stroking patterns of the mother, not simply her presence, triggered the increase in the growth-promoting hormones in the pups. To test this hypothesis, mother's licking behavior was simulated by stroking the pups with a wet paintbrush. Those pups who were stroked heavily had the greatest increase in growth-promoting hormone levels. In contrast, pups who were stroked lightly, deprived of stroking, or pinched showed little to no increase in growth-promoting hormones. Schanberg's (1995) results provides general support for two postulates underlying family-centered and rooming-in programs—specifically, that maternal presence facilitates the development of the newborn and that appropriate tactile stimulation of the infant by a caregiving individual promotes infant growth and well-being.

One form of tactile stimulation, called *kangaroo care,* is used in many hospital individualized care and family-centered programs for infants. Kangaroo care, also known as *skin-to-skin contact,* consists of the mother (or father) holding the infant beneath her clothing, against her skin and between her breasts or on one breast (Anderson, 1995). It can be introduced minutes after the infant is born, if the infant is medically stable. Kangaroo care can also be accommodated to serve infants who need oxygen, are on a ventilator, or who have episodes of apnea or bradycardia. It is also utilized in rooming-in programs for preterm infants because it facilitates on-demand breastfeeding. Skin-to-skin contact appears to enhance the infant's self-regulatory access to a mother's milk and is used to introduce infants who are gavage fed to the practice of breast-feeding (see Anderson, 1995, for a more complete discussion of this procedure).

In reviews of current research, using a variety of methodologies ranging from randomized clinical trials to the use of case studies, Anderson (1991, 1995) suggested that infants exposed to kangaroo care manifested greater regularity in their heart rate and respiration, better regulation of their body temperature, superior oxygenation of their blood, and a greater degree of deep sleep. They also appeared more alert, cried less, had reduced levels of infection, greater weight gain, less need of incubators and were discharged earlier from the hospital. Mothers who provided kangaroo care breast-fed more, appeared to experience a stronger attachment with their infant, and felt more confidence in providing care for them.

Postnatal Influences: The Caretaker–Child Interaction

In the previous section, the importance of parents in hospital-based treatment programs for newborns and medically compromised infants was highlighted. In this section, we examine how mothers in home settings influence infant health, the importance of tactile stimulation for infant growth, the influence of sleeping arrangements on infant physical functioning, and the possible roles the social-caretaking environment plays in SIDS and failure to thrive syndrome (FTT). Space prevents discussion of a variety of other important topics relating to infant health. For example, little is said here about fathers or infant abuse. Whereas little research has investigated the effect of fathers on infant health, considerable attention has been given in the literature to infant abuse. Recent statistics indicate that one third of all abuse victims are younger than 1 year. Abuse, including shaken baby syndrome, is a major cause of hospitalization in infants (Osofsky, 1994). Moreover, physical abuse is the leading cause of death in infants, with more than 50% of children dying from abuse-related causes being younger than 1 year. The main perpetrators of violence toward infants are in the home—and the agents typically are the child's caretakers or parents. Although research on the causes and consequences of infant abuse is being actively pursued, our understanding of how caretakers more generally influence the infant's physical well-being is only beginning.

Maternal Influences on Infant Health. A major key to understanding infant health and illness is the mother–infant relationship. From a biopsychoenvironmental perspective, the mother provides the biological environment from which the infant emerges. The phenotypic expression of the infant's genetic structure is influenced early on by the uterine environment of the mother, and especially through the umbilical connection. Although we do not typically think of the mother as constructing this biological environment, she certainly influences it through her lifestyle, including her eating, sleeping, and exercise habits, her use of medical care, her management of stress, and her overall knowledge of fetal development. After the baby's birth, the mother typically continues to exert a major environmental influence on the infant through the social umbilicus of her relationship to her baby. The mother in our society usually plays a major role in establishing the child's physical sleeping arrangements, controls the amount, nature, and type of physical contact the baby has with her, influences eating regimens and schedules, and controls, at least partially, the access of the social environment, including the father, to the infant. She also provides basic care through changing diapers and making available appropriate clothing. In addition, she provides stimulation to the child through touch, speech, as well as the other sensory modalities. These social and physical arrangements in turn influence the infant's health, growth, level of stress, socioemotional development and cognitive life. Although the child's biological characteristics (e.g., temperament) play a role in what is a reciprocal interactive relationship with mother, the mother's control of the direction of this relationship is considerable and provides a major context for understanding infant health.

Early on during pregnancy, a reciprocal bond starts to form between the mother and fetus that continues, under typical circumstances, to be strengthened after the birth of the baby. Although specific attachments of the baby to the mother are commonly thought not to occur before the second half of the child's first year of life, the baby clearly recognizes and shows preference for mother before that time, suggesting that this bond gradually forms over time. Studies examining the interaction patterns of nonclinical populations of mothers with their newborn, full-term infants indicate how actively involved mothers, as well as other caretakers, are in looking and touching their babies. For example, Tronick (1995), reporting the results of a naturalistic observational study, indicated that 3- to 18-week infants among the Efe, a community of foragers living in the Ituri Forest of Zaire, are in almost constant social contact with caretakers (97% of the time during the day) and older infants at 1 year of age are the frequent recipients of "affectionate" touch

(50% of the observational intervals) from those around them. Tronick (1995) also cited laboratory data concerning American mothers' indications of how actively involved they are with their 6-month-old infants through touching, stroking, holding, and kissing. Research by Klaus (1995) yields a similar profile.

The importance of this relationship is suggested by work examining infant–mother separation. Research suggests that infants separated from their mothers may experience adverse effects ranging from anaclitic depression and failure to thrive to mental retardation (Harlow, 1958; Hunt, 1961; Schanberg, 1995). In recent controlled laboratory research, Schanberg (1995) described what happens when 8-day-old rat pups are deprived of their mothers for short periods. The pups switch to what Schanberg referred to as a survival mode. According to Schanberg, physiological effects experienced by the rat pups include a marked decrease in the activity of an enzyme (ODC) that provides an index of cell differentiation and replication, a reduction in DNA synthesis in most organ tissues, increasing corticosterone secretion, and decreasing growth hormone secretion. In other words, the rat pups are stressed and cease growing.

Schanberg (1995) also discussed the role of β-endorphin, a neuropeptide, which, when injected into the rat pups, mimics the physiological effects of maternal separation. He believes that β-endorphin is a central mediator of what he labeled the *touch deprivation syndrome.* He suggested that a decreased tactile sensory signal leads to a decrease in afferent input to the brain, which in turn results in a release of β-endorphin in the brain. Schanberg (1995) stated, "I believe that the brain reacting to the environment can reach its long arm right down into the middle of a cell and regulate genes that . . . can be considered the basic units of life itself" (p. 78). Thus, Schanberg suggested that the environment influences the expression of a genotype.

Research on maternal depression indicates that infants do not have to be physically separated for long periods of time to suffer adverse effects. Field (1995a), reviewing research in the area of maternal depression, pointed out that depressed mothers spend relatively little time looking at, touching, and talking to their infants. These mothers generally display negative rather than positive facial expressions. Their infants in turn have lower activity levels, vocalize less, and show signs of stress as well as general evidence of physiological dysregulation, including sleep problems, lower vagal tone, and higher norepinephrine levels, symptoms which if prolonged can lead to a variety of health problems.

Field (1995a) suggested that therapies directed at both the mother and infant can improve maternal mood states and reduce signs of infant physiological dysregulation. Interventions designed to alter the mother's mood states have included the use of music, relaxation, and physical massage. Intervention directed at infants have involved altering mother's behaviors toward the infant, such as overstimulation, understimulation, and intrusive touching. Infants of depressed mothers also have been successfully treated through interventions administered by other nondepressed people familiar to the infant, such as nursery teachers and fathers (see

Field, 1995a, for a further discussion of this research). Field (1995a) emphasized beneficial effects of massage for infants of depressed mothers. As suggested earlier in discussing the research by Schanberg (1995), certain kinds of tactual stimulation seem to have pronounced effects on early growth. A variety of other research suggests that touch is related to the functioning of the infant immune system (see discussions by Reite, 1990; Suomi, 1995). The exact pathway or pathways by which touch influences the immune response is less clear. Touch might affect infant response to stress, which, in turn, affects the immune system. For example, touch might reduce serum cortisol, which is a potent immune suppressor. Reite (1990) also suggested that touch might influence the function of the immune system via modulation of arousal and associated central nervous system hormonal activity. More specifically, touch interventions might affect the immune system by reducing the infant's expenditure of energy through decreasing heart rate, activity level, and crying, making available more calories for growth and the development of infant behaviors for self-regulating stress.

The potential benefits of maternal presence, tactile interactions and touch interventions are also suggested by research on co-sleeping, SIDS, and FTT are discussed in the next sections.

Co-Sleeping and SIDS. McKenna (1993) suggested that in modern Western cultures an ethos has developed that encourages the early physical separation of mother and infant. This separation is perhaps most evident in parent–infant sleeping practices, which tyically involve placing the infant in its own bed that is often located in a separate room. McKenna (1993) pointed out that in preindustrial societies infants commonly sleep between or in reach of their parents at night and often during the day nap in a sling or pouch tied to mother's back or chest. He argued that what he called *co-sleeping* (children sleeping in close proximity to their parents) makes good evolutionary sense. Reviewing research on the effects of parent–infant contact and separation, he pointed out the many apparently related benefits of infants being in close physical contact with their parents or caretaker (e.g., improved access to food, regulation of physiological responses, including temperature maintenance, and increased maternal affectionate behavior) and the potential adverse effects of separation (e.g., anxious attachment, abuse, increase in adrenal secretions and plasma cortisol levels, decrease in antibodies, disturbed sleep, lack of growth, and anaclitic depression). McKenna (1993) suggested that in our culture co-sleeping is uncommon because of cultural taboos, irrational fears, discouragement by pediatricians, and inconvenience. Emphasizing the potential advantages of co-sleeping and close parent–infant physical contact, McKenna and Mosko (1993) suggested a possible relation between infant sleeping environment and SIDS.

Sudden infant death sydrome, or crib death, is a major cause of death in infants between 1 and 12 months of age in the United States, with an incidence rate of more than 1 victim per 1,000 live births. The peak incidence occurs between 2 and

4 months of age, with 90% occurring before 6 months of age. There is a seasonal relationship in SIDS, with more deaths occurring in the winter and spring. Children who are diagnosed as having died from SIDS apparently simply stop breathing, almost always while sleeping. After a complete postmortem examination, the specific cause of deaths diagnosed as SIDS remains unexplained. Speculations about the cause(s) of SIDS vary considerably and include reference to immaturity of the central or autonomic nervous system, respiratory disorders, sleep apnea, hyperthermia, and gastrointestinal problems (Lipsett, 1982; Zylke, 1989).

Risk factors associated with SIDS include poor prenatal maternal health, having an adolescent mother, maternal smoking, prenatal drug exposure, inadequate prenatal care, low socioeconomic status, low birthweight, and high parity. The nature of these risk factors suggest that the physical and social environment plays a critical role in SIDS. Lipsett (1982) offered an intriguing and as yet untested hypothesis, specifically, that although there is probably a congenital predisposition, the proximal cause of SIDS might be related to a failure of the infant to learn appropriate defensive responses that are needed to replace unlearned protective reflexes that disappear with maturation.

Although there is no definitive treatment for SIDS, the American Academy of Pediatrics Task Force on Infant Positioning and SIDS (1992) suggested that healthy infants be placed on their side or back when being put down for sleep. Neonatologists and pediatricians also sometimes recommend that families of infants at risk for SIDS use infant sleep monitors to alert them if their infant stops breathing. In light of earlier discussions in this chapter on the benefits of tactile and kinesthetic stimulation and co-sleeping, it is interesting to note that McKenna and Mosko (1993), in discussing SIDS, argued for the potential protective benefits of co-sleeping. They suggest that due to natural physiological vulnerabilities, some infants, particularly those in deeper sleep states, might have difficulty regulating their breathing. They further argue that co-sleeping offers certain advantages to such infants by entraining infant rhythms and arousals to their co-sleeping mothers, thereby catalyzing more frequent state transitions in infants and thus reducing the length of their deep sleep states. In this regard, McKenna (1990) noted that co-sleeping infants spend most of their sleeping time on their sides facing their mothers.

In summary, recent research on SIDS, like work in the area of maternal depression, suggests the importance of close contact between mother and infant. Another syndrome that may be affected by the mothers' interactional style and physical presence is nonorganic failure to thrive (NFIT).

Nonorganic Failure to Thrive. The FTT syndrome is used to describe children with a growth deficiency, that is, children who are more than two standard deviations below the mean in weight, specifically those below the fifth percentile. There are two basic types of FTT; one type is organic failure to thrive (OFTT), which is caused by specific physical conditions, such as lactose intolerance or a cardiac disorder, and the other type is NFTT, for which no medical cause can be demonstrated. Researchers and clinicians have shown that NFTT is frequently due to psychosocial factors such as parental neglect, emotional deprivation, and parental psychopathology. The primary cause of the growth deficiency that is labeled FTT is malnutrition. In most instances, children diagnosed with FTT gain weight when given appropriate food, suggesting that most FTT is of a nonorganic type (see Drotar, 1995; Heffer & Kelley, 1994, for a general discussion of this disorder).

Although most children with what appears to be NFTT can be treated through the appropriate provision of food, it is critical to determine the reasons the infant is not getting the food or benefiting from food given. The most common reasons for NFTT probably are limited food availability, deliberate food restriction, inappropriate diet, faulty feeding practices, family stress, and parent–child conflict. Drotar (1995) reviewed research and suggested that FTT might be due to an array of linked factors including relationship stress, maternal psychological adjustment problems, and insecure child attachments to their mother. A provocative but preliminary investigation by Polan and Ward (1994) suggests that children with FTT have less physical contact with their mothers. Although research evidence is lacking, it may also be that some FTT children may be under greater stress, due to relational or other external factors, and as a consequence might not be able to grow even with appropriate amounts of food. Close physical and affectional contact with the mother or primary caretaker might protect, or at least buffer, the infant from the effects of such stressors.

Future research needs to examine the distinctiveness of OFTT and NFFT and whether psychosocial factors might also contribute to the severity of some FTT disorders thought to have an organic cause. Moreover, more attention needs to be given to whether different etiologies exist in the general NFTT category, such as neglect versus abuse, as well as how specific psychosocial factors, such as child temperament, might moderate the effects of other psychosocial factors related to NFTT, such as incompetent feeding practices. Implementation of effective prevention and intervention strategies depend on the systematic and comprehensive evaluation of these as well as other factors purported to be responsible for NFTT.

FINAL THOUGHTS

In this century, dramatic changes have occurred in our understanding how biological factors influence infant health. In contrast, an understanding of how social and environmental factors affect the infant's physical well-being is only beginning. Ironically, in this latter regard, more is known about hospital settings than home environments. In part the reason for this uneven advance is related to the fact that infants in hospitals, particularly sick infants, are closely monitored and opportunities to evaluate infant–environmental relations can occur more easily. Systematic research in the home or laboratory settings is still at a rudimentary stage but is starting to evolve through the efforts of researchers such as Field and McKenna. Ultimately for such research to succeed fully, the biological factors that mediate the influence of the social and physical environment on infant health must be understood. Such knowledge would allow interventions to be implemented at either the more molar environmental or the biological level.

There has been little discussion in this chapter of how characteristics of the infant might be associated with illness. Although developmental psychologists studying infant behavior have focused considerable attention on the emergence of the cognitive, temperament and motor systems and how they affect one another, there has been relatively little empirical examination of how these three systems might influence infant health. However, these types of relations are beginning to be more actively discussed and investigated. For example, Skuse, Pickles, Wolke, and Reilly (1994) suggested that as a result of cognitive impairments, an infant may not be able to integrate or coordinate sensory inputs. Consequently, crucial tasks, such as breastfeeding, might become extremely difficult or even impossible for an infant to accomplish and place the infant at risk for undernourishment, reduced somatic growth, and future illnesses.

Motor deficits also might contribute to feeding disorders. For example, an infant's food intake may decrease significantly if its impaired motor abilities prevent it from communicating hunger to a caregiver (Batshaw & Perret, 1992; Skuse et al., 1994). More generally, motor functioning may be related to infant illness through activity level. Infants who are more active tend to be more resilient and to cope better with illness and stressful environments (Priel, Henik, Dekel, & Tal, 1990). Physical activity is beneficial because it strengthens muscles and bones and enhances motor skills (Batshaw & Perret, 1992). Conversely, lack of activity due to motor deficits or restrictive physical and social environments may contribute to the deterioration of the motor system as well as to an increased risk of infant problems, such as respiratory disorders.

Carey (1995), in discussing temperament, also suggested a relation between activity and health problems. For example, infants with difficult temperaments tend to be involved in more accidents because of their higher activity levels. More generally, Carey (1995) pointed out that a variety of physical problems, including colic, functional abdominal pain, restless sleep patterns, constipation, obesity, low weight gain, hypertension, allergies, and enuresis, are related to temperamental dispositions (Carey, 1995).

Temperament can influence infant health in diverse ways. For instance, ill infants who are more reactive and intense might receive treatment sooner because they cry until their parents recognize that they have a problem. However, parents might have more difficulty distinguishing between crying due to an illness and crying due to an infant's temperamental disposition. In contrast, easygoing infant dispositions, although less of a burden to parents, make presence of an illness harder for parents to detect. Thus, treatment might be delayed. Easy-tempered infants have also been found to exhibit poor hunger communication cues along with a low motivation to feed, thus placing them at risk for undernourishment (Skuse et al., 1994).

Research has also suggested that rhythmicity, another component of temperament, may be related to asthma in infants. Priel et al. (1990), comparing a group of wheezy infants with a group of acutely ill infants who did not have asthma, found that rhythmicity (i.e., maternal perceptions of an infant as predictable in biological functioning) was associated with asthma. Infants with higher levels of rhythmicity were better able to regulate their airways and to cope more effectively with the stressor of wheeziness. Priel et al. (1990) pointed out that mothers with rhythmic infants might be better able to recognize deviations in infant health status, thus enabling them to seek more timely medical attention.

Future research needs to examine further the direct role that infant temperament, motor and cognitive processes play in health and illness. Moreover, empirical investigations into how parenting might serve to moderate and mediate the influence of these processes on infant health are needed. For example, infants who are more reactive to environmental stimulation and not able to self-regulate their emotional responses easily might be more likely to develop health problems if they have parents who are less sensitive to their distress signals and less competent in providing emotional support. Syndromes, such as FTT and SIDS might in part be a function of a poor fit between specific infant characteristics and parenting behavior. As these types of relations become better understood, more effective intervention and prevention programs can be designed.

REFERENCES

Als, H. (1994). Individualized developmental care for the very low-birth weight preterm infant. *Journal of the American Medical Association, 272,* 853–858.

Als, H., & Gilkerson, L. (1995). Developmentally supportive care in the neonatal intensive care unit. *Zero to Three, 15,* 1–10.

American Academy of Pediatrics. (1992). Positioning and SIDS. *Pediatrics, 89,* 1120–1126.

Anderson, G. C. (1989). Risk in mother-infant separation postbirth. *IMAGE: The Journal of Nursing Scholarship, 21,* 196–199.

Anderson, G. C. (1991). Current knowledge about skin-to-skin (Kangaroo) care for preterm infants. *Journal of Perinatology, 11,* 216–226.

Anderson, G. C. (1995). Touch and the kangaroo care method. In T. M. Field (Ed.), *Touch in early development* (pp. 35–52). Mahwah, NJ: Lawrence Erlbaum Associates.

Batshaw, M. L., & Perret, Y. M. (1992). *Children with disabilities: A medical primer* (3rd ed.). Baltimore, MD: P. H. Brooks.

Brazelton, T. B. (1984). *Neonatal Behavioral Assessment Scale.* London: Spastics International Medical Publications.

Brazelton, T. B., & Field, T. M. (1990). Introduction. In N. Gunzenhauser (Ed.), *Advances in touch: New implications in human development* (pp. xiii–xvii). Skillman, NJ: Johnson & Johnson Consumer Products.

Carey, W. (1995). Temperament and pediatric practice. In S. Chess & A. Thomas (Eds.), *Temperament and clinical practice* (pp. 218–239). New York: Guilford.

Children's Defense Fund. (1994). *The state of America's children yearbook.* Washington, DC: Author.

Drotar, D. (1995). Failure to thrive (growth deficiency). In M. C. Roberts (Ed.), *Handbook of pediatric psychology* (pp. 516–536). New York: Guilford.

Field, T. M. (1980). Supplemental stimulation of preterm neonates. *Early Human Development, 4*(3), 301–314.

Field, T. M. (1995a). Infants of depressed mothers. *Infant Behavior and Development, 18,* 1–13.

Field, T. M. (Ed.). (1995b). *Touch in early development.* Mahwah, NJ: Lawrence Erlbaum Associates.

Field, T., Schanberg, S., Scafidi, F., Bower, C., Vega-Lahr, N., Garcia, R., Nystrom, J., & Kuhn, C. M. (1986). Tactile/kinesthetic stimulation effects on preterm neonates. *Pediatrics, 77,* 654–658.

Forsythe, P. (1995). Changing the ecology of the NICU. *Institute for Family-Centered Care: Designing for Child Health, 3,* 11–14.

Harlow, H. (1958). The nature of love. *American Psychologist, 13,* 673–685.

Heffer, R. W., & Kelley, M. L. (1994). Nonorganic failure to thrive: Developmental outcomes and psychosocial assessment and intervention issues. *Research in Developmental Disabilities, 15,* 247–268.

Hunt, J. M. (1961). *Intelligence and experience.* New York: Ronald Press.

Johnson, B. H. (1995). Newborn intensive care units pioneer family-centered charge in hospitals across the country. *Zero to Three, 16* 11–17.

Kawakami, K., Takai-Kawakami, K., Kurihara, H., Shimizu, Y., & Yanaihara, T. (1996). The effect of sounds on new born infants under stress. *Infant Behavior and Development, 19,* 375–379.

Klaus, M. H. (1995). Touching during and after birth. In T. M. Field (Ed.), *Touch in early development* (pp. 19–34). Mahwah, NJ: Lawrence Erlbaum Associates.

Lipsitt, L. P. (1982). Perinatal indicators and psychophysiological precursors of crib death. In J. Belsky (Ed.), *In the beginning: Readings on infancy* (pp. 74–82). New York: Columbia University Press.

McKenna, J. J. (1990). Evolution and sudden infant death syndrome. *Human Nature, 1,* 145–177.

McKenna, J. J. (1993). Co-sleeping. In M. A. Carskadon (Ed.), *Encyclopedia of sleep and dreaming* (pp. 143–148). New York: Macmillan.

McKenna, J. J., & Mosko, S. (1993). Evolution and infant sleep: An experimental study of infant-parent co-sleeping and its implications for SIDS. *Acta Pædiatrics Supplement, 389,* 31–36.

McKusick, V. A. (1994). *Mendelian inheritance in man: A catalogue of human genes and genetic disorders.* Baltimore, MD: Johns Hopkins University Press.

Miller, C. L., White, R., Whitman, T. L., O'Callaghan, M. F., & Maxwell, S. E. (1995). The effects of cycled versus noncycled lighting on growth and development in preterm infants. *Infant Behavior and Development, 18,* 87–95.

Mouradian, L. E., & Als, H. (1994). The influence of neonatal intensive care unit caregiving practices on motor functioning of preterm infants. *American Journal of Occupational Therapy, 48,* 527–533.

Osofsky, J. D. (1994). Caring for infants and toddlers in violent environments: Hurt, healing and hope. *Zero to Three, 3–7.*

Polan, H. J., & Ward, M. J. (1994). Role of the mother's touch in failure to thrive: A preliminary investigation. *Journal of the American Academy of Child and Adolescent Psychiatry, 33,* 1098–1105.

Priel, B., Henik, A., Dekel, A., & Tal, A. (1990). Perceived temperamental characteristics and regulation of physiological stress: A study of wheezy babies. *Journal of Pediatric Psychology, 15,* 197–209.

Reite, M. (1990). Effects of touch on the immune system. In N. Gunzenhauser (Ed.), *Advances in touch: New implications in human development* (pp. 22–31). Skillman, NJ: Johnson & Johnson Consumer Products.

Santrock, J. W. (1996). *Children.* Madison, WI: Brown & Benchmark.

Schanberg, R. S. (1995). The genetic basis for touch effects. In T. M. Field (Ed.), *Touch in early development* (pp. 67–80). Mahwah, NJ: Lawrence Erlbaum Associates.

Skuse, D., Pickles, A., Wolke, D., & Reilly, S. (1994). Postnatal growth and mental development: Evidence for a "sensitive period." *Journal of Child Psychology and Psychiatry, 53,* 521–545.

Suomi, S. J. (1995). Touch and the immune system in rhesus monkeys. In T. M. Field (Ed.), *Touch in early development* (pp. 89–104). Mahwah, NJ: Lawrence Erlbaum Associates.

Tronick, E. Z. (1995). Touch in mother-infant interaction. In T. M. Field (Ed.), *Touch in early development* (pp. 53–66). Mahwah, NJ: Lawrence Erlbaum Associates.

White, R. D. (1996). Enhanced neonatal intensive care design: A physiological approach. *Journal of Perinatology, 16*, 381–384.

Zylke, J. W. (1989). Sudden infant death syndrome: Resurgent research offers hope. *Journal of the American Medical Association, 262*, 1565–1566.

7

Endogenous and Exogenous Factors in Childhood Health and Disease

Julia M. Braungart-Rieker
Antonia L. Guerra
University of Notre Dame

HISTORICALLY, clinical assessment and treatment of children have often been insensitive to developmental issues (Ferrari, 1990). In recent years, however, disciplines such as behavioral pediatrics, pediatric medicine, developmental psychology and psychopathology have emphasized the importance of developmental issues in child health and disease. Childhood is a period of rapid growth. Children are constantly changing physically, mentally, socially, and emotionally. For example, the differences between two children aged 5 and 7 can be quite incredible, in terms of their motor skills, their mental reasoning abilities, the social network that they experience, and their emotionality. Even at a particular age, however, children's development across domains can be uneven. For example, motor skills might be quite advanced and energy and curiosity levels might be high, but children's ability to make sound judgments could be lacking. Such a combination of ability and inability might lead children to be particularly vulnerable to health problems such as accidental injury. Indeed, injury is the primary cause of death in children in the United States (Budnick & Chaiken, 1985).

Not only should parents, clinicians, and psychologists be aware that childhood is a time of great risk for certain health problems, but the treatment of children with injuries, chronic diseases, or other medical disorders also should be developmentally appropriate. Research on children who must deal with illness, hospitalization, and medical treatments shows that such children are at risk for emotional and psychosocial adjustment problems (Ferrari, 1990). Thus, gaining a better understanding of how to treat children is crucial not only in managing physical trauma but also in circumventing psychological problems as well.

In addition to recognizing that children are different from adults in many ways, clinicians need to be sensitive to the wide variation in skills even within age groups. For example, some children might be less cautious, more impulsive, and have poorer judgment than others, increasing their risk for injury. The family environments that children experience also can be vastly different. For example, some children receive adequate care and supervision for their age and skill level, whereas others are neglected. Thus, individual differences in endogenous characteristics, such as children's temperamental style, cognitive abilities, and genetic risk for certain diseases, as well as exogenous factors, such as their living conditions, family dynamics, school, or peer experiences might be critical in preventing or treating a health problem.

This chapter focuses on health and disease during childhood (approximately 3–12 years) and is divided into five sections. The first four sections review empirical studies pertaining to particular aspects of health and disease. More specifically, childhood injury, obesity, juvenile diabetes, and enuresis are addressed by examining how endogenous or exogenous factors relate to children's individual differences in child health and disease. The final section of the chapter provides suggestions for future research.

The physical disorders reviewed in this chapter certainly are not meant to be comprehensive. Rather, each topic is chosen for a specific reason. First, accidental injury is the primary cause of death in children (Budnick & Chaiken, 1985). Second, obesity is a problem that not only appears to be growing in prevalence (Gortmaker, Dietz, Sobol, & Wehler, 1987), but also seems to serve as a risk factor for other physical and psychological problems (Rocchini, 1993) and is highly predictive of adult obesity (Stark, Atkins, Wolff, & Douglas, 1981). Third, juvenile diabetes is chronic and has long-lasting implications. Finally, nocturnal enuresis is often viewed as more psychological than physical, whether or not that assumption is empirically validated (Scharf, Pravda, Jennings, Kauffman, & Ringel, 1987).

ACCIDENTAL INJURIES

During childhood, injuries cause more deaths to children than all other factors combined (Budnick & Chaiken, 1985). For example, in the 5- to 9-year-old age group, motor vehicle occupant accidents account for the largest number of deaths, followed by pedestrian injuries, drowning, fire injuries, homicide, bicycle injuries, unintentional firearm use, and poisoning (Rivara, 1995). What makes these deaths so traumatic is that the vast majority are preventable. Indeed, accidents do not appear to occur at random (Boyce, 1992). For example, in a study of school-related injuries, 1% of 55,000 school children were responsible for almost 20% of all injuries in a 3-year period (Boyce, Sobelewski, & Schaefer, 1989).

Studies that attempt to account for the disproportionate child injury rates examine the role of environmental risk factors or individual characteristics of the children, although not usually both simultaneously. This section reviews studies that examine the role of two exogenous factors, socioeconomic status (SES; and related variables) and parental behavior, and two endogenous characteristics, developmental delay and temperament.

Exogenous Factors

Socioeconomic Status. Most studies found that poverty is associated with childhood injury (see Rivara, 1995, for a review). For example, in a study of pedestrian injuries and demographic parameters in Memphis, a greater proportion of injuries occurred in poorer neighborhoods—as indexed by lower median family income, higher proportion of families headed by women, lower housing values, and more crowding (Rivara & Barber, 1985). Similarly, Pless, Verreault, Arsenault, Frappier, and Stulginskas (1987) found that children from low-income areas in Montreal had higher rates of traffic injury than did children from middle- or upper-income areas.

A distal variable, such as SES, might be related to childhood injury due to differences in the environment that directly surrounds the child. Children from poorer neighborhoods might experience heavier traffic conditions and less vigilant adult supervision and have parents who focus less on safety issues. A study on bicycle helmets, for example, indicated that parents with more education (and perhaps with greater incomes) are more likely to own bicycle helmets than parents who are less educated (DiGuiseppi, Rivara, & Koepsell, 1990). Another study found that physical features in the child's environment were related to injury; specifically, greater levels of noise and confusion were associated with higher rates of injury in children aged 1 to 3, and homes that were lower in adequacy (social and material features) placed children (aged 1–3 and 6–9) at greater risk for injury (Matheny, 1987). Interestingly, the Matheny study (1987) suggests that child characteristics become increasingly important as a predictor of injury as children develop. Factors that seem to contribute to childhood injury are discussed later in further detail.

Families in poverty may also be at risk for medical problems because they experience more stress and negative life events (e.g., loss of job, death in the family) than middle- and upper class families do (Attar, Guerra, & Tolan, 1994). Indeed, families who experience more negative life events experience a greater number of injuries (Padilla, Rohsenow, & Bergman, 1976). Such findings suggest that the effects of SES often might be mediated by more proximal environmental factors.

Parental Characteristics. Environmental factors that are perhaps even more proximal to the child than socioeconomic status and physical features in the environment are parental characteristics. An examination of parental personality reveals that mothers who were low in activity, vigor, stability, and reflectiveness had young children (aged 1–3) who were more at risk for accidents—although these characteristics were not predictive of injury in elementary-aged children (Matheny, 1987). Paternal characteristics also served as predictors of child injury: Young children who had more injuries had fathers who were less dominant and less social, whereas school-aged children with more injuries had fathers who were higher in impulsivity (Matheny, 1987). These age-related differences in prediction are interesting and warrant further investigation. Why would characteristics such as low maternal activity and vigor be more salient in the prediction of injury for younger children than for older children?*

Perhaps parental personality characteristics are linked with supervisory behavior. For example, a mother who is low in activity and vigor might have trouble mustering enough energy to supervise her curious and roving toddler adequately, whereas the same kind of energy might be adequate for supervising older children. Thus, certain maternal characteristics may be less salient as predictors of child injuries as children get older. Indeed, younger children are at more risk for certain kinds of injuries, such as poisonings or burns—events that more often occur in the home—whereas older children are more likely to experience accidents outside of the home (e.g., pedestrian accidents; Rivara, 1995).

Parental expectations about their children's skills also might be important in determining the degree to which parents supervise their children. Injuries such as pedestrian accidents might result from parents' poor judgments regarding their children's skills. In a study of parents of children in kindergarten through Grade 4, most parents perceived 5- to 6-year-old children as unable to cross streets alone (Rivara, Bergman, & Drake, 1989). Yet, one third allowed kindergarten-aged children to cross quiet residential streets by themselves. Notable is that parents who allowed their young children to cross the street also perceived their children as being "above average" in intelligence (Rivara et al., 1989). Relatedly, Yarmey and Rosenstein (1988) found that although parents overestimate their children's safety knowledge at all ages (5, 8, and 12), the extent of this overestimation was greatest for children in the youngest age groups. Taken together, these results again suggest that the age of the child is an important factor in determining the extent to which parental characteristics are related to children's risk for injury.

Endogenous Factors

In addition to factors that are considered external to the child, such as features in the home and parental supervision style, characteristics in the child, such as temperament and cognitive functioning, are particularly relevant in the study of accidental injury.

Temperament. Temperament has been described in terms of early appearing observable behavioral characteristics that are at least partly genetically influenced (Goldsmith et al., 1987). Temperament refers to the "how" of behavior, rather than the "what" or the "why." For example, children differ in their emotional reactions to novel, frustrating, and social situations, and such reactions can be observed in the first few months of life (Matheny, Riese, & Wilson, 1986). Infants are labeled as *difficult* when they show highly intense responses, predominantly negative mood, high activity level, low adaptability; conversely, infants with the opposite pattern are considered to be *easy* (Thomas & Chess, 1977). Such differences in children have been found to predict later outcomes, such as behavioral problems (Garrison & Earls, 1987).

Several studies also demonstrate links between temperament and injury; however, most studies do not find that a single dimension of temperament, for example, activity level, is solely responsible for differences in accident rates. For example, Nyman (1987) identified two groups of children under age 5—those that were hospitalized due to accidental injury and those that were hospitalized for other reasons. Nyman (1987) found that the type of outcome (general hospitalization vs. hospitalization due to an accident) differed depending on children's temperament. Specifically, children hospitalized for nonaccident reasons were more likely to have been rated as higher in negative mood and intensity of responding, whereas those in the accident group were rated as more persistent, higher in activity level, and more negative in their response to novel situations. Similarly, Matheny (1987) found that children who were higher in activity, rated as difficult, and directed attention less optimally were more likely to be injured than children who were less reactive, more easygoing, and more attentive.

In an extensive, prospective longitudinal study in New Zealand (Langley, Silva, & Williams, 1987), child temperament and personality characteristics were the sole predictors of injury rate (as assessed at age 5). That is, of the 90 variables examined, only emotional activity and activity level at age 3 and attention span and "naughty behavior" at age 5 were significantly associated with rate of injury. However, neither temperamental characteristics, nor family, behavioral, and developmental variables significantly predicted injury at ages 7, 9, and 11. Thus, it is important for researchers to consider whether different etiological factors account for child injury, depending on the age at which the child is being studied.

Researchers have also suggested that an interactional relationship between factors may predict child injury. In a study of 144 children age 3 to 5 years, Boyce (1996) found that the group with the highest rates of injuries were those children who had high reactivity, as assessed by cardiovascular responses to several semistressful conditions and who had experienced a greater number of negative events in their child care setting (e.g., changes in daily routine, losing a toy, etc.). Interestingly, those children that were highly reactive and had fewer negative experiences had the lowest number of injuries (Boyce, 1996).

Developmental Delay. In addition to behavioral differences, children with cognitive deficits might be at more risk for injury than those who are average or above average. Research on the relation between developmental delay and childhood injury is fairly sparse, however, and has yielded somewhat contradictory findings. For example, Baird and Sadovnick (1988) found that the rate of death due to trauma for patients with Down syndrome was no different than that in the general population.

In contrast, other researchers have found differences in injury-related mortality rates for disabled versus nondisabled populations. A study by Angle (1975) shows that children with poor locomotor skills had an increased risk of injuries. Moreover, Dunne, Asher, and Rivara (1993) found that preschool children with developmental disabilities had significantly higher rates of injuries than controls, although differences in children aged 6 to 17 were nonsignificant. However, an interesting interaction between developmental disabilities and sex emerged for children in this age range. The rate of injury for control versus developmentally disabled males was similar, but the rate of injuries of females with developmental disabilities was greater, compared to that of controls. In fact, the rate of injury for girls with developmental disabilities was similar to the rates for boys with and without developmental delay. All of this research in combination suggests the importance of a variety of factors for understanding child injury in developmentally delayed popoulations, including types of disability, age, and gender.

The mechanisms and processes mediating the link between developmental delay and risk of injury is unclear from the research. For example, it is possible that children with developmental disabilities live in an environment that is less supervised—particularly if such children are living in group homes. Alternatively, children with delays might show poorer judgment in situations that are dangerous.

OBESITY

The general criterion for a determination of obesity is 20% above the ideal weight for a person's age, body frame, and gender, although not all studies use this criterion (Harlan, 1993). Recent estimates suggest that as many as 25% of school-age children are obese (Harlan, 1993), although studies report obesity rates for children that range from 6% to 40% (LeBow, 1984). Such variability in the reporting of rates of obesity is probably in part a function of the specific definitions of obesity employed (LeBow, 1984). Nevertheless, according to Gortmaker et al. (1987), the prevalence of childhood obesity does seem to be increasing.

Obesity can create serious physical problems for children, such as increased risk for cardiovascular and renal disease (Freedman et al., 1985), as well as pediatric hypertension (Rames, Clark, & Connor, 1978; Rocchini, 1993). A study of school-aged children (5–18 years old) who were followed for 40 to 52 years links mortality to relative weight during childhood (Nieto, Szklo, & Cemstock, 1992). Substantial evidence also exists demonstrating that obese children become obese adults (Stark et al., 1981). Some studies report that as many as 80% of children who were obese at ages 10 through 13 were also found to be obese at age 30 (Abraham, Collins, & Nordsieck, 1971).

In addition to physical problems, children who are obese are at more risk for psychological and social problems. Studies on children's attitudes towards obesity show that children view obesity quite negatively (Lerner & Korn, 1972; Reaves & Roberts, 1983). This disparaging peer opinion of obese children can influence the self-concept of obese children. Sallade (1973) found that obese children in elementary school had lower self-image ratings than did children of normal weight. Internalization of the negative stereotypes, such as that fat children are lazy, have poor self-control, and eat too much, can lead children to develop feelings of self-hatred (Stunkard, 1976). In addition to self-esteem issues, childhood obesity might be related to more severe psychological disorders. For example, Mills and Andrianopoulous (1993) found that adults who developed obesity in childhood were more likely to display psychopathology than were individuals who became obese during adulthood. The next sections address studies that focus on exogenous or endogenous factors that might contribute to childhood obesity. Understanding the etiology of childhood obesity is crucial if appropriate prevention and intervention strategies are to be developed.

Exogenous Factors

Socioeconomic Status. Studies have found that social class is inversely related to obesity, with those from lower SES groups being more at risk for obesity (Brownell & Stunkard, 1978; Gerald, Anderson, Johnson, Hoff, & Trimm, 1994; Saltzer & Golden, 1985). Also, because children from single-parent households are typically of lower SES, they are more likely to be obese than are children from two-parent households (Gerald et al., 1994).

Parental Behavior. Several reasons might explain the link between SES and obesity. First, different standards for acceptable body weights might vary according to race and class. For example, Thompson, Corwin, and Sargent (1997) found that females and Whites experience more body dissatisfaction and weight concerns than males and African Americans—even at the young age of 9. Kleseges, Malott, Boschee, and Weber (1986) found that parents who encourage their preschoolers to be active had children who weighed less. Conversely, parents who encouraged their children to eat more had children who ate for longer periods of time and weighed more.

Families also might differ in their knowledge about nutrition. For example, families from lower SES backgrounds might serve foods that are higher in fat content and less nutritious (Zigler, 1995). Children naturally prefer foods that are high in sugar and fat, but if they are rewarded for eating healthier foods, including food such as fruits with natural sugars, children can show increases in choosing more nutritious snacks (Birch, Zimmerman, & Hind, 1980).

Television Viewing. Long hours of television viewing are considered a predictor of obesity, as this involves little activity and invites snacking while watching (Kolata, 1986; Locard et al., 1992). In addition to the relation between long hours of television viewing, inactivity, and obesity, the content of television commercials strongly influences children. The average child sees more than 11,000 low-nutrition "junk" food ads per year on television (Balfour, McLellearn, & Fox, 1982). Given young children's cognitive limitations, it is not surprising that younger children are more likely to believe that television ads were telling the truth (Ward & Wackman, 1972). Thus, younger children might be at particular risk for being "under the influence" of commercial propaganda.

The frequency with which children ask for certain foods also seems to parallel those foods that were advertised (Taras, Sallis, Patterson, Nader, & Nelson, 1989). Moreover, children whose weekly television viewing hours were greater were more likely to make a larger number of food requests from their mothers (Taras et al., 1989). In summary, there are links between hours of TV viewing, number of foods that were advertised, food requested by the child, and then purchased (and, presumably, consumed; Taras et al., 1989).

Endogenous Factors

Genetics. In chapter 3, behavioral genetic studies on obesity across the life span were reviewed. In general, substantial evidence indicates that heredity plays a large role in body weight, with the exception of weight assessed during infancy. For example, using longitudinal twin data, Wilson (1976) found that body weight was about 60% heritable from ages 12 months to 6 years, as indicated by greater correlations for identical twins than for fraternal twins. Adoption designs are also helpful for examining the extent to which similarities in the family environment influence body weight. Results from the Colorado Adoption Project on parent–child similarities in body mass index (weight, relative to height) revealed no significant effects due to shared environment but significant effects due to heritability—after age 3. More specifically, correlations among parents and their adopted children were near zero, whereas correlations among biological parents and adopted-away offspring were signficant (Cardon, 1994).

It is important to keep in mind that behavioral genetic results just reported do not mean that environment is unimportant; rather, it means that environmental effects might operate in a nonshared manner (Plomin, 1986). In other words, differential experience in children's lives might substantially affect a characteristic such as obesity. Also important is that substantial effects due to heredity do not mean that the pathway to obesity is unavoidable for some children. Heritability is a static estimate because it is based on findings from a certain population at a given time. Different heritability estimates could be obained from samples whose individuals have vastly different experiences. For example, even if heritability were 100% for body weight, children growing up under starvation conditions will not reach their genetic potential for body mass. Such an environmental condition becomes an overpowering influence on body weight and the influence of genetic differences becomes less important. In summary, even though genetics has considerable influence on body weight, it is still important to look at nongenetic factors that might influence obesity.

Temperament. Because weight gain involves behavior (e.g., the act of eating, decreased physical exercise, or inability to adhere to a weight reduction regimen), a child's behavioral style might be important to consider. Due to Carey's (1986) small, albeit significant, finding that infant fussiness, a temperamental characteristic, was related to obesity during infancy, Carey (1988) examined whether temperamental dimensions during middle childhood were related to obesity and rapid weight gain during this same period. Carey (1988) found that obese children were less predictable and less persistent but more approaching (e.g., sociable) in temperament than matched controls. Relatedly, children who have problems adhering to or remaining in obesity treatment are more likely to have difficult behavioral styles (Spence, 1986). Taken together, these results suggest that temperamental characteristics are related to the etiology as well as success in the treatment of obesity.

JUVENILE DIABETES

Insulin-dependent diabetes mellitus (IDDM), also referred to as Type I diabetes, is one of the more common chronic diseases in childhood; about 1 in every 600 children born in the U.S. has IDDM (LaPorte & Tajima, 1985). The risk of developing IDDM is equal to that of all childhood cancers combined and is greater than that of other well-known diseases of childhood including cystic fibrosis, rheumatoid arthritis, and muscular dystrophy (LaPorte & Cruickshanks, 1985). Despite its prevalence, the etiology of IDDM is still not entirely clear, although genetic factors have been implicated. For example, relatives of IDDM patients are more likely to develop the disease than nonrelatives (Johnson, 1995a). However, genetic effects are not the sole causes, because even when one member of an identical twin pair develops IDDM, 40% of the remaining co-twins do not (Barnett, Eff, Leslie, & Pyke, 1981). The major goal of this portion of the chapter is not to discuss the etiology of IDDM; rather, it focuses on individual differences that are likely relevant to the control and treatment processes of childhood diabetes.

Prior to the discovery of insulin in 1922, children with diabetes had a life expectancy of less than 2 years (Johnson, 1995a). In the 1990s, diabetes is considered to be a chronic disease in which life expectancy is about 75% of a normal life span (Travis, Brouhard, & Schreiner, 1987). Most diabetologists believe that adherence to treatments for maintaining blood glucose levels in the near-normal range is crucial in preventing, delaying, or minimizing the effects of IDDM (Johnson, 1995a). Thus, obtaining a better understanding of why some children succeed in performing this task, whereas others fail, is critical.

Exogenous Factors

Socieoeconomic Status and Family Structure. Recently, Auslander, Anderson, Bubb, Jung, and Santiago (1990) found links between family structure and two outcome indicators for diabetic children. Children with diabetes living with single mothers had poorer metabolic control compared to children with diabetes living in two-parent households (Auslander et al., 1990). However, it is important to note that family structure was also correlated with SES and race, making it impossible to disentangle demographic effects. In a study by Overstreet et al. (1995) however, diabetic children who varied in family structure were matched on SES and race with a control group, thus enabling the examination of the effect due to family structure, per se. Overstreet et al. (1995) found that nontraditional family structure was more disruptive for children with diabetes than for children in the control group and was related to poorer metabolic control. Interestingly, parents in nontraditional families—in both the diabetes and control groups—reported lower levels of organization, a quality that might be particularly important in the lives of diabetic children (Overstreet et al., 1995).

Parental Involvement. Several studies have found that children adhere better to treatment regimens for IDDM than adolescents (e.g., Ingersoll, Orr, Herrold, & Golden, 1986; Johnson et al., 1992). This association may be due to less parental involvement in treatment as diabetic children develop into adolescents. Using a longitudinal design, Johnson (1995b) found that parents become less strict in their care of their children's diabetes and supervise their children less as the children get older. However, the role of parental supervision is complex. For example, Johnson (1995b) found that greater supervision was related to better adherence by the child to an insulin injection regimen and to amount of exercise. However, increased parental supervision was also associated with certain negative dietary behaviors, such as consumption of total calories, sweets, and fat (Johnson, 1995b).

Family Lifestyle. The health climate in a family—even prior to diabetes diagnosis—might be important to children's adherence to treatment regimens. Johnson (1995a) suggested that children with existing healthy lifestyles in terms of exercise and diet might adapt more easily to treatment protocols than do children from families who have a less healthy lifestyle.

Family Conflict. In addition to lifestyle, the emotional climate of the family might be important in children's adherence to treatment. Families with low conflict and high organization have children with better IDDM management (Bobrow, AvRuskin, & Siller, 1985; Hauser et al., 1990). In addition, children whose families are more adaptable, flexible, and show more frequent diabetes-specific supportive behaviors, adhere better to treatment regimens (Hanson, DeGuire, Schinkel, & Henggeler, 1992).

Stress. Studies of stress indicate that even in both IDDM and non-IDDM patients, stress seems to result in energy mobilization, which increases glucose availability to body and brain (for a review, see Surwit, Schneider, & Feinglos, 1992). Thus, stress appears to have a direct effect on glycemic control. Stress also could have an indirect effect on glycemic control in that stress might affect children's adherence behaviors negatively. In addition, children might change their eating and exercising habits when faced with stressful circumstances. Self-report data suggests that diabetic patients believe that stress adversely influences glycemic control (Cox, Taylor, Nowacek, Holloey-Wilcox, & Pohl, 1984); however, laboratory controlled studies have not documented strong links between psychologically induced stress and hyperglycemia (Gilbert, Johnson, Silverstein, & Malone, 1989).

The age of the IDDM patient might be important in finding links between stress and glycemic control. For example, Chase and Jackson (1981) found that the number of major life events (e.g., parent divorce) predicted metabolic control in adolescent IDDM patients, but not in younger or older patients. These results suggest that perception of stress as well as available coping skills and social supports for dealing with stressful events, domains that may be, in part, age-dependent, mediate connections between actual stress and glucose control.

Endogenous Factors

Temperament. In a study of children with IDDM and their healthy siblings, Rovet and Ehrlich (1988) found that, although there were no overall mean differences between diabetic and nondiabetic siblings on temperament characteristics, temperament in the diabetic groups was predictive of metabolic control. Diabetic children who had higher activity levels, greater rhythmicity, a higher threshold of reaction (i.e., greater stimulation is necessary to cause a reaction), greater distractibility, and who were higher in negative mood had better glycemic control. Although Rovet and Ehrlich (1988) did not examine behavioral compliance to treatment regimen, behavioral compliance to proper medical regimens might mediate the effect of temperament on glycemic control.

Garrison, Biggs, and Williams (1990), examined links among temperament, metabolic control, and behavioral compliance to treatment. They found that children who were lower in general and sleep activity levels and who had greater attention spans and rhythmicity were more likely to be considered compliant in their treatment protocol. In predicting actual metabolic control, children who were more negative in mood and who had higher attention spans had better overall metabolic control (Garrison et al., 1990). Although it is not clear why different temperament dimensions would predict metabolic control versus behavioral compliance, it appears that temperament affects diabetes at multiple levels.

NOCTURNAL ENURESIS

Nocturnal enuresis refers to bedwetting. According to the Diagnostic and Statistical Manual of Mental Disorders (American Psychiatric Association, 1994), children with nocturnal enuresis urinate while asleep at least twice a week for at least 3 months. The child's chronological age must be at least 5 years. Children with developmental delays must have a mental age of least 5 years. However, clinicians often disagree on the frequency with which urination must occur and the age at which enuresis is diagnosed. Some have argued that children need to be older than 6 years, whereas others diagnose at 3 years (Friman & Christophersen, 1986). Still others have recommended that a child should be treated for enuresis when bedwetting begins to interfere with social, emotional, or cognitive development (Cohen, 1975).

Despite differences in definitions, which affect estimates of prevalence, enuresis is believed to be a fairly common clinical problem. For 5-year-old males, the prevalance rates are 7% and for females, 3%; at age 10 years, the prevalence rates are 3% and 2% for males and females, respectively (American Psychiatric Association, 1994). However, some have estimated that 25% of all elementary school children exhibit the problem at least once (Wright, Schaefer, & Solomons, 1979). Approximately 10% of the cases of enuresis may be attributed to organic causes, such as urinary tract obstruction, infections, neurological disease, and distal urethral stenosis (Wright et al., 1979). However, the majority of cases appear to have a more complex etiology.

Exogenous Factors

Socioeconomic Status. There is an increased proportion of enuresis in families of lower SES (Gross & Dornbusch, 1983; Wright et al., 1979). However, other variables associated with SES might be tied in more directly with enuresis. For example, Gross and Dornbusch (1983) suggested that families with lower SES have less time to spend with their children, which might affect children already at risk for enuresis in particular. To promote continence, children with a family history of enuresis likely require increased time and attention.

Family Characteristics. Historically, nocturnal enuresis has been attributed primarily to psychological problems in the child's home (Wright et al., 1979). For example, Sears, Maccoby, and Levin (1957) believed that enuresis was caused by three factors: severity of toilet training, lack of maternal warmth, and the mother's sex-related anxiety. Others suggested that sibling rivalry, dislike of school, peer difficulties, and instability in the parent–child relationship contribute to bedwetting (Benjamin, Stover, Geppert, Pizer, & Burdy, 1971). However, little research supports a link between emotional turmoil and nocturnal enuresis (Walker, 1995). Currently, researchers seem to agree that psychological stressors are more of consequence than the cause of enuresis. That is, psychological problems and conflict appear to be the result of parents' responses to bedwetting (Scharf, et al., 1987).

Endogenous Factors

Genetic Influence. Several studies demonstrate that a child is more likely to have enuresis when family members were enuretic as children. Bakwin (1973) found that 43% of the children with one enuretic parent and 77% of the children with two enuretic parents became enuretic themselves. In contrast, only 15% of children with no enuretic parents developed enuresis. Similarly, twin studies indicate greater concordance rates for identical than fraternal twins (e.g., Abe, Oda, & Hatta, 1984)—a pattern indicative of genetic influence. Finally, in a study of 161 children raised in a kibbutz, in which children slept separately from their parents and were toilet trained by someone other than their parents, 67% of enuretic children had enuretic siblings, compared with 22% of the continent children (Kaffman & Elizur, 1977). In general, these studies suggest the importance of genetics rather than just family environments in the etiology of nocturnal enuresis.

Physiological Problems. Generally, research findings on physiological roots of enuresis are divergent. For example, Scharf et al. (1987) found that bedwetters experienced more frequent and intense contractions of the primary detrusor muscle and also experienced greater bladder pressure than control participants. Another recent study found that only 3% to 5% of patients with nocturnal enuresis had unstable bladders (Eiberg, Berendt, & Mohr, 1995). A decreased functional bladder capacity (volume of urine voided after micturition has been postponed for as long as possible) has also been suggested to relate to enuresis. Ullom-Minnich (1996) hypothesized that the small functional bladder capacity might result from inadequate cortical inhibition of the bladder and also might be related to developmental delay. An interesting alternative hypothesis is that low functional bladder capacity might be a consequence of the child's micturition habits, rather than a cause (Houts, 1991). In other words, enuretic children might not become accustomed to holding larger volumes of urine because they are unable to hold urine for long periods of time at night. The low functional bladder capacity, then, becomes a consequence, rather than the cause of bedwetting.

Sleep disorders have also been proposed to cause bedwetting. Wille (1994) hypothesized that children with enuresis either spend more time in deeper sleep or are more difficult to arouse from sleep, but many sleep studies do not support this hypothesis (Ullom-Minnich, 1996). However, in one longitudinal study, Fergusson, Horwood, and Shannon (1986) found that children who had slept for longer periods of time at ages 1 to 2 years were slower to achieve bladder control later on.

Developmental or Cognitive Deficits. Some clinicians and researchers have suggested that children who are developmentally delayed are more at risk for enuresis. Modest support for this hypothesis is found in that some studies have shown that enuretic children reach certain developmental milestones (e.g., language onset) later than nonenuretic children (MacKeith, 1972). Other research has supported the idea that enuretic children are somewhat less intelligent that nonenuretics (Iester et al., 1991); however, at least one study has not found such an association (Steinhausen & Gobel, 1989). Walker (1995) suggested that learning differences, even a learning disability specific to mastering urination skills, rather than a lack of intellectual capacity, is more at the root of the problem. Indeed, many children of superior intelligence have been enuretic (Walker, 1995).

CONCLUSIONS AND DIRECTIONS
FOR FUTURE RESEARCH

It seems clear that most childhood physical disorders or health problems are complex; no one variable adequately explains the reasons some children are injured more frequently, some children become obese, some children are less successful at keeping diabetes under control, or some become enuretic. Thus, future research needs to examine multiple systems in children's lives simultaneously to gain a better understanding of the etiology of childhood health problems. Understanding more completely the etiology of disease in turn increases the efficacy of of treatment or prevention programs. For example, family and genetic history (Wilson, 1976), temperament (Carey, 1986), opportunities for proper food selection (Birch, Zimmerman, & Hind, 1980), and amount of television viewing (Locard et al., 1992) are related to the development of childhood obesity. More articulated prevention or intervention strategies need to take into consideration which and how many of these characteristics are relevant to a program for a particular child.

Moreover, through multivariate analyses, potential interactions or processes can be explored. For example, given certain genetic predispositions, how do differences in parenting behavior affect children's risk for becoming obese? It is likely that not all children are affected by certain exogenous factors in the same way. Endogenous and exogenous factors increase children's risk for poor health in main effects, moderational, and mediational manners. In each model, endogenous (e.g., child temperament) and exogenous factors (e.g., stress, parental supervision) affect the health of the child (e.g., child injury). Figure 7.1a depicts a main effects model, Fig. 7.1b portrays a moderational model, and Figure 7.2a and 7.2b present two examples of a mediational model.

In the main effects model, endogenous (difficult temperament) and exogenous factors (parental supervision) serve as risk factors in health outcome (injury). As shown in Fig. 7.1a, children with difficult temperaments are more likely to get hurt than children with easy temperaments. Likewise, children whose parental super-

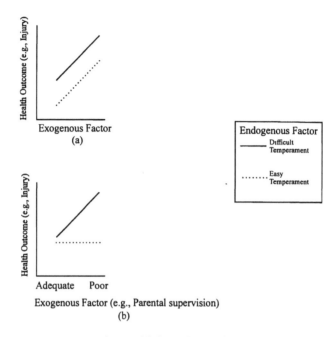

FIG. 7.1.   (a) Main effects model. (b) Moderational or interactional model.

vision is poor are more likely to become injured than children's whose parental supervision is adequate. Having both of these risk factors—difficult temperament and poor parental supervision—places children at greatest risk for injury in the sense that risk factors are additive or cumulative.

In a moderational or interactional model, however, the effects of one risk factor are moderated or influenced by the the other factor. For example, Fig. 7.1b shows that difficult temperament places children at risk for greater injury, but only when the parents of such children do not provide adequate supervision. Stated differently, having an easy temperament would render poorly supervised children resilient from the negative effects of poor parenting. This moderational model is similar to one proposed by Garmezy, Masten, and Tellegen (1984), in which certain factors (e.g., endogenous characteristics) either protect the child or make them more vulnerable to stressful environmental conditions. However, in the Garmezy et al. (1984) model, psychological rather than physical problems serve as the potential outcome.

Research in the area of child health might also profit by evaluating health problems through mediational models in which one or a set of factors is found to affect outcome indirectly through another characteristic (Baron & Kenny, 1986). Such models provide us with an examination of the processes that take place during the development of a problem. A mediational model tests the degree to which one factor mediates the relation between two other factors. Three conditions must be met in order for a mediational model to be revealed (Baron & Kenny, 1986):

1. The outcome variable is predicted by two separate factors when each factor is examined alone.
2. When both predictors are included in a model (typically multiple regression), the explanatory power of one of the factors becomes nonsignificant (preferably drops to 0, as in a standardized beta coefficient).
3. The remaining significant predictor can be explained by variation in the now-nonsignificant original predictor term.

Figure 7.2 depicts two potential mediational models that involve endogenous and exogenous factors in the prediction of child health.

In Fig. 7.2a, poor parenting accounts for greater rates of child injury; however, if child factors, such as child judgment, are considered, the amount of variance explained by poor parenting becomes nonsignificant. If variation in child judgment is explained by differences in poor parenting, a mediational model is suggested. In other words, parents with poor supervision skills have children who develop poor judgment skills. In turn, children who do not learn how to assess whether a situation is potentially dangerous, put themselves at greater risk for injury (see Fig. 7.2).

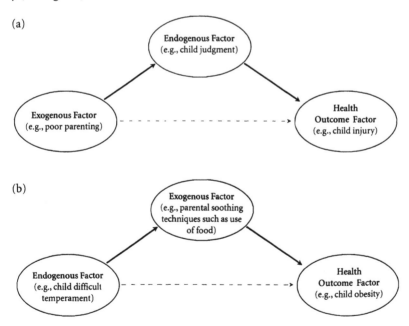

FIG. 7.2. (a) Mediational model in which the endogenous factor mediates the association between the exogenous and outcome factors. (b) Mediational model in which the exogenous factor mediates the association between the endogenous and outcome factors.

In Fig. 7.2b, in which child obesity serves as the outcome variable, exogenous factors mediate the link between endogenous characteristics and obesity. For example, as temperamental difficulty increases, parents use increasingly ineffective strategies for soothing children, such as offering high-fat foods, which then results in their children becoming overweight.

If empirically validated, such models could be used to guide the development of intervention and prevention strategies. For example, if poor parenting is at the root of the problem in the prediction of child injury, preventions could be designed to target and teach parents to provide their children with better judgment skills. Such specific prevention efforts might involve efficient and relatively inexpensive ways to alleviate potentially traumatic and expensive childhood injuries.

In summary, future research evaluating the influences on childhood health needs to focus to a greater extent on multiple factors in children's lives that place children at risk or protect them from health problems. Moreover, greater attention needs to be paid to how these factors might interact or mediate one another so that a better understanding of the processes involved in health and disease can be obtained. Such processes would suggest more efficient strategies for avoiding or alleviating certain problems. In addition, such research models, if used in conjunction with longitudinal designs, could provide a greater understanding of when certain processes might ensue and when certain treatments might prove more effective.

REFERENCES

Abe, K., Oda, N., & Hatta, H. (1984). Behavioural genetics of early childhood: Fears, restlessness, motion sickness, and enuresis. *Acta Genetica Medica Gemellogica, 33,* 303–306.

Abraham, S., Collins, G., Nordsieck, M. (1971). Relationship of childhood weight status to morbidity in adults. *Public Health Reports, 86,* 273–284.

American Psychiatric Association. (1994). *Diagnostic and statistical manual of mental disorders* (4th ed.). Washington, DC: Author.

Angle, C. R. (1975). Locomotor skills and school accidents. *Pediatrics, 56,* 819–822.

Attar, B. K., Guerra, N. B., & Tolan, P. H. (1994). Neighborhood disadvantage, stressful life events, and adjustment in urban elementary-school children. *Journal of Clinical Child Psychology, 23,* 391–400.

Auslander, W. F., Anderson, B. J., Bubb, J., Jung, K. C., & Santiago, J. V. (1990). Risk factors to health in diabetic children: A prospective study from diagnosis. *Health and Social Work, 15,* 133–142.

Bakwin, H. (1973). The genetics of enuresis. In I. Kolvin, R. C. MacKeith, & S. R. Meadow (Eds.), *Bladder control and enuresis* (pp. 73–77). Philadelphia: Lippincott.

Balfour, J. D., McLellearn, R. W., & Fox, D. T. (1982). The development of children's eating habits: The role of television commercials. *Health Education Quarterly, 9,* 174–189.

Baird, P. A., & Sadovnick, A. D. (1988). Causes of death to age 30 in Down syndrome. *American Journal of Human Genetics, 43,* 239–248.

Barnett, A., Eff, C., Leslie, R., & Pyke, D. (1981). Diabetes in identical twins. *Diabetologia, 20,* 87–93.

Baron, R. M., & Kenny, D. A. (1986). The moderator-mediator variable distinction in social psychological research: Conceptual, strategic, and statistical considerations. *Journal of Personality and Social Psychology, 51,* 1173–1182.

Benjamin, L. S., Stover, D. O., Geppert, T. V., Pizer, E. F., & Burdy, J. (1971). The relative importance of psychopathology, training procedure, and urological pathology in nocturnal enuresis. *Child Psychiatry and Human Development, 1,* 215–232.

Birch, L. L., Zimmerman, S. I., & Hind, H. (1980). The influences of social-affective context on the formation of children's food preferences. *Child Development, 51,* 856–861.

Bobrow, E., AvRuskin, R., & Siller, J. (1985). Mother-daughter interaction and adherence to diabetes regimens. *Diabetes Care, 8,* 146–151.

Boyce, W. T. (1992). The vulnerable child: New evidence, new approaches. *Advanced Pediatrics, 39,* 1–33.

Boyce, W. T. (1996). Biobehavioral reactivity and injuries in children and adolescents. In M. H. Bornstein & J. L. Genevro (Eds.), *Child Development and Behavioral Pediatrics* (pp. 35–58). Mahwah, NJ: Lawrence Erlbaum Associates.

Boyce, W. T., Sobolewski, S., & Schaefer, C. (1989). Recurrent injuries in school-age children. *American Journal of Diseases of Children, 143,* 338–342.

Brownell, K. D., & Stunkard, A. J. (1978). Behavioral treatment of obesity in children. *American Journal of Diseases of Children, 132,* 403–412.

Budnick, L. D., & Chaiken, B. P. (1985). The probability of dying of injuries by the year 2000. *Journal of the American Medical Association, 254,* 3350–3352.

Cardon, L. R. (1994). Height, weight, and obesity. In J. C. DeFries, R. Plomin, & D. W. Fulker (Eds.), *Nature and nurture during middle childhood* (pp. 165–172). Oxford: Blackwell.

Carey, W. B. (1986). The difficult child. *Pediatrics in Review, 8,* 39–45.

Carey, W. B. (1988). A suggested solution to the confusion in attention deficit diagnoses. *Clinical Pediatrics, 27,* 348–349.

Chase, J., & Jackson, G. (1981). Stress and sugar control in children with insulin dependent diabetes mellitus. *Journal of Pediatrics, 98,* 1011–1013.

Cohen, M. W. (1975). Enuresis. *Pediatric Clinics of North America, 22,* 545–560.

Cox, D., Taylor, A., Nowacek, G., Holley-Wilcox, P., & Pohl, S. (1984). The relationship between psychological stress and insulin-dependent diabetic blood glucose control: Preliminary investigations. *Health Psychology, 3,* 63–75.

DiGuiseppi, C. G., Rivara, F. P., & Koepsell, T. D. (1990). Attitudes toward bicycle helmet ownership and use by school-age children. *American Journal of Diseases in Children, 144,* 83–86.

Dunne, R. G., Asher, K. N., & Rivara, F. P. (1993). Injuries in young people with developmental disabilities: Comparative investigation from the 1988 National Health Interview Survey. *Mental Retardation, 31,* 83–88.

Eiberg, H., Berendt, I., & Mohr, J. (1995). Assignment of dominant inherited nocturnal enuresis (ENUR1) to chromosome 13q. *Nature Genetics, 10,* 354–356.

Fergusson, D. M., Horwood, L. J., & Shannon, F. T. (1986). Factors related to the age of attainment of nocturnal bladder control: An 8-year longitudinal study. *Pediatrics, 78,* 884–890.

Ferrari, M. (1990). Developmental issues in behavioral pediatrics. In A. M. Gross & R. S. Drabman (Eds.), *Handbook of clinical behavioral pediatrics* (pp. 29–47). New York: Plenum.

Freedman, D. S., Burke, G. L., Harsha, D. W., Srinivasan, S. R., Cresanta, J. L., Webber, L. S., & Berenson, G. S. (1985). Relation of changes in obesity to serum lipid and lipoprotein changes in childhood and adolescence. *Journal of the American Medical Association, 254,* 515–520.

Friman, P. C., & Christophersen, E. R. (1986). Biobehavioral prevention in primary care. In N. A. Krasnegor, J. D. Aresteh, & M. F. Cataldo (Eds.), *Child health behavior: A behavioral pediatrics perspective* (pp. 254–280). New York: Wiley.

Garmezy, N., Masten, A. S., & Tellegen, A. (1984). The study of stress and competence in children: A building block for developmental psychopathology. *Child Development, 55,* 97–111.

Garrison, W. T., Biggs, D., & Williams, K. (1990). Temperament characteristics and clinical outcomes in young children with diabetes mellitus. *Journal of Child Psychology and Psychiatry, 31,* 1079–1088.

Garrison, W. T., & Earls, F. J. (1987). *Temperament and child psychopathology.* Newbury Park: Sage.

Gerald, L. B., Anderson, A., Johnson, G. D., Hoff, C., & Trimm, R. F. (1994). Social class, social support and obesity risk in children. *Child Care, Health, and Development, 20,* 145–163.

Gilbert, B., Johnson, S., Silverstein, J., & Malone, J. (1989). Psychological and physiological responses to acute laboratory stressors in insulin-dependent diabetes mellitus adolescents and non-diabetic controls. *Journal of Pediatric Psychology, 14,* 577–591.

Goldsmith, H. H., Buss, A. H., Plomin, R., Rothbart, M., Thomas, A., Chess, S., Hinde, R., & McCall, R. (1987). Roundtable: What is temperament? *Child Development, 58,* 505–529.

Gortmaker, S. L., Dietz, W. H., Sobol, A. M., & Wehler, C. A. (1987). Increasing pediatric obesity in the United States. *American Journal of Diseases of Children, 141,* 535–540.

Gross, R. T., & Dornbusch, S. M. (1983). Enuresis. In M. D. Levine, W. B. Carey, A. C. Crocker, & R. T. Gross (Eds.), *Developmental-Behavioral Pediatrics* (pp. 573–586). Philadelphia: Saunders.

Harlan, W. R. (1993). Epidemiology of childhood obesity: A National perspective. In C. L. Williams & S. Y. S. Kimm (Eds.), *Prevention and treatment of childhood obesity. Vol. 699: Annals of the New York Academy of Sciences* (pp. 1–5). New York: The New York Academy of Sciences.

Hanson, C., DeGuire, M., Schinkel, A., & Henggeler, S. (1992). Comparing social learning and family systems correlates of adaptation in youths with IDDM. *Journal of Pediatric Psychology, 17,* 555–572.

Hauser, S., Jacobson, A., Lavori, P., Wolfsdorf, J., Herskowitz, R., Milley, J., & Bliss, R. (1990). Adherence among children and adolescents with insulin-dependent diabetes mellitus over a four-year longitudinal follow-up: II. Immediate and long-term linkages to family milieu. *Journal of Pediatric Psychology, 15,* 527–542.

Houts, A. C. (1991). Nocturnal enruesis as a biobehavioral problem. *Behavior Therapy, 22,* 133–151.

Iester, A., Marchesi, A., Cohen, A., Iester, M., Bagnasco, F., & Bonelli, R. (1991). Functional enuresis: Pharmacological versus behavioral treatment. *Child's Nervous System, 7,* 106–108.

Ingersoll, G., Orr, D., Herrold, A., & Golden, M. (1986). Cognitive maturity and self-management among adolescents with insulin-requiring diabetes mellitus. *Journal of Pediatrics, 108,* 620–623.

Johnson, S. B. (1995a). Insulin-dependent diabetes mellitus in childhood. In M. C. Roberts (Ed.), *Handbook of pediatric psychology* (2nd ed., pp. 263–285). New York: Guilford.

Johnson, S. B. (1995b). Managing insulin dependent diabetes mellitus: A developmental perspective. In J. Wallander & L. Siegel (Eds), *Adolescent health problems: Behavioral perspectives* (pp. 265–288). New York: Guilford.

Johnson, S. B., Kelly, M., Henretta, J., Cunningham, W., Tomer, A., & Silverstein, J. (1992). A longitudinal analysis of adherence and health status in childhood diabetes. *Journal of Pediatric Psychology, 17,* 537–553.

Kaffman, M., & Elizur, E. (1977). Infants who become enuretics: A longitudinal study of 161 Kibbutz children. *Monographs of the Society for Research in Child Development, 42,* 2–12.

Kleseges, R. C., Malott, J. M., Boschee, P. F., & Weber, J. M. (1986). The effects of parental influences on children's food intake, physical activity, and relative weight. *International Journal of Eating Disorders, 5,* 335–346.

Kolata, G. (1986). Obese children: a growing problem. *Science, 232,* 20–21.

Langley, J., Silva, P. A., & Williams, S. M. (1987). Psychosocial factors in childhood injuries: Results from a longitudinal study. *Journal of Safety Research, 18,* 73–89.

LaPorte, R., & Cruickshanks, K. (1985). Incidence and risk factors for insulin-dependent diabetes. In M. Harris & R. Hamman (Eds.), *Diabetes in America* (NIH Publ. No. 95-1468, pp. III: 1–2). Bethesda, MD: National Institutes of Health.

LaPorte, R., & Tajima, N. (1985). Prevalence of insulin-dependent diabetes. In M. Harris & R. Hamman (Eds.), *Diabetes in America* (NIH Publ. No. 95-1468, pp. III: 1–2). Bethesda, MD: National Institutes of Health.

LeBow, M. D. (1984). *Child obesity: A new frontier of behavior therapy.* New York: Springer.

Lerner, R. M., & Korn, S. J. (1972). The develoment of body-build stereotypes in males. *Child Development, 43,* 908–920.

Locard, E., Mamelle, N., Billete, A., Miginiac, M., Munoz, F., & Rey, S. (1992). Risk factors of obesity in a five year old population: Parental versus environmental factors. *International Journal of Obesity Related Metabolic Disorders, 16,* 721–729.

MacKeith, R. C. (1972). Is maturation delay a frequent factor in the origins of primary nocturnal enu-
    resis? *Developmental Medicine and Child Neurology, 14*, 217–223.
Matheny, A. P., Jr. (1987). Psychological characteristics of childhood accidents. *Journal of Social Issues,
    43*, 45–60.
Matheny, A. P., Jr., Riese, M. L., & Wilson, R. S. (1986). Rudiments of infant temperament: Newborn to
    9 months. In S. Chess & A. Thomas (Eds.), *Annual Progress in Child Psychiatry and Child Develop-
    ment* (pp. 355–369). New York: Bruner/Mazel.
Mills, J. K., & Andrianopolous, G. D. (1993). The relationship between childhood onset obesity and psy-
    chopathology in adulthood. *Journal of Psychology, 127*, 547–551.
Nieto, F. J., Szklo, M., & Cemstock, G. W. (1992). Childhood wieght and growth rate as predictors of
    adult mortality. *American Journal of Epidemiology, 136*, 201–213.
Nyman, G. (1987). Infant temperament, childhood accidents, and hospitalization. *Clinical Pediatrics,
    26*, 398–404.
Overstreet, S., Goins, J., Chen, R. S., Holmes, C. S., Greer, T., Dunlap, W. P., & Frentz, J. (1995). Family
    environment and the interrelation of family structure, child behavior, and metabolic control for
    children with diabetes. *Journal of Pediatric Psychology, 20*, 435–447.
Padilla, E. R., Rohsenow, D. J., & Bergman, A. B. (1976). Predicting accident frequency in children. *Pedi-
    atrics, 58*, 223–226.
Pless, I. B., Verreault, R., Arsenault, L., Frappier, J. Y., & Stulginskas, J. (1987). The epidemiology of road
    accidents in childhood. *American Journal of Public Health, 77*, 358–360.
Plomin, R. (1986). *Development, genetics, and psychology*. Hillsdale, NJ: Lawrence Erlbaum Associates.
Reaves, J. Y., & Roberts, R. (1983). The effect of type of information on children's attraction to peers.
    Child Development, 54, 1024–1031.
Rivara, F. P. (1995). Developmental and behavioral issues in childhood injury prevention. *Developmen-
    tal and Behavioral Pediatrics, 16*, 362–370.
Rivara, F. P., & Barber, M. (1985). Demographic analysis of childhood pedestrian injuries. *Pediatrics, 76*,
    375–381.
Rivara, F. P., Bergman, A. B., & Drake, C. (1989). Parental attitudes and practices toward children as
    pedestrians. *Pediatrics, 89*, 1017–1021.
Rocchini, A. P. (1993). Hemodynamic and cardiac consequences of childhood obesity. In W. L. Williams
    & S. Y. S. Kimm (Eds.), *Prevention and treatment of childhood obesity. Vol. 699: Annals of the New York
    Academy of Sciences* (pp. 46–56). New York: The New York Academy of Sciences.
Rovet, J. F., & Ehrlich, R. (1988). Effect of temperament on metabolic control in children with diabetes
    mellitus. *Diabetes Care, 11*, 77–82.
Sallade, J. (1973). A comparison of psychological adjustment of obese vs. non-obese children. *Journal of
    Psychosomatic Research, 17*, 89–96.
Saltzer, E. B., & Golden, M. P. (1985). Obesity in lower and middle socio-economic mothers and their
    children. *Research in Nursing and Health, 8*, 147.
Scharf, M. B., Pravda, M. F., Jennings, S. W., Kauffman, R., & Ringel, J. (1987). Childhood enuresis. A
    comprehensive treatment program. *Psychiatric Clinics of North America, 10*, 655–666.
Sears, R. R., Maccoby, E. E., & Levin, J. (1957). *Patterns of child rearing*. New York: Harper & Row.
Spence, S. H. (1986). Behavioral treatment of childhood obesity. *Journal of Child Psychology and Psychi-
    atry, 27*, 447–453.
Stark, O., Atkins, E., Wolff, O. H., & Douglas, J. W. B. (1981). Longitudinal study of obesity in the Na-
    tional Survey of Health and Development. *British Medical Journal, 283*, 13–17.
Steinhausen, H. C., & Gobel, D. (1989). Enuresis in child psychiatric clinic patients. *Journal of the Amer-
    ican Academy of Child and Adolescent Psychiatry, 28*, 279–281.
Stunkard, A. J. (1976). *The pain of obesity*. Palo Alto, CA: Bull Press.
Surwit, R., Schneider, M., & Feinglos, M. (1992). Stress and diabetes mellitus. *Diabetes Care, 15*, 1413–
    1422.

Taras, J. L., Sallis, J. F., Patterson, T. L., Nader, P. R., & Nelson, J. A. (1989). Television's influence on children's diet and physcial activity. *Journal of Developmental Behavioral Pediatrics, 10,* 176–180.

Thomas, A., & Chess, S. (1977). *Temperament and development.* New York: Bruner/Mazel.

Thompson, S. H., Corwin, S. J., & Sargent, R. G. (1997). Ideal body size beliefs and weight concerns of fourth-grade children. *International Journal of Eating Disorders, 21,* 279–284.

Travis, L., Brouhard, B., & Schreiner, B. (1987). *Diabetes mellitus in children and adolescents.* Philadelphia: Saunders.

Ullom-Minnich, M. R. (1996). Diangosis and management of nocturnal enuresis. *American Family Physician, 54,* 2259–2266.

Walker, C. E. (1995). Elimination disorders: Enuresis and encopresis. In M. C. Roberts (Ed.), *Handbook of pediatric psychology* (2nd ed., pp. 537–557). New York: Guilford.

Ward, S., & Wackman, D. B. (1972). Children's purchase influence attempts and parental yielding. *Journal of Marketing Research, 9,* 316–321.

Wille, S. (1994). Nocturnal enuresis: Sleep disurbance and behavioural patterns. *Acta Pædiatricae, 83,* 772–774.

Wilson, R. S. (1976). Concordance in physical growth for monozygotic and dizygotic twins. *Annals of Human Biology, 3,* 1–10.

Wright, L., Schaefer, A. B., & Solomons, G. (1979). *Encyclopedia of Pediatric Psychology.* Baltimore, MD: University Park Press.

Yarmey, A. D., & Rosenstein, S. R. (1988). Parental predictions of their children's knowledge about dangerous situations. *Child Abuse and Neglect, 12,* 355–361.

Zigler, E. (1995). Can we "cure" mild mental retardation among individuals in the lower socioeconomic stratum? *American Journal of Public Health, 85,* 302–304.

8

Adolescent Development
and Health

Dawn M. Gondoli
University of Notre Dame

ADOLESCENCE is a period in the life span with great potential for wellness. Adolescents, who have survived infancy and early childhood, are not yet vulnerable to the major killers of adulthood. As part of pubertal maturation, adolescents gain increased strength and stamina. Gains in cognitive development give adolescents a more sophisticated understanding of physiology and health, and gains in autonomy and independence set the stage for adolescents to take increasing responsibility for their well-being. From a medical perspective, great strides have been made in reducing adolescent mortality from illness and disease: As a result of improved public health practices, gains in medical technology, and better health care delivery, adolescent deaths due to natural causes dropped 90% between 1935 and 1985 (Fingerhut & Kleinman, 1989).

Given contemporary adolescents' potential for good health, it is unfortunate that they face a number of significant health problems, the most pressing of which stem from accidents, lifestyle choices, and problematic environments that undermine health. For example, the primary causes of morbidity during adolescence are injuries from the use of motor and recreational vehicles, and health problems stemming from substance abuse and sexually transmitted infections (Irwin & Millstein, 1992). Other major causes of morbidity include depression, eating disorders, oral health problems, and problems associated with adolescent pregnancy and parenting (Gans, Blyth, & Elster, 1990; Irwin, Brindis, Brodt, Bennett, & Rodriguez, 1991; U.S. Department of Health and Human Services, 1991). The primary causes of mortality in adolescence are motor vehicle accidents, homicide, and suicide (Fingerhut & Kleinman, 1989; Gans et al., 1990; Hingson & Howland, 1993; Rosenberg, Ventura, & Maurer, 1995).

Morbidity and mortality among contemporary adolescents also vary as functions of gender, race, and socioeconomic status. Males are more likely to be injured
or to die from accidents, are more likely to be homicide victims, and are more likely
to commit suicide than are females. Minority teens are more likely than their non-
minority peers to be victims of homicide. Gender also interacts with race in accounting for adolescent deaths; White males aged 15 to 24 years have the highest
suicide rates among youth, whereas non-White males aged 15 to 24 years have the
highest homicide rates (National Center for Education Statistics, 1993). Adolescents in poverty (who are often minority adolescents) have the double burden of
poorer health and poorer access to health care in comparison with their more ad-
vantaged peers (Lieu, Newacheck, & McManus, 1993).

Given that the major causes of morbidity and mortality in adolescence have
shifted from natural to psychosocial causes, the focus of adolescent health care has
shifted from the traditional medical management of disease to health promotion.
Health promotion efforts for adolescents emphasize community-oriented, educational strategies designed to foster healthy behaviors and reduce unhealthy behaviors. As part of the shift to health promotion, health care providers have recognized
that a life-span developmental perspective is necessary if effective interventions for
adolescents are to be developed (for discussion, see Millstein, Petersen, & Nighten-
gale, 1993).

In part, the life-span perspective encourages researchers to view adolescence as
an important transitional period when health-related behaviors become established and set the stage for health outcomes that might not become apparent until
later in life. For instance, atherosclerosis begins in childhood and adolescence and
eventually causes more than half of all deaths (Kaplan & Stamler, 1983). Adolescents who do not have adequate calcium intake and who do not exercise are more
likely to develop osteoporosis later in life (National Research Council, 1989). The
age distribution of AIDS deaths also indicates a menacing sleeper effect: In 1995,
AIDS was the sixth leading cause of death for adolescents and young adults aged 15
to 24 years, killing 643 individuals (Rosenberg et al., 1995). During the same year,
however, AIDS was the primary cause of death for adults aged 25 to 44 years,
killing 30,465. Given the long incubation period between exposure to HIV and the
development of AIDS-related symptoms and eventual death, it is apparent that
substantial numbers of young adults are exposed to the virus during adolescence.

The life-span perspective also encourages recognition that adolescence is more
than just a transitional period. Adolescence is a unique developmental period during which youngsters experience changes in multiple overlapping domains (Hill,
1983). Adolescents experience puberty, show gains in cognitive development, make
a number of important social transitions (e.g., the move from elementary school
to junior high school), and experience changes in their relationships with parents
and peers. Although important throughout the life span, several psychosocial issues become especially prominent during adolescence, including the expression of
sexuality and the development of identity.

From a life-span perspective, a contextual approach is likely to benefit research and intervention efforts (see Lerner, Ostrom, & Freel, 1997; Schulenberg, Maggs, & Hurrelman, 1997). According to the contextual approach, the health effects of bio-logical, cognitive, and socioemotional development during adolescence depend on the environments in which these changes take place. More specifically, adolescent well-being is the product of interactions among individual characteristics and en-vironmental conditions. Applying the contextual approach to adolescent develop-ment and health, Schulenberg et al. (1997) noted the following:

> In thinking about how developmental transitions may be linked with health risks and opportunities, we believe it is more productive to focus on "interactions" rather than "main effects" (cf. Bronfenbrenner, 1979). That is, rather than questioning whether a given developmental transition contributes to health risks or opportunities, a more illuminating question would be: What are the individual and contextual conditions under which a given developmental transition contributes to a given health risk or health opportunity? (p. 7)

This chapter provides an overview of pubertal, cognitive, and social develop-ment during adolescence, and links development in each of these domains to health-related behaviors and health outcomes. The chapter concludes with sugges-tions for future research and intervention efforts.

PUBERTAL DEVELOPMENT

Broadly, the term *puberty* refers to a series of hormonal and somatic changes that adolescents experience as they attain reproductive capacity. Increases in the sex hormones (androgens and estrogens) and increases in thyroid and growth hor-mones lead to the development of reproductive capability, rapid body growth, and the development of an adult appearance. In girls, key changes of puberty include breast development, pubic and axillary hair growth, and menarche. In boys, key changes include genital development, pubic and axillary hair growth, deepening of the voice, and the emergence of facial hair. Both girls and boys experience a "growth spurt" in height and weight. Gender differences in the distribution of fat and muscle emerge such that boys put on relatively less fat and more muscle than do girls. For both genders, however, muscle development and growth of the heart and lungs lead to greater strength, stamina, and tolerance for exercise (for a de-tailed discussion of pubertal development, see Brooks-Gunn & Reiter, 1990, and Tanner, 1972).

Although all normal adolescents go through puberty, there is great variation among individuals in terms of when they begin puberty (pubertal timing) and the speed at which they progress through pubertal changes (pubertal tempo). Normal puberty may begin as early as 8 years in girls and 9.5 years in boys, or as late as 13 years in girls and 13.5 years in boys. Among girls, the length of time between the onset of puberty and complete maturation can be as short as 1.5 years or as long as 6 years. Among boys, a normal interval can range from 2 to 5 years (Tanner, 1972). In concrete terms, variation in pubertal timing and tempo means that some adolescents will have completed puberty before other adolescents of the same age experience the first pubertal changes.

A large body of research has examined adolescents' adjustment to puberty, yielding information on the impact of puberty on adolescent health. Of particular relevance to this chapter are a number of studies that have examined relations between puberty and dimensions of the self-image and relations between puberty and risky behavior (e.g., Magnusson, Stattin, & Allen, 1985; Simmons & Blyth, 1987). Review of this research reveals three themes. First, puberty appears to have little direct effect on physical health. Rather, puberty affects adolescents' self-image and also affects how others in the social environment view them. In turn, these changing perceptions are linked to adolescents' health behaviors, and, ultimately, to their physical well-being. Second, adolescents' adjustment to puberty, health-related behaviors, and eventual physical well-being are more affected by pubertal timing than by the mere occurrence of puberty. Third, the social context in which puberty occurs moderates the impact of pubertal processes on adolescent emotional and behavioral health, and physical well-being.

Puberty and the Self-Image

Because puberty results in dramatic changes in one's appearance, it is reasonable to believe that adolescents' self-images would be greatly affected by pubertal development. A number of studies have focused on the connections between pubertal processes and dimensions of the self-image (e.g., global self-esteem, body image). In the main, these studies have indicated that puberty has only modest effects on global self-image or self-esteem (e.g., Simmons & Blyth, 1987).

Robust relations, however, have been found between pubertal processes and specific aspects of the self-image, such as body image. It is important to consider body image at adolescence because of the connection between low body image and eating disorders (Attie & Brooks-Gunn, 1989). Several studies have indicated that girls maturing early have lower body image than on-time and late-maturing girls (Simmons & Blyth, 1987; Smolak, Levine, & Gralen, 1993). The dissatisfaction that early maturing girls feel about their bodies appears to stem from their unhappiness with their weight (Simmons & Blyth, 1987). Just prior to puberty, girls' body fat increases rapidly. As a result of this body fat increase, many girls become overly concerned with their weight, even if their weight is normal for their height and age (Smolak et al., 1993). Early maturing girls appear to be especially concerned with this body fat increase, most likely because they experience the increase while their on-time and late-maturing peers maintain much leaner physiques (Smolak et al., 1993). Although dieting is common among adolescent girls, early maturing girls are especially likely to diet and to show patterns of disordered eating (Smolak et al., 1993). Thus, early maturing girls appear to be at heightened risk for the development of eating disorders such as anorexia and bulimia.

In contrast, early maturing boys appear more satisfied with aspects of their appearance than their later maturing peers (Simmons & Blyth, 1987). Early maturing boys feel positive about their height and muscle development, although they also might show some concerns about their weight (Simmons & Blyth, 1987). In accounting for the body image differences between early adolescent girls and boys, Simmons and Blyth (1987) suggested that early puberty might rush youngsters into adolescence before they are emotionally ready to cope with this transition. These authors further note that early maturing girls might be especially rushed, as they mature so much sooner than their peers, including early maturing boys. On the average, early maturing boys reach puberty about 1 year after early maturing girls, giving them more time to get ready for the change.

Simmons and Blyth (1987) also noted, however, that cultural values about the ideal body types for women and men might lead early maturing girls to feel unhappy about their development, while leading early maturing boys to feel happy about their development. These authors have noted that with pubertal development, girls are moving away from a body type that is culturally valued (i.e., the skinny fashion model), whereas boys are moving toward a body type that is culturally valued (i.e., the tall and muscular hunk; see also Brooks-Gunn & Reiter, 1990).

In addition to the effect of the larger culture, smaller cultures, or *microsystems* in Bronfenbrenner's (1979) terms, might moderate the effect of pubertal development on body image and associated risks of eating disorders. Richards, Boxer, Petersen, and Albrecht (1990), for example, compared body image and satisfaction with weight among pubertal adolescents from two school districts that served middle-class, suburban youngsters. Consistent with previous research, Richards et al. (1990) found that boys were more satisfied with their bodies than were girls. In addition, boys in the two school districts did not differ in regard to body image. In contrast, girls in one district reported greater satisfaction with their bodies. The differences in girls' satisfaction between the districts appeared to be the result of differences in school climate. Specifically, the more satisfied girls described their schools as less "cliquish" and also described themselves as more involved in school activities, including sports. When the school climate differences were controlled in multivariate analyses, school district differences in body and weight satisfaction were eliminated or substantially reduced. In interpreting these patterns of findings, the authors suggested that participation in sports and other activities helps girls feel more competent and more positive about their bodies. The authors also suggested that when peer acceptance is perceived as uncertain or unstable (as in very cliquish schools), girls might become preoccupied with controlling other aspects of their lives, including their weight.

Puberty and High-Risk Behaviors

Another focus of the literature on puberty and adjustment has been on the connections between pubertal processes and adolescent's involvement in high-risk behaviors. Similar to the less favorable relations between early puberty and body image, it appears that early maturing youngsters show greater involvement than their
on-time and late-maturing peers in risky behaviors that often compromise health,
including delinquency, truancy, conduct problems in school, and use of alcohol
and other drugs (e.g., Caspi & Moffitt, 1991; Magnusson et al., 1985). The higher
rates of problem behavior among early maturing youngsters appears to arise because early maturers tend to develop friendships with older peers (especially older
boys) who expose them to behaviors more common in an older crowd, such as alcohol and drug use and minor delinquency. The negative effects of engaging in
such behaviors are heightened for young adolescents, who lack the maturity to experiment with these behaviors in a safer manner, or in moderation. Engaging in
behaviors that are more normative for older adolescents also appears to have the
effect of "hurrying" young teens through adolescence, making it difficult for them
to negotiate this period successfully (Baumrind & Moselle, 1985; Newcomb &
Bentler, 1988).

Again, however, the social context appears to moderate the connection between
early pubertal timing and behavioral problems. What seems important for the link
to occur between early maturation and health-risking behaviors is that youngsters
are exposed to environments that provide opportunities to engage in problem behavior. Caspi, Lynam, Moffitt, and Silva (1993), for example, found that early maturing girls had higher levels of behavior problems than on-time or late-maturing
girls only when they attended mixed-sex schools. In all-girls schools, early maturing girls did not have higher levels of problem behavior than their on-time or late-
maturing peers. In addition, this longitudinal study found that problem behavior
was more stable among girls who attended mixed-sex schools. These patterns of
findings led the authors to conclude that problem behavior among girls is much
more likely if pubertal maturation occurs in settings that provide opportunities
and reinforcements for deviance (i.e., settings that contain boys).

The link between early pubertal maturation and risky behaviors also appears to
be moderated by the presence or absence of behavioral problems during childhood. Consistent with prior studies, Caspi and Moffitt (1991) found that early
maturation among girls was associated with higher levels of problem behavior,
such as aggression. However, when the early maturing girls in their sample were
grouped according to degree of problem behavior shown during childhood, an interesting pattern emerged: Early maturation was associated with increased problem behavior only among girls with high levels of problem behavior during childhood. Early maturing girls without childhood behavior problems were no more
likely than on-time and late-maturing girls to show problem behaviors during
adolescence.

COGNITIVE DEVELOPMENT

In addition to the biological changes of puberty, adolescents experience a number of changes in cognitive skills. Compared to children, adolescents think in ways that are more sophisticated, efficient, and effective. Most adolescents become increasingly able to understand abstract concepts, use formal logic, think hypothetically, and consider several sides of a problem or situation simultaneously. Adolescents are also more self-reflective than are children and are more likely than children to see issues and situations as relative, rather than absolute (Keating, 1990).

The cognitive gains of adolescence have implications for health-related behaviors and health status. Compared to children, most adolescents are better able to understand mechanisms of illness and disease as well as the mechanisms of health-promoting behaviors, such as good nutrition and exercise. In addition, adolescents have a much more sophisticated set of cognitive tools for making health-related decisions. Because many of the most serious health problems among adolescents stem from the lifestyle choices that they make, it is important to consider adolescent decision-making skills in more detail.

Why do many adolescents decide to engage in health-risking behaviors? One possibility is that despite their relative cognitive sophistication, adolescents lack decision-making competence. A number of studies, however, have indicated that at least by age 15 or 16, most youngsters do not differ from adults on various indicators of competence (e.g., understanding of the relevant facts, using a reasonable decision-making process; for review, see Melton, 1983). Adolescents also appear to use the same basic cognitive processes in decision making as do adults, such as identifying alternative choices and the consequences that follow each choice (Fischhoff, 1992).

A second and frequently discussed explanation for the high levels of adolescent risk-taking is that adolescents are more likely than adults to believe in the personal fable, that is, to hold the erroneous belief that they are unique and therefore will not be harmed by behaviors and experiences that are potentially harmful (see Elkind, 1967). There is little empirical support, however, for the idea that adolescents believe they are particularly invulnerable to harm. Quadrel, Fischhoff, and Davis (1993), for example, compared adolescents and adults on perceived invulnerability across a range of events, including events that reflected some of the primary sources of mortality and morbidity for teens (e.g., auto accident injury, unplanned pregnancy). Results from this effort indicated that although adolescents and adults tended to underestimate their own risks, adolescents actually viewed themselves as more vulnerable than did adults.

Thus, adolescents do not appear to differ appreciably from adults in regard to decision-making competence, the process of decision making, or perceptions of personal vulnerability. Nevertheless, many adolescents do engage in risky behaviors that are likely to compromise physical health. Surveys have found that many sexually active teens use contraceptives inconsistently, if at all (e.g., Hayes, 1987). Binge drinking (defined as having more than five drinks in a row) is common among adolescents (Johnston, Bachman, & O'Malley, 1993), as are risky driving practices such as speeding, lack of seat belt use, and driving while intoxicated (Hingson, Howland, Schiavone, & Damiata, 1991). Teens also take risks while engaging in exercise, turning a potentially health-promoting activity into a health-compromising one; one recent study found that nearly 80% of boys and 60% of girls take unnecessary risks while skateboarding or riding bikes (Millstein et al., 1992).

If adolescents have the potential to be competent decision makers, why do they often behave in excessively risky ways? One likely possibility is that risky behavior often serves important developmental needs and goals. As discussed by Maggs, Schulenberg, and Hurrelmann (1997), risky behaviors such as smoking and drinking can help fulfill goals such as having fun, admission to and acceptance by the peer group, identity exploration, assertion of autonomy from adult influence, and demonstration of a more adultlike social status. A short-term longitudinal study focused on college students' drinking, for example, found that students were more likely to binge drink if they believed that drinking was fun, felt accepted by their peers, and ranked social goals, such as making new friends, as important (Maggs, 1997). Similarly, Silbereisen and Noack (1988) found that cigarette smoking helped adolescents approach potential friends (e.g., going over and asking for a light; offering a match or a smoke).

PARENT–ADOLESCENT RELATIONSHIPS

In addition to biological and cognitive changes, adolescents also experience changes in their relationships with parents. These relationship changes have implications for health behaviors, and, ultimately, for physical health.

Influenced by the psychoanalytic tradition (e.g., Blos, 1970; Freud, 1958) the parent–adolescent relationship was once viewed as inevitably stormy. Over time, empirical studies have accumulated that indicate that during adolescence, most families do not experience severe conflict, rebellion, or deterioration in the parent–adolescent relationship. In the main, adolescents continue to feel close to their parents, and feel that they can turn to their parents for advice and help (for review, see Silverberg, Tennenbaum, & Jacob, 1992).

At the same time, however, most families do experience increased parent–adolescent conflict, notably around the apex of pubertal change—or the time at which pubertal change is most rapid (Hill, Holmbeck, Marlow, Green, & Lynch, 1985a, 1985b). Most conflict revolves around mundane issues, such as chores and matters of style rather than around serious ideological differences. Conflict between parents and adolescents diminishes as teens progress beyond the apex of puberty, perhaps because parents and teens have adjusted to changes in both the teen and the family system. For example, with pubertal and cognitive maturation, adolescents might come to see themselves as more mature and as more deserving of a say in family decisions and household rules. Conflict might increase temporarily, as parents learn to deal with the newly assertive adolescent. Once the family system has adjusted (e.g., the adolescent is now consulted about the details surrounding a family vacation; parents now knock on the teen's bedroom door before coming in), conflict diminishes.

In addition to experiencing more conflict with parents, most adolescents also experience a decrease in parental supervision. During adolescence, youngsters spend progressively more time in activities that take them away from their parents, whether these activities are extracurricular activities, part-time work, or socializing with friends. Increases in single-parent families and maternal employment have also resulted in more adolescents' being responsible for their own care before and after school. As contact with parents has decreased, time spent with peers has increased; contemporary adolescents spend twice as much time each week with peers as with parents or other adults, even considering time spent in the company of teachers at school (Brown, 1990). Much of this time spent with peers is spent away from direct adult supervision.

Many studies have examined the connections between aspects of the parent–adolescent relationship and adolescent emotional and behavioral adjustment. Although this research has not explicitly compared direct versus indirect effects of the parent–adolescent relationship on adolescent health, the research base does suggest that the parent-adolescent relationship has a largely indirect effect on adolescent physical health; that is, aspects of this relationship affect adolescents' emotional well-being and health-related behaviors, which, in turn, affect adolescent physical health.

The clearest finding in the literature is that when parents can maintain a warm and involved relationship with their children during the teenage years, adolescent health is promoted. More specifically, an authoritative parenting style, reflecting high levels of warmth, reasonably democratic decision making, and firmness, is associated with emotional and behavioral well-being in adolescents (for review, see Silverberg et al., 1992). Adolescents with authoritative parents tend to have high self-esteem, low levels of depression and anxiety, and low levels of problem behavior such as substance abuse. Focus on the components of authoritativeness suggest, not surprisingly, that warmth, affection, and democratic family management practices help adolescents to develop a positive sense of self and positive emotional tone, both of which are important for reducing the risk of depression, and the physical health risks that accompany depression, such as the risk of suicide and eating disorders. In contrast, parental firmness, which includes limit setting and monitoring, helps teens to avoid high levels of health-risking behaviors. Indeed, monitoring is the single most effective way for parents to help minimize their child's involvement in risky behavior, including substance use, early sexual behavior, and aggression (e.g., Blum & Rinehart, 1997; Patterson & Stouthamer-Loeber, 1984).

PEER RELATIONSHIPS

In addition to changes in relationships with parents, adolescents' relationships with peers also undergo a number of important transitions that have implications for health-related behaviors and for emotional and physical health. This section focuses on three features of adolescent peer relations that have particular relevance for adolescent health: the development of emotionally supportive friendships, the initiation of romantic relationships, and the emergence of peer crowds.

Childhood friendships are based on shared activities, with *friends* defined as individuals that one likes to play with. Adolescent friendships are also based on shared interests, but they emphasize affective characteristics, such as perceived emotional supportiveness. During adolescence, *friends* are defined as people who are fun to be with, and who are supportive, trustworthy, and loyal (Hartup, 1983).

Although platonic, opposite-sex friendships occur in adolescence, most best friends are still same-sex friends. Added to these same-sex chumships, however, are new romantic relationships. Heterosexual romantic relationships develop slowly across adolescence, moving from a burgeoning interest in the opposite sex during early adolescence to the active pursuit of romantic relationships in middle and late adolescence (Blyth, Hill, & Thiel, 1982; Furman & Wehner, 1994).

While experiencing changes in the nature of their close friendships, adolescents also experience the emergence of peer crowds. During high school, adolescents begin to classify themselves and other students as belonging to crowds, or groups of adolescents who share similar appearance, attitude, and behavior. Crowds help adolescents to organize the often large peer system that exists in high schools; contemporary U.S. high schools typically contain crowds such as "jocks," "brains," "nerds," "druggies," and so on. Assignment to a particular crowd is often based on reputation and stereotype rather than on actual interaction. In other words, adolescents may be classified as belonging to a particular crowd because they look and act like the stereotypical representation of that crowd and not because they have close relationships with other members of their crowd (Brown, 1990).

A number of studies have examined connections between the features of adolescent peer relations and adolescent well-being. Interestingly, this body of research indicates that adolescents' friends can both promote and undermine health. First, evidence shows that friend support can bolster emotional well-being yet undermine behavioral well-being. Cauce, Mason, Gonzales, Hiraga, and Liu (1994), reported that perceived social support from friends was associated with lower depression among adolescents, and Windle (1992) reported that the absence of friend support was associated with higher depression among adolescents. Windle (1992) also found, however, that high friend support was positively associated with adolescent girls' alcohol problems (e.g., drinking until passing out, having legal and school problems as a result of drinking). Chassin, Presson, Sherman, Montello, and McGrew (1986) reported that adolescents who had tried cigarettes and had supportive friends were more likely to become regular smokers than those who had unsupportive friends.

Involvement in romantic relationships also appears to have positive and negative effects on adolescent health. On the one hand, adolescents may gain social status from dating which can benefit self-esteem. In addition, the development of romantic relationships might afford adolescents new contexts in which intimacy can be expressed. On the other hand, involvement in romantic relationships can expose adolescents to new sources of anxiety and disappointment, which can undermine emotional well-being. Larson and Asmussen (1991) reported that from preadolescence to adolescence, girls and boys experienced increases in negative emotions (e.g., worry, sadness, or anger) stemming from their interactions with friends. Additional analyses revealed that almost all of the increase in negative emotions stemming from friend interactions actually derived from opposite-sex interactions.

Opposite-sex involvement has also been associated with risky behavior. One of the most important predictors of sexual intercourse among adolescents is involvement with a steady boyfriend or girlfriend (Small & Luster, 1994). To the extent that adolescents do not use contraceptives reliably, such sexual involvement exposes them to greater risk of pregnancy and sexually transmitted diseases. Dating is also associated with higher levels of delinquency and substance use, especially among younger adolescents (e.g., Brown, Dolcini, & Leventhal, 1997; Magnusson et al., 1985). One reason for this association is that young teens who date are likely to have older friends who expose them to activities such as substance use (Magnusson et al., 1985). Adolescents who date may also be especially popular, peer-oriented youngsters who spend a large amount of unsupervised time with peers and thus have more opportunities for deviance that occurs in the peer context.

Recently, authors have begun to discuss the effects of crowd affiliation on health-related behaviors and health outcomes. As noted by Brown et al. (1997), there are reciprocal connections between crowds and adolescents' health-related behaviors. Moreover, depending on an adolescent's crowd affiliation, his or her health can be promoted or undermined. For instance, an adolescent who uses drugs encourages peers to associate him or her with the drug-using crowd. Once identified with the "druggies" or "burnouts" such an adolescent is likely to experience more opportunities and reinforcements for drug use, and can also use his or her particular crowd label as a way of defining a public image or identity. Of course, more health-promoting systems may operate in other crowds such as the "brains." Because of the relations between crowd association and health, suggesting that adolescent health could be promoted by changing adolescents' crowd affiliations from less healthy to more healthy crowds is tempting. It is extremely difficult, however, for adolescents to shift their crowd affiliations. Downs, Flanagan, and Robertson (1985/1986), for example, identified a crowd whose members had high levels of drinking, had low levels of school achievement and school involvement, and who were relatively isolated from the other school crowds. Some adolescents from the drinking/isolated crowd eventually decreased their drinking to the low or moderate levels found in some of the other crowds. However, peers from the other crowds still avoided associating with these youngsters, making it virtually impossible for them to change their drinking/isolated label, and, presumably, making it harder for them to maintain their change in lifestyle (for further discussion of crowds as barriers to health promotion see Brown et al., 1997).

DIRECTIONS FOR FUTURE RESEARCH AND INTERVENTION

Although much has been learned about adolescent development and health, much also remains to be examined. In regard to the connections between pubertal development and health, more attention needs to be directed to individual differences and contextual conditions that moderate adolescents' adjustment to puberty. In particular, more attention should be directed to early-maturing adolescents with good adjustment, that is, who are resilient in the face of this stressful, "off-time" transition. Understanding more about the personal and social resources of youngsters who are doing well despite the challenge of early puberty would help us to develop more effective intervention programs to help guide adolescents through this period of physical and social changes.

In regard to puberty and health promotion, adolescents at puberty would benefit greatly from education about proper nutrition and exercise. Young adolescents need to be educated about the problems of dieting and should be encouraged to eat well and to exercise, with emphasis placed on physical fitness rather than on weight. Health interventions in adolescence—whether focused on diet and exercise or other health behaviors—should recognize adolescents' sophisticated cognitive skills (e.g., the ability to think abstractly and hypothetically and to consider several sides of an issue simultaneously). Adolescents are likely to benefit by interventions that provide information, encourage discussion about options and values, and help youngsters to improve their interpersonal skills while focusing on specific health-related decisions, such as whether to become sexually active or use alcohol.

Interventions aimed at improving decision making, however, should also take into account that risky behavior can serve important developmental goals. For instance, adolescence is culturally defined as a time of curiosity, exploration, and experimentation, all in the service of "finding oneself." Although many adolescents experiment in ways that are health-promoting, many also explore risky behaviors, especially those behaviors defined as adult (e.g., substance use and sexual activity). Although we rightly worry about the harm that might follow risky behavior, engaging in some risk does appear to serve identity development. Furthermore, teens who explore their identities—which sometimes involves risk—appear to have better mental health than those who do not (for a review, see Maggs et al., 1997).

With this in mind, a prevention goal might be to reduce rather than completely eliminate risk (see Baumrind, 1987). Programs with this goal might focus on (a) helping adolescents avoid excessively risky behavior; (b) helping young adolescents delay activities such as drinking and sexual intercourse; and (c) helping adolescents meet important needs, such as peer affiliation and identity exploration through nonrisky behaviors (for a discussion of prevention and intervention programs, see Maggs et al., 1997).

In addition to physical and cognitive development, adolescents experience changes in their relationships with parents. Although adolescents gain emotional and behavioral autonomy vis-à-vis parents, and although parents and adolescents experience increases in conflict and distancing, parents continue to play very important roles in adolescent health. Parents who are able to combine warmth and firmness, and who are involved in their adolescents' lives, promote well-being. Perhaps most important for future research and intervention is to consider the individual, familial, and contextual factors that promote or impede appropriate parenting. In a recent report, the Carnegie Council on Adolescent Development (1996) stated that reengaging parents with their adolescent children should be a main priority in the United States. The report noted a number of factors that limit parents' involvement during this crucial time, including a lack of knowledge about adolescent development, job demands, rigid boundaries between home and work, and normative demands from aging parents and younger children. Recommendations to help parents with these issues included extending the family friendly workplace policies now in place for families with young children to families with adolescents (e.g., flextime, job sharing, telecommuting, and part- time work with benefits), and an extension of the child care tax credit from its current ceiling age of 10 to at least age 14, thereby providing some assistance for working parents who want to provide supervision for their adolescents after school and in the early evening hours.

Adolescents also experience substantial changes in their peer relationships. Most notably, adolescents begin to experience friendships as emotionally supportive, begin romantic relationships, and define themselves and their peers as belonging to peer crowds. More research is necessary to understand the effects of each of these changes on health. For instance, more systematic study is needed on the relative impact of friend and parent support on emotional well-being and physical health. Research to date suggests that adolescents might benefit most when they have high levels of friend and parent support, but more research evaluating this possibility is necessary. Interactions between friend and parent support also might occur. When parent support is low, for example, adolescents may benefit emotionally from high levels of friend support (Barrera & Garrison-Jones, 1992). Exclusive reliance on friend support, however, also might be associated with greater involvement in risky behavior.

More research is also needed on the health consequences of involvement in romantic relationships. Most research in this area is focused on contraceptive behav-

160   GONDOLI

ior and the physical health consequences that may follow sexual involvement, such as sexually transmitted diseases and pregnancy. It is also important, however, to focus on the emotional impact of romantic involvement, especially the effect of relationship dissolution on adolescents' emotional well-being and physical health. Larson and Asmussen argued that "disappointments in love represent one of the major sources of distress, strain, and perhaps psychiatric disorder in adolescence" (p. 38; see also Brown et al., 1997). A contextual perspective would help to understand who is at most risk of emotional and physical health problems following relationship loss. The effect of relationship loss on emotional well-being, for example, might be moderated by individual coping styles, other sources of social support, and dating and relationship norms in schools and communities.

In reviewing the impact of crowds on adolescent health, Brown et al. (1997) noted several important issues for designing health intervention programs. One is to consider is that health-compromising behaviors (e.g., smoking, drinking, and recklessness) help define certain crowds. Asking crowd members to stop these behaviors is equivalent to asking them to give up their crowd membership, which may result in feelings of loneliness and alienation and decreased emotional and physical well-being. As illustrated by Downs et al. (1985/1986), adolescents who "reform" are also not likely to be accepted into a new, healthier crowd. Interventions aimed at curbing unhealthy or risky behaviors might be more successful if they also helped teens to develop the kinds of social skills and activities that would enable them to form new social identities (see Brown et al., 1997, for further discussion).

In general, research and intervention efforts are likely to be most useful and effective when they reflect a life-span, contextual approach. Adolescence is a bridge between childhood and adulthood and is a unique developmental period in its own right. Adolescent health is affected by individual development and personal behavior, yet it is also affected by features of the environment and by interactions between the individual and various social contexts. In regard to health, contemporary adolescence is the best and worst of times. The challenge for society is to build on adolescents' considerable strengths while addressing the individual and environmental factors that compromise psychological and physical well-being.

REFERENCES

Attie, I., & Brooks-Gunn, J. (1989). Development of eating problems in adolescent girls: A longitudinal study. *Developmental Psychology, 25,* 70–79.
Barrera, M., & Garrison-Jones, C. (1992). Family and peer social support as specific correlates of adolescent depressive symptoms. *Journal of Abnormal Child Psychology, 20,* 1–16.
Baumrind, D. (1987). A developmental perspective on risk taking in contemporary America. In C. E. Irwin, Jr. (Ed.), *Adolescent social behavior and health* (pp. 93–125). San Francisco, CA: Jossey-Bass.
Baumrind, D., & Moselle, K. A. (1985). A developmental perspective on adolescent drug use. *Advances in Alcohol and Substance Use, 5,* 41–67.

Blos, P. (1970). *The adolescent passage.* New York: International Universities Press.

Blum, R. W., & Rinehart, P. M. (1997). *Reducing the risk: Connections that make a difference in the lives of youth.* Minneapolis, MN: Division of General Pediatrics and Adolescent Health, University of Minnesota.

Blyth, D. A., Hill, J. P., & Thiel, K. S. (1982). Early adolescents' significant others: Grade and gender differences in perceived relationships with familial and nonfamilial adults and young people. *Journal of Youth and Adolescence, 11,* 425–450.

Bronfenbrenner, U. (1979). *The ecology of human development.* Cambridge, MA: Harvard University Press.

Brooks-Gunn, J., & Reiter, E. O. (1990). The role of pubertal processes. In S. S. Feldman & G. R. Elliot (Eds.), *At the threshold: The developing adolescent* (pp. 16–53). Cambridge, MA: Harvard University Press.

Brown, B. B. (1990). Peer groups and peer cultures. In S. S. Feldman & G. R. Elliot (Eds.), *At the threshold: The developing adolescent* (pp. 171–196). Cambridge, MA: Harvard University Press.

Brown, B. B., Dolcini, M. M., & Leventhal, A. (1997). Transformations in peer relationships at adolescence: Implications for health-related behavior. In J. Schulenberg, J. L. Maggs, & K. Hurrelmann (Eds.), *Health risks and developmental transitions during adolescence* (pp. 161–189). Cambridge, UK: Cambridge University Press.

Carnegie Council on Adolescent Development (1996). *Great transitions: Preparing adolescents for a new century.* Washington, DC: Carnegie Council on Adolescent Development.

Caspi, A., Lynam, D., Moffitt, T. E., & Silva, P. A. (1993). Unraveling girls' delinquency: Biological, dispositional, and contextual contributions to adolescent misbehavior. *Developmental Psychology, 29,* 19–30.

Caspi, A., & Moffitt, T. E. (1991). Individual differences are accentuated during periods of social change: The sample case of girls at puberty. *Journal of Personality and Social Psychology, 61,* 157–168.

Cauce, A. M., Mason, C., Gonzales, N., Hiraga, Y., & Liu, G. (1994). Social support during adolescence: Methodological and theoretical considerations. In F. Nestman & K. Hurrelmann (Eds.), *Social networks and social support in childhood and adolescence* (pp. 89–108). Hillsdale, NJ: Lawrence Erlbaum Associates.

Chassin, L., Presson, C. C., Sherman, S. J., Montello, D., & McGrew, J. (1986). Changes in peer and parent influence during adolescence: Longitudinal versus cross-sectional perspectives on smoking initiation. *Developmental Psychology, 22,* 327–334.

Downs, W. R., Flanagan, J. C., & Robertson, F. (1985/1986). Labeling and rejection of adolescent heavy drinkers: Implications for treatment. *Journal of Applied Social Sciences, 10,* 1–19.

Elkind, D. (1967). Egocentrism in adolescence. *Child Development, 38,* 1025–1034.

Fingerhut, L. A., & Kleinman, J. C. (1989). *Trends and current status in childhood mortality, United States, 1900–85.* Vital and Health Statistics, Series 3, No. 26 (DHHS Pub. No. PHS 89–1410). Hyattsville, MD: National Center for Health Statistics.

Fischhoff, B. (1992). Risk-taking: A developmental perspective. In J. Yates (Ed.), *Risk-taking behavior* (pp. 133–162). New York: Wiley.

Freud, A. (1958). Adolescence. *Psychoanalytic Study of the Child, 13,* 255–278.

Furman, W., & Wehner, E. A. (1994). Romantic views: Toward a theory of adolescent romantic relationships. In R. Montemayor, G. R. Adams, & T. P. Gullotta (Eds.), *Personal relationships during adolescence* (pp. 168–195). Thousand Oaks, CA: Sage.

Gans, J. E., Blyth, D. A., & Elster, A. B. (1990). *America's adolescents: How healthy are they?* Chicago: American Medical Association.

Hartup, W. W. (1983). Peer relations. In E. M. Hetherington (Ed.), *Handbook of child psychology* (Vol. 4, pp. 103–196). New York: Wiley.

Hayes, C. (1987). *Risking the future: Adolescent sexuality, pregnancy, and childbearing, Volume I.* Washington, DC: National Academy Press.

Hill, J. (1983). Early adolescence: A framework. *Journal of Early Adolescence, 3,* 1–21.

Hill, J. P., Holmbeck, G. N., Marlow, L., Green, T. M., & Lynch, M. E. (1985a). Menarcheal status and parent–child relations in families of seventh-grade girls. *Journal of Youth and Adolescence, 14,* 301–316.

Hill, J. P., Holmbeck, G. N., Marlow, L., Green, T. M., & Lynch, M. E. (1985b). Pubertal status and parent–child relations in families of seventh-grade boys. *Journal of Early Adolescence, 5,* 31–44.

Hingson, R., & Howland, J. (1993). Promoting safety in adolescents. In S. G. Millstein, A. C. Petersen, & E. O. Nightingale (Eds.), *Promoting the Health of Adolescents: New Directions for the Twenty-First Century* (pp. 305–327). New York: Oxford University Press.

Hingson, R., Howland, J., Schiavone, T., & Damiata, M. (1991). The Massachusetts saving lives program: Six cities widening the focus from drunk driving to speeding, reckless driving, and failure to wear safety belts. *Journal of Traffic Medicine, 18,* 123–132.

Irwin, C. E., Jr., Brindis, C., Brodt, S., Bennett, T., & Rodriguez, R. (1991). *The health of America's youth: Current trends in health status and utilization of health services.* Rockville, MD: Bureau of Maternal and Child Health and Resources Department, Public Health Service.

Irwin, C. E., Jr., & Millstein, S. G. (1992). Risk-taking behaviors and biopsychosocial development during adolescence. In E. J. Susman, L. V. Feagans, & W. J. Ray (Eds.), *Emotion, cognition, health, and development in children and adolescents* (pp. 75–102). Hillsdale, NJ: Lawrence Erlbaum Associates.

Johnston, L. D., Bachman, J., & O'Malley, P. (1993). *Monitoring the future: Questionnaire responses from the nation's high school seniors, 1992.* Ann Arbor, MI: Institute for Social Research.

Kaplan, N. M. & Stamler, J. (Eds.). (1983). *Prevention of coronary heart disease: Practical management of risk factors.* Philadelphia: Saunders.

Keating, D. P. (1990). The role of pubertal processes. In S. S. Feldman & G. R. Elliot (Eds.), *At the threshold: The developing adolescent* (pp. 16–53). Cambridge, MA: Harvard University Press.

Larson, R., & Asmussen, L. (1991). Anger, worry, and hurt in early adolescence: An enlarging world of negative emotions. In M. E. Colten & S. Gore (Eds.), *Adolescent stress: Causes and consequences* (pp. 21–41). New York: Aldine De Gruyter.

Lerner, R. M., Ostrom, C., & Freel, M. A. (1997). Preventing health-compromising behaviors among youth and promoting their positive development: A developmental contextual perspective. In J. Schulenberg, J. L. Maggs, & K. Hurrelmann (Eds), *Health risks and developmental transitions during adolescence* (pp. 498–521). Cambridge, UK: Cambridge University Press.

Lieu, T., Newacheck, P., & McManus, M. (1993). Race, ethnicity, and access to ambulatory care among U.S. adolescents. *American Journal of Public Health, 83,* 960–965.

Maggs, J. L. (1997). Alcohol use and binge drinking as goal-directed action during the transition to postsecondary education. In J. Schulenberg, J. L. Maggs, & K. Hurrelmann (Eds), *Health risks and developmental transitions during adolescence* (pp. 345–371). Cambridge, UK: Cambridge University Press.

Maggs, J. L., Schulenberg, J., & Hurrelmann, K. (1997). Developmental transitions during adolescence: Health promotion implications. In J. Schulenberg, J. L. Maggs, & K. Hurrelmann (Eds), *Health risks and developmental transitions during adolescence* (pp. 522–545). Cambridge, UK: Cambridge University Press.

Magnusson, D., Stattin, H., & Allen, V. L. (1985). Biological maturation and social development: A longitudinal study of some adjustment processes from mid-adolescence to adulthood. *Journal of Youth and Adolescence, 14,* 267–283.

Melton, G. (1983). Toward "personhood" for adolescents: Autonomy and privacy as values in public policy. *American Psychologist, 38,* 99–103.

Millstein, S. G., Irwin, C. E., Jr., Adler, N., Cohn, L., Kegeles, S., & Dolcini, M. (1992). Health-risk behaviors and health concerns among young adolescents. *Pediatrics, 3,* 422–428.

Millstein, S. G., Petersen, A. C., & Nightingale, E. O. (1993). Adolescent health promotion: Rationale, goals, and objectives. In S. G. Millstein, A. C. Petersen, & E. O. Nightingale (Eds.), *Promoting the Health of Adolescents: New Directions for the Twenty-First Century* (pp. 3–10). New York: Oxford University Press.

National Center for Education Statistics. (1993). *Youth indicators 1993: Trends in the well-being of American youth.* Washington, DC: U.S. Government Printing Office.

National Research Council. (1989). *Diet and health: Implications for reducing chronic disease risk.* Washington, DC: National Academy Press.

Newcomb, M. D., & Bentler, P. M. (1988). *Consequences of adolescent drug use: Impact on the lives of young adults.* Newbury Park, CA: Sage.

Patterson, G., & Stouthamer-Loeber, M. (1984). The correlation of family management practices and delinquency. *Child Development, 55,* 1299–1307.

Quadrel, M., Fischhoff, B., & Davis, W. (1993). Adolescent (in) vulnerability. *American Psychologist, 48,* 102–116.

Richards, M. H., Boxer, A. M., Petersen, A. C., & Albrecht, R. (1990). Relations of weight to body image in pubertal girls and boys from two communities. *Developmental Psychology, 26,* 313–321.

Rosenberg, H. M., Ventura, S. J., & Maurer, J. D. (1995). Births and deaths: United Sates, 1995. *Monthly vital statistics report: Vol. 45, No. 3, supp. 2* (p. 31). Hyattsville, MD: National Center for Health Statistics.

Schulenberg, J., Maggs, J. L., & Hurrelmann, K. (1997). Negotiating developmental transitions during adolescence and young adulthood: Health risks and opportunities. In J. Schulenberg, J. L. Maggs, & K. Hurrelmann (Eds.), *Health risks and developmental transitions during adolescence* (pp. 1–19). Cambridge, UK: Cambridge University Press.

Silbereisen, R. K., & Noack, P. (1988). On the constructive role of problem behavior during adolescence. In N. Bolger, A. Caspi, G. Downey, & M. Moorehouse (Eds.), *Persons in context: Developmental processes* (pp. 152–180). Cambridge, UK: Cambridge University Press.

Silverberg, S. B., Tennenbaum, D. L., & Jacob, T. (1992). Adolescence and family interaction. In V. B. Van Hasselt & M. Hersen (Eds.), *Handbook of social development: A lifespan perspective* (pp. 347–370). New York: Plenum.

Simmons, R. G., & Blyth, D. A. (1987). *Moving into adolescence: The impact of pubertal change and school context.* New York: Aldine de Gruyter.

Small, S., & Luster, T. (1994). Adolescent sexual activity: An ecological, risk-factor approach. *Journal of Marriage and the Family, 56,* 181–192.

Smolak, L., Levine, M., & Gralen, S. (1993). The impact of puberty and dating on eating problems among middle school girls. *Journal of Youth and Adolescence, 22,* 355–368.

Tanner, J. M. (1972). Sequence, tempo, and individual variation in growth and development of boys and girls aged twelve to sixteen. In J. Kagan & R. Coles (Eds.), *Twelve to sixteen: Early adolescence* (pp. 1–24). New York: Norton.

U.S. Department of Health and Human Services. (1991). *Healthy people 2000.* Washington, DC: United States Government Printing Office.

Windle, M. (1992). A longitudinal study of stress buffering for adolescent problem behaviors. *Developmental Psychology, 28,* 522–530.

9

Chronic Illnesses in Childhood

Penny J. Miceli
Jane F. Rowland
Thomas L. Whitman
University of Notre Dame

THIS BOOK emphasizes understanding the role that psychological, biological, and environmental factors play in the development of illness. In contrast to this focus, this chapter discusses the ways children's chronic illnesses affect their lives as well as the lives of those around them. During childhood, rapid physical, cognitive, emotional, and social development normally occurs. Although childhood is viewed in terms of its potential as a period of growth, for children with chronic illnesses the obstacles to development sometimes seem to outweigh the opportunities. The experience of living with a chronic childhood illness also presents very real obstacles for the families of ill children. Just as children are challenged by their medical condition, so too are their families who often must make considerable changes in their living patterns to accommodate the special needs of their children. The presence of a chronic childhood illness affects not only long-term goals and planning for the family but also day-to-day decisions and activities. At one extreme, some families of chronically ill children have had to relocate to be geographically closer to needed medical services. Although beneficial for the child, such a change often comes at considerable financial, personal, and emotional expense for the entire family. At a more mundane level, routine tasks with which most families have little difficulty, such as finding child care or an occasional baby-sitter, can become seemingly insurmountable chores for the family of a chronically ill child.

Although the presence of a chronic illness can be debilitating for some children and their families, it becomes a growth-engendering event for others. For example, although siblings of children with chronic conditions often experience negative effects, such as increased responsibilities and decreased parental attention, they also report positive effects, such as an increased appreciation of the uniqueness of other individuals, tolerance for differences, increased compassion, and high self-esteem (Powell & Gallagher, 1993). Perhaps the clearest finding from the literature on the effects of chronic childhood illness is that the degree of success that children and their families experience as they adjust to life with a chronic illness varies greatly. This chapter is directed at understanding what contributes to this variability in adjustment.

Some of the more common chronic illnesses and conditions in childhood include arthritis, asthma, autism, cerebral palsy (CP), cleft lip or palate, congenital heart disease, cystic fibrosis (CF), diabetes mellitus, Down syndrome, hearing or visual impairment, hemophilia, leukemia, mental retardation, muscular dystrophy, spina bifida, sickle cell anemia, and seizure disorders. Although the incidence (new cases) and prevalence (new plus existing cases) of any one of these disorders is relatively low, in combination their overall frequency is considerable. As many as 11 million children have a chronic illness, with perhaps around 1 million children having severe chronic illnesses (Thompson & Gustafson, 1996). Although there is no convincing evidence for change in the incidence of existing chronic childhood diseases, the prevalence of this group of disorders might be increasing due to improved health care that in turn results in lower mortality as well as the development of new conditions, such as childhood AIDS. Suffice it to say that chronic childhood illness presents a major treatment challenge to society and the medical establishment.

This chapter examines the effects of chronic illness on children and the reasons the effects are so diverse, and presents relevant conceptual models and research. In particular, the chapter emphasizes understanding the reasons some children are so resilient when confronted by medical stressors, whereas other children display serious developmental and adjustment problems. It should be noted at the outset that the purpose of this chapter is not to provide an exhaustive literature review (for an excellent overview the reader is referred to a recent book by Thompson & Gustafson, 1996). Instead, our goal is to stimulate more sophisticated ways of thinking about and investigating the effects of chronic illness on children and their families. In pursuit of this goal, we highlight the potential value of investigating factors that moderate and/or mediate the effects of chronic illness. Although moderational and mediational factors are frequently alluded to in the literature on chronically ill children, they are often misunderstood and seldom examined in empirically adequate ways. Finally, the implications of these types of factors for the development of intervention programs and social policy are discussed.

ADJUSTMENT IN CHILDREN WITH CHRONIC ILLNESS

The literature on adjustment of children with chronic conditions or illnesses makes obvious the fact that although this population has been the focus of much empirical attention, agreement on key conceptual issues is lacking. For example, it is often unclear what *adjustment* encompasses. The literature on adjustment of chronically ill children is heavily weighted toward examining socioemotional outcomes, such as internalizing and externalizing problems. In contrast, studies have seldom focused on biological outcomes, such as the emerging course of the disease. Moreover, the impact of a chronic illness on the child's developmental progression in other domains has been neglected. For example, Troster and Brambring (1993) found that motor development in children with blindness was significantly delayed, not only in visually guided skills such as toy manipulation but also in skill areas that seem independent from vision, such as postural control and sitting. Those authors suggested that visual stimulation serves as an important general elicitor of motor activity during the first year of life. They also stressed the importance of caregivers' providing compensatory opportunities for infants with blindness to practice motor skills to curtail developmental delay. More generally, familial adjustment to the unique demands of a child with a chronic condition, such as blindness, likely influences the extent to which the illness has a negative effect on developmental outcomes in the social, cognitive, or motor domains. It is also likely that the trajectory of an illness is related not only to the disease itself but also to a variety of social and personal factors, including the child and family's ability to adjust and cope with the disease.

Another research issue that has not been fully addressed is whether chronically ill children should be conceptualized as a single group, or, conversely, whether children with different conditions should be studied separately. Some argue that illnesses vary so greatly that they necessarily have very different implications for the child and family. Others argue, however, that there are common concerns that children and families face regardless of the nature of the disorder and that chronic illness should be considered unitary. Still others advocate a compromise of sorts, focusing on key dimensions across illnesses, such as etiology, symptomatology, course, and treatment (Thompson & Gustafson, 1996). These unresolved issues regarding key conceptual and definitional points often prevent researchers from drawing clear conclusions about the impact of chronic illness on children and their families.

With these caveats in mind, what can be said regarding the adjustment of children with chronic illness? Children experiencing various chronic illnesses are at increased risk for adjustment difficulties, particularly psychosocial problems. For example, Thompson and colleagues found that 60% to 62% of a sample of children with CF (Thompson, Gustafson, Hamlett, & Spock, 1992) and 50% to 64% of a sample of children with sickle cell disease (Thompson, Gil, Burbach, Keith, & Kinney, 1993) showed increased evidence of problems, such as internalizing (e.g., depression) and externalizing (e.g., aggression) behaviors, when compared to the general population. Similarly, higher rates of internalizing behavior problems have been found in children with asthma (Austin & Huberty, 1993; MacLean, Perrin, Gortmaker, & Pierre, 1992). In a sample of children with either CP or spina bifida, Wallander, Hubert, and Varni (1988) also reported more internalizing and externalizing problems as well as lower social competence. Although major psychiatric disorders do not seem to be common, chronically ill children appear at risk for anxiety disorders and attention deficit hyperactivity disorder (Cadman, Boyle, Szatmari, & Offord, 1987).

Responses to chronic childhood illness, however, are quite diverse (Thompson & Gustafson, 1996). Perrin, Ayoub, and Willett (1993) found that although healthy children are perceived overall as being better adjusted, most children with a chronic illness do function well. For example, Reid, Dubow, and Carey (1995) found that children and adolescents with diabetes were generally functioning in the normal range on measures of depression and school performance. Spaulding and Morgan (1986) reported self-concept scores for children with spina bifida that were *higher* than reported norms. Other researchers have reported no differences between children with chronic illnesses and matched peers with respect to self-reported loneliness, depression, social acceptance, athletic competence, physical attractiveness, scholastic competence, behavioral conduct, and global self-worth (Krusac, Passo, Hovanitz, Taylor, & Noll, 1997). Based on a meta-analytic study, Lavigne and Faier-Routman (1992) concluded that although children with chronic illness are at increased risk for overall adjustment problems, the results of individual studies regarding adjustment vary considerably, even when considering children in a single diagnostic category. In this regard, O'Dougherty, Wright, Garmezy, Loewenson, and Torres (1983) found a disproportionate number of children with heart defects scoring in both the lower *and* higher ends of the IQ continuum. Such inconsistent findings raise questions about the ways a chronic illness influences child adjustment.

UNDERSTANDING ADAPTATION
TO CHRONIC CHILDHOOD ILLNESS

Many conceptual models have been proposed regarding adaptation to chronic illness. Although these models vary in their specifics, most share a similar view of chronic illness as a stressor, as well as a systems perspective regarding factors influencing the process of adjustment (Kazak, 1989). Most models suggest that adjustment to chronic illness is influenced by a number of variables, including those related to the nature of the specific illness, the sick individual's personal characteristics, the characteristics and resources of the family, and the broader social context in which the family is embedded. For example, Pless and Pinkerton's (1975) integrated model of adjustment to chronic illness emphasizes the characteristics of individuals with chronic illness, including their self-concepts, coping styles, and intelligence, along with characteristics of the specific disease and the familial and societal response to the person's illness. In a similar vein, Moos and Tsu's (1977) life crisis model of adjustment to chronic illness includes a focus on the specific illness and social environmental factors, while also emphasizing as key concepts the chronically ill individual's cognitive appraisals, coping skills, and the importance of adaptive tasks, such as symptom management and working with health professionals. Wallander, Varni, Babani, Banis, and Wilcox (1989) also included illness, individual, and environmental parameters in their disability-stress-coping model. Chronic illness is hypothesized to place individuals at risk for adjustment problems not only because of their illnesses but also because of the other stressors in their lives. Resistance to the stress (i.e., resilience) emerges as a result of intrapersonal and social ecological factors. Thompson and Gustafson (1996) noted that existing models of adjustment operate mainly at the descriptive level, delineating factors that might be associated with adjustment but do not articulate the reasons such relations exist or how they exert their influence. In the following sections, the major parameters contained in these models are discussed, along with related research.

Illness-Related Parameters

Chronic illness has been characterized as having a protracted course, either progressive and fatal or nonprogressive in nature, and involving impaired physical or mental functioning (Mattsson, 1972). Because chronic illness is not a single entity, its etiology, severity of symptomatology, treatment, treatability, degree of chronicity, course, and implications for day-to-day activities vary considerably. Some chronic illnesses have genetic origins, whereas others are environmentally caused. Some illnesses involve multiple severe physical and mental symptoms, whereas the symptomatology of others is mild and basically invisible. Some conditions are relatively short term; others are lifelong. For some chronic illnesses the prognosis is relatively favorable; for others it might involve a succession of acute phases, progressive decline, and death. Because of this diversity it is not surprising that illness parameters have been systematically examined by researchers trying to understand individual differences in child adjustment to chronic illness. Such investigations have most commonly focused either on type of illness (i.e., comparisons across diagnostic categories) or severity of illness symptomatology.

Research examining the impact of type of illness on child adjustment supports the assumption that different illnesses vary in their implications for child adjustment. Generally speaking, illnesses involving the brain are associated with greater adjustment difficulties. For example, Walker, Ortiz-Valdes, and Newbrough (1989) investigated behavior problems in children with diabetes, CF, mental retardation, or no physical illness. Mothers of children with mental retardation were more likely to report behavior problems in their children than were mothers of children with diabetes or CF. Similarly, Austin and Huberty (1993) found that mothers of children with epilepsy rated their children as showing significantly more behavior problems and depression than did mothers of children with asthma. In an investigation of adjustment in children with seizure disorders, CP, orthopedic conditions, or no physical illness, Perrin et al. (1993) found that children with orthopedic conditions tended to be rated as having fewer adjustment difficulties than children in the other diagnostic categories. These authors suggested that children with orthopedic conditions might have fared better because their illness, in addition to not involving the brain, was more openly visible to others. Perrin et al. suggested that children might be more effective at coping with disorders that have clearly defined statuses rather than illnesses that are comparatively nonvisible and easily mistaken for other problems. Children in this study who had petit mal seizures were rated by teachers as less well adjusted than children with other illnesses. Teachers, less likely to be aware of the child's condition, might have been more inclined to consider the child inattentive and poorly adjusted (Perrin et al., 1993). This type of social evaluation seems bound to adversely affect how chronically ill children perceive themselves.

Investigations examining the relation of severity of physical symptoms of a disease and child adjustment have yielded conflicting results. For example, O'Dougherty et al. (1983) found that a cumulative medical risk score was negatively related to standard achievement and perceptual-motor test scores in children with congenital heart disease, with children experiencing greater medical risk functioning at a less optimal level. However, those same authors found no relation between medical risk and behavioral ratings for the children. DeMaso et al. (1991) similarly found no relation between their measure of medical severity and behavioral ratings for children with congenital heart disease. Such results suggest that among children with congenital heart disease, adjustment varies depending on the specific domain assessed. Studying children with epilepsy and asthma, Austin and Huberty (1993) found an association between the severity of the child's illness and illness-related attitudes. Children experiencing more frequent illness episodes were more likely to have negative attitudes about their illness, and in turn, more negative attitudes were associated with poorer self-concept. Among children with sickle cell disease (Thompson et al., 1993) and CF (Thompson et al., 1992), severity did not differentiate between good versus poorly adjusted children. Results by Perrin et al. (1989) suggest that the relation between severity of illness and child adjustment might not always be linear. They found that children with moderate asthma symptoms were better adjusted than children with either mild or severe symptoms. Children with mild illness, whose symptoms may be overlooked by others, and children with very severe symptoms, might have greater difficulty soliciting adequate social supports.

In summary, it should be noted that although meta-analytic data suggests that illness-related characteristics are significantly correlated with child adjustment, this parameter is less predictive of adjustment than child characteristics and family-related variables (Lavigne & Faier-Routman, 1993). Thus, examining the relative importance of these latter factors becomes crucial to understanding children's adjustment to chronic childhood illness.

Child Characteristics

Characteristics of the chronically ill child that are important for adjustment fall into two broad categories—those that are age-related, which most children of a certain age have in common (such as advances in cognitive-developmental level and reasoning ability); and those that involve individual differences that are unique to the child and set him or her apart from same-age peers (such as personality, temperament, or IQ). As noted by Perrin and Gerrity (1984), the types of adjustment difficulties encountered by chronically ill children likely differ depending on age, because different ages have unique developmental tasks that the child and family must confront. Infancy, for example, is characterized as a time for building close bonds between child and parent, with the child having to learn to trust that caregivers will consistently meet his or her needs in a sensitive and timely manner. The presence of a chronic illness during this time might interfere with the development of this trust as a consequence of ill-timed treatments and hospitalizations. Conversely, for similar reasons, the parents' bonding to the child might be disrupted. For a toddler or preschool-aged child, issues of mastery and independence become more salient. At a time when exercising one's own control over choices and activities becomes paramount, the presence of a chronic illness and associated treatment regimens might impose unusual external demands and restrictions on the child. Middle childhood and adolescence also bring their own developmental issues, including peer acceptance and the need to be "just like everyone else." For chronically ill children, their conditions might constantly remind them and others that they are different, making them feel less acceptable. Thus, because of the changes with age in the child's issues and agenda, adjustment to chronic illness is best considered within a developmental framework.

In addition to changes in the developmental tasks that a child and family face, children of different ages think very differently about illness (Perrin & Gerrity, 1984). Such age-related cognitive changes likely have implications for the child's ability to understand the illness, to communicate about it with adult caregivers and medical professionals, and to cope actively with it. Burbach and Peterson's (1986) review of studies that examined children's conceptualizations of illness revealed that children's understanding evolves in a sequence congruent with Piaget's stages of cognitive development. For example, less cognitively mature children often hold misconceptions about the causes of illness, attributing illness to factors simply because they co-occur with the illness, or engage in circular reasoning, such as the notion that you are "sick" because "you have a cough." In addition, less cognitively mature children often overemphasize the role of contagion. It is only as children become more cognitively advanced that they understand and can articulate the role of specific physiological causes of illness (e.g., viruses), and how they act on the body to produce illness. The child's understanding of the illness, emotional response to it, and ability to take an active role in its treatment might be critical both to the overall course of the illness as well as to the child's general development and adjustment.

Because of the potential importance of developmental factors, age of the child is often included in examinations of adjustment to chronic illness, typically as a covariate. Results regarding age effects are mixed, with some investigations reporting a significant relation of child age and adjustment, and others showing no such relation (DeMaso et al., 1991; Lavigne & Faier-Routman, 1993; Thompson et al., 1992; Walker et al., 1989). Support for an age effect comes from Reid et al. (1995), who found age-related differences in coping style in a sample of children and adolescents with diabetes. Although children and adolescents did not differ in their usage of avoidance-coping strategies (such as distancing one's self from the problem), children used approach-coping strategies (such as seeking support of others) more than adolescents. An approach-coping style was associated with more positive adjustment. Although studies such as this underscore the age-related developmental changes operating in the lives of chronically ill children, individual investigations often include a limited range of ages, thus making it more difficult to detect an age effect. In their meta-analysis across studies with children of different ages, Lavigne and Faier-Routman (1993) found a significant relation between child age and adjustment, such that older age was associated with greater maladjustment. Ideally, research needs to examine age-related characteristics rather than age per se across a wide range of ages and conditions so that a clearer and more refined understanding of the dynamic and developmental nature of adjustment to chronic illness can be obtained.

In addition to age-related characteristics, individual differences in children of the same age also might affect adjustment to chronic illness. For example, individual differences in intelligence have been investigated in relation to the child's ability to detect illness symptoms, an important consideration if the child is to take an active role in illness-management. Fritz, McQuaid, Spirito, and Klein (1996) found that children who were more intelligent than their peers were better able to perceive symptoms relating to asthma. The ability to accurately assess their current symptoms was in turn related to general functioning, as reflected in measures such as the number of days of missed school. Thus, day-to-day management of a chronic illness might differ from one child to another based on the children's other unique characteristics.

Past research shows temperament to be an important individual difference parameter contributing to child adjustment. Children who are temperamentally difficult, for example predisposed toward negative affective states or poor self-regulation (relative to their age mates), might react very differently to the onset and presence of a chronic illness than do temperamentally easy children. In a study of children with myelomeningocele, Lavigne, Nolan, and McLone (1988) found that children with difficult temperaments were rated as showing more internalizing and externalizing behavior problems. In addition, children in that study who were less distractible tended to show more problematic behavior as well. Although being highly distractible would seem like a negative temperamental characteristic, it might be advantageous for chronically ill children who must endure considerable discomfort associated with their illness. Other research suggests that differences in a dimension of temperament also might predispose the chronically ill child to adjustment problems. For example, Wallander et al. (1988) found internalizing behaviors to be more common in chronically ill children scoring high on the activity dimension of temperament, whereas externalizing behaviors were more common in those scoring high in reactivity.

Socio-Environmental Factors

In addition to child characteristics, caregiver, familial, and other environmental factors have been examined as important correlates of child adjustment to chronic illness. For example, maternal personality factors have been associated with child behavioral adjustment. More specifically, higher maternal rhythmicity (i.e., lack of flexibility) has been associated with greater internalizing and externalizing behavior problems in children with physical disorders (Wallander et al., 1988). O'Dougherty et al. (1983) found a negative relation between current life stress of the parent and adjustment in the child. Similarly, DeMaso et al. (1991) found a positive relation between behavior problem ratings of children with congenital heart disease and parenting stress of their mothers. In addition, Thompson and colleagues found significant relations between maternal adjustment measures, such as anxiety and depression, and child behavior problems in samples of children with sickle cell disease and CF. In particular, behavioral maladjustment in the child was associated with greater anxiety and depression in the mother (Thompson et al., 1992; Thompson et al., 1993). In conjunction, these types of studies suggest that parents who are highly stressed or experiencing adjustment problems might be less equipped to provide caregiving environments that provide support to their children who must cope with chronic illness.

At a more molar level, the structure of the family with a chronically ill child appears to function as a risk/protective factor. For example, Gortmaker, Walker, Weitzman, and Sobol (1990) found that children with diverse chronic illnesses who had only one biological parent present in the family were at greater risk for behavior problems compared to children with intact biological families. Moreover, family cohesion has been associated with better adjustment in the child (Lavigne et al., 1988; Lavigne & Faier-Routman, 1993). Perrin et al. (1993) found that the quality of the home environment was a strong predictor of child adjustment across different types of illness (mental retardation, seizure disorders, orthopedic condition, or healthy) regardless of who was rating the child's adjustment (child, parent, or teacher). These types of findings underscore the importance of including family as well as caregiver parameters in models trying to explain individual differences in children's adjustment to chronic illness.

In addition to caregiver and family characteristics, the broader social context surrounding the family unit must also be considered. For example, the quality and availability of medical and social supports plays an important role in the progression of a disease, which in turn affects a child's adjustment to chronic illness. In part, the nature and availability of these supports is a function of the type of illness. Some diseases are well understood and those with the disease have a wider range of effective treatment options available. For example, with early diagnosis and proper dietary support the progression of symptoms associated with phenyl-ketonuria can be curtailed. For other disorders, such as CF, symptoms commonly associated with the disorder can be controlled. For other disorders, such as autism, critical supports are both educational and medical in nature. The extent to which supports from medical and other formal agencies are available to a family some-times depends on where the family resides. For example, smaller or rural commu-nities might not have the same types of sophisticated support agencies available as do larger metropolitan communities (Perrin & Ireys, 1984). The availability of for-mal supports also depends in part on whether community and government agen-cies perceive a need for such supports. Certain diseases, such as AIDS, because they are prevalent or have persuasive advocacy groups, have attracted political and pub-lic support for research, treatment, and education programs not available for other diseases. In addition, the medical and social supports available to children in school settings likely affect their adjustment to their illness. As noted by Walker (1984), adequate care of the chronically ill child requires education and training for school personnel. Without such education and training, the ability of teachers and other personnel to provide essential supports might be greatly diminished.

Also critical to the chronically ill child are the informal supports provided by extended family and friends. Whereas some children and their families are sur-rounded by a large and tightly connected group of supportive individuals, others might function in relative isolation. Unfortunately, relatively little research has been conducted on the role of social support in the adjustment of chronically ill children. Perrin et al. (1993) found no relation between the size of the mother's social network and adjustment in the child. However, social supports available to mothers of children with physical disorders have been linked to differences in pa-rental functioning. For example, Dyson and Fewell (1986) examined the relation between social support and maternal stress in a sample of children with a variety of disorders. Although failing to reach statistical significance (perhaps due to small sample size and low power), a negative trend was found such that mothers report-ing greater social support tended to experience less stress. In addition, in a mixed sample of children with spina bifida, CP, and muscular dystrophy, a more intru-sively controlling parenting style was associated with larger social networks, and with more frequent contacts with network members (Jennings, Stagg, Connors, & Ross, 1995). Research on social support in populations other than families of chronically ill children suggests that support-related factors other than size might be important predictors of parent and child functioning, such as the relative de-gree of support satisfaction the mother perceives (Crnic & Greenberg, 1987) and type of support (Crnic, Greenberg, Ragozin, Robinson, & Basham, 1983). Crnic et al. (1983) found that intimate support (i.e., from spouse or partner) was related to maternal life satisfaction, whereas community-based support was important for maternal interactive behavior with newborn infants. Future research efforts need to examine how these different social support indices influence the adjustment of chronically ill children and their families.

NEGLECTED CONCEPTUAL ISSUES: MODERATING AND MEDIATING INFLUENCES

As suggested, individual responses to chronic childhood illnesses can be quite diverse. Although sometimes conflicting, research is beginning to explicate the various factors that are associated with adjustment to chronic illness. Because there is not a straightforward correspondence between chronic illness and maladjustment, understanding the circumstances under which adverse effects are likely to emerge, and how or why they emerge, is essential for both researchers and clinicians. To this end, we draw attention to conceptual issues that have been largely neglected in the empirical work on adjustment to chronic childhood illness: moderating and mediating influences, and the distinction between the two. To the extent that *moderating* and *mediating influences* have been discussed in regards to the adjustment of chronically ill children, these terms have often been used interchangeably or incorrectly. By making the distinction between them clear, we hope to provide a more useful way of thinking about the processes involved in adjustment to chronic childhood illness, and to stimulate more precise empirical work in the field. Although we provide the basic conceptual distinctions between moderators and mediators in our discussion, the interested reader is referred to Baron and Kenny (1986) for a more complete handling of this topic, including statistical approaches for distinguishing moderating and mediating influences.

As discussed by Baron and Kenny (1986), a *moderator variable* alters the nature or strength of the relation between a predictor variable (such as chronic illness) and an outcome variable (such as child adjustment). Moderator variables might be qualitative (e.g., type of illness afflicting the child, or child gender) or quantitative (e.g., income of the family, age of the child) and are often helpful in understanding inconsistent or discrepant findings reported in the literature. As noted in the previous sections, studies that report adjustment problems in children experiencing a chronic illness are often accompanied by other studies showing no adjustment problems. Moderator variables, such as the age of the child at diagnosis or cognitive level of the child, might help explain seemingly inconsistent findings from sample to sample, as well as the reasons subgroups in a larger sample seem more or less prone to adjustment difficulties.

A *mediator variable,* on the other hand, represents an intervening mechanism by which a predictor variable (such as chronic illness) exerts its influence on an outcome variable (such as child adjustment; Baron & Kenny, 1986). For example, in the case of the relation between illness severity and child adjustment, one way that severity of the child's condition might influence child adjustment is via its impact on other important psychosocial factors, such as parenting stress. That is, children with more severe symptoms might show more behavior problems as a result of stressed parent–child relationships that the added demands of severe illness bring to the family. Thus, parenting stress might be a critical part of the process through which illness affects child adjustment. By identifying important mediators, one is better able to understand the *processes* involved in adjustment to chronic illness, and the direct and indirect methods of influence, rather than simply describing the range of potential outcomes associated with chronic illness.

In sum, "moderator variables specify *when* certain effects will hold, [whereas] mediators speak to *how or why* such effects occur" (italics added; Baron & Kenny, 1986, p. 176). Both moderators and mediators are essential to understanding individual differences in child adjustment to chronic illness. In addition, it should be noted that some variables, by their very nature, can serve only as moderators because they are static measures that cannot be altered by the illness (or any other process). If for example, the rate of adjustment difficulties associated with a given disorder differed markedly for males versus females, then the effect of chronic illness on adjustment depends on an immutable child characteristic, in this case, sex. Other variables, however, might function as moderators in one instance, and mediators in another. For example, the financial situation of the family at the time of onset of a chronic illness in the child might moderate the impact of the illness on child and family adjustment, such that those with ample financial resources are less adversely affected than those who are already financially strained. However, the financial situation of the family also might be *altered* by the presence of a chronic illness *over time,* due to lengthy hospital stays and medical treatments. These *changes* in financial status might be important mechanisms through which chronic illness exerts its influence on the child and family over the long term. This is just one example of how a variable may function as a moderator initially, and a mediator over time. One can easily imagine the same sort of dual-influence for other variables, such as parenting stress. In summary, we must bear in mind that the existence of one type of influence (moderating or mediating) does not necessarily preclude the the existence of the other.

MODERATORS OF THE IMPACT
OF CHRONIC CHILDHOOD ILLNESS ON ADJUSTMENT

This section examines factors that might act to moderate the impact of chronic illness on child adjustment. That is, the focus is on research that goes beyond simple correlations between predictors and child adjustment, addressing instead the issue of the circumstances that foster different effects and relations. To date, such research has been sparse. However, the literature available suggests moderating influences and the unique ways in which illness, child characteristics, and family variables come together to influence adjustment.

As discussed earlier, illness severity has at times proven to be a significant predictor of child adjustment, but at other times is found to be unrelated to child outcomes. Research by Silver, Stein, and Dadds (1996) examining the illness–adjustment relation under differing family conditions sheds light on when this relation is likely to be present. They found that severity of illness was associated with child maladjustment, and this relation was strongest if the mother was living with a spouse or partner who was not biologically related to her child. Conversely, the relation between severity of illness and psychological maladjustment of the child was weakest in two-parent (both biologically related to child) families and in families consisting of the mother and other adult relatives. In families in which mothers were raising a chronically ill child alone, the strength of the relation between severity of illness and psychological maladjustment was somewhere between that of the other types of families. Thus, family composition seemed to moderate the severity–adjustment relation.

In a study of the relation between child attitudes toward illness and adjustment, Washington, Janus, and Goldberg (1997) found evidence of the moderating role of type of illness. Specifically, the relation between child illness-related attitudes and adjustment varied depending on whether the child was diagnosed with CF or congenital heart disease. The authors found that more negative attitudes regarding the illness were associated with poorer behavioral adjustment among children with congenital heart disease but not among children with CF. This suggests that interventions aimed at improving the way children think and feel about their chronic illness might be more necessary for certain conditions, like congenital heart disease, than others.

Characteristics of the chronically ill child also might serve to moderate the influence of illness on adjustment. Speltz, Endriga, Fisher, and Mason (1997) examined attachment in children with cleft lip and/or palate and found that although these children did not differ overall in their rates of insecurity as compared to children without clefts, child characteristics, such as sex, played a significant role in determining which children with clefts would show attachment difficulties. Specifically, girls with clefts were more likely to be insecurely attached than boys with clefts. Interestingly, sex did not predict security of attachment in a comparison group of children without clefts.

In one of the few studies specifically exploring moderating influences, Perrin et al. (1993) examined the relations between illness, child characteristics, family factors, and child adjustment. The role of one child factor, intelligence, yielded particularly interesting findings. Although the simple correlation between child intelligence (as measured by the Peabody Picture Vocabulary Test; Dunn & Dunn, 1981) and self-reported child adjustment was nonsignificant, the interaction of intelligence and diagnosis predicted adjustment. That is, the nature of the relation between intelligence and adjustment depended on the child's diagnosis. Specifically, intelligence was related to child adjustment for children with orthopedic or seizure disorders, with more intelligent children perceiving themselves as better adjusted, but intelligence was unrelated to adjustment for healthy children and children with CP. When examining maternal perceptions of child adjustment, the importance of child intelligence was again evident for at least one subgroup of the sample. Specifically, the relation between child intelligence and adjustment varied as a function of the mother's health locus of control, but only for children with CP. When mothers of children with CP held an internal locus of control, perceiving illness as controllable, there was a strong relation between child intelligence and adjustment. Mothers of more intelligent children rated them as better adjusted. When mothers of children with CP held an external locus of control, their ratings of child adjustment did not vary as a function of child intelligence. For other diagnostic categories, such as orthopedic conditions, the relation between child intelligence and adjustment was the same regardless of the mother's health locus of control.

MEDIATORS OF THE IMPACT OF CHRONIC
CHILDHOOD ILLNESS ON ADJUSTMENT OVER TIME

We now move from a discussion of moderating variables that describe *when* a particular relation between chronic illness and child adjustment might occur to focus on *how* chronic illness might influence child adjustment over time. In other words, we examine potential mediators of the relation between chronic illness and child adjustment. To facilitate discussion of a potentially complex web of relations, we categorize mediating influences into two general classes: characteristics of the family (e.g., financial status) and characteristics of support systems outside the immediate family (e.g., attitudes of classmates toward a chronically ill child). Components of each of these two broad categories most likely differ in the degree to which they serve as mediating variables. Moreover, to the extent that these components influence one another, in addition to mediating the influence of chronic illness on child adjustment, a more complicated network of mediating influences exists. Our discussion focuses primarily on how family characteristics or extrafamilial social supports might be influenced by chronic illness and, in turn, facilitate or hinder child adjustment. We might have included in our discussion child characteristics (e.g., attitudes toward illness) as another mediating parameter. Although the empirical literature suggests that family characteristics and social support systems are important contributors to child adjustment and are themselves influenced by the onset of a chronic illness, few studies have looked at their role as mediators.

The first category of mediating variables we consider is that of family characteristics. These characteristics, which might change with the onset of an illness, include financial status, employment status and performance, attitudes, stress level, and parenting style. For example, families might be financially challenged when medical costs associated with the care of the chronically ill child become extensive. Moreover, additional child-care responsibilities might force a parent to reduce working hours or to quit a job altogether, thereby further decreasing the family's ability to make ends meet. Barnett and Boyce (1995) found that married mothers of children with Down syndrome reduced the time dedicated to paid work by roughly 7 hours a week (compared to an 11-hour reduction for single mothers), and increased the time devoted to child care by approximately 9 hours per week.

Clearly, the families of children with a chronic illness might need to make some major life changes due to their child's requirements and the family's financial problems. Parents of children with chronic illnesses likely will experience cognitive and behavioral changes as well. For example, when faced with an illness they know very little about, parents might begin educating themselves to gain a sense of control over what is happening and to assist in their child's treatment at home. Furthermore, parents might alter their expectations about their child's future, for example by coming to grips with the possibility that their child with Down syndrome might never be able to function independently as an adult, or that their child with leukemia or CF might not survive into adulthood.

The stress level of family members also might be altered by the onset of a chronic illness. The additional caretaking and financial burdens, loss of leisure time, and uncertainty about the child's future health might produce tension between family members and increase the normal stress associated with raising a child. Parents might react to the child's illness with grief, anger, or even guilt, and perhaps withdraw from their child emotionally. If the child begins asking difficult questions about his or her illness in an attempt to understand it, parents might feel uncomfortable and try to avoid the topic. Marital relationships might suffer as well. Discussing parents' reactions to CF, Myer (1988) suggested that anticipation of their child's death might lead spouses to isolate themselves from each other, displaying a decrease in communication, sharing, and trust.

Although the myriad of stressors and life changes seem to present almost insurmountable obstacles to families of an ill child, families often demonstrate surprising resiliency and adaptation in response to an illness. Some researchers have found no differences in parenting attitudes, stress, overall functioning (Spaulding & Morgan, 1986), or marital satisfaction (Klinnert, Gavin, Wamboldt, & Mrazek, 1992) between families of children with chronic illnesses and matched comparison families without ill children. Barnett and Boyce (1995) found that although mothers and fathers of children with Down syndrome reported more time spent in child-care activities, they gave similar estimates for the amount of time spent sleeping, devoted to personal care, passive leisure, shopping, and educational activities. In an attempt to explain a lack of relation between chronic illness and marital distress, Klinnert et al. (1992) provided three possible explanations. First, increased time and attention directed toward the child might leave parents with less time to spend in direct conflict with one another. Second, through caring for an ill child, one parent may derive a great deal of satisfaction that enables him or her to act differently toward his or her spouse, so the positive feelings and attitudes of one parent might spill over into the marital relationship. Third, the additional burden of caring for a child with an illness might encourage some couples to draw on one another for support, thereby enriching their relationship (Klinnert et al., 1992). Thus, the onset of a chronic illness may have wide-ranging effects on a family system. For some, it can be a source of considerable emotional strain, whereas for others it may foster interpersonal growth and lead to enhanced relations between family members.

180 MICELI, ROWLAND, WHITMAN

Families not only are affected differently by a child's illness, but they also might change their response to their child's illness over time. Perrin et al. (1993) suggested that by spending greater amounts of time tending to their ill child's physical needs, the extra responsibilities and added stress might leave parents with few emotional resources to respond sensitively to their child's emotional needs. They further suggested that chronically ill children might be unable to provide the social feedback that parents find so rewarding, and parent–child interaction might suffer as a result. As a consequence, a child's attachment to the parent might be affected. Goldberg, Simmons, Newman, Campbell, and Fowler (1991), comparing healthy children to children with congenital heart disease, found evidence of more insecure avoidant attachments in the latter group. In addition, attachment was predicted not by severity of illness early on, but by the change in medical condition over time, with secure infants demonstrating improving health. This latter finding suggests that perhaps parents are more able to provide sensitive care once they see evidence of the child's recovery and begin to have more positive expectations. In conjunction, the studies by Perrin et al. (1993) and Goldberg et al. (1991) suggested that family characteristics might be changed by the onset and also the course of a chronic illness and that these changes, in turn, might influence child adjustment. In other words, these studies suggest that family characteristics might serve as mediators of the influence of chronic illness on child adjustment.

A second category of possible mediating variables between child chronic illness and child adjustment is the extrafamilial support system, which includes specific individuals with whom the immediate family is likely to have close contact, such as doctors, nurses, friends, neighbors, and relatives, the broader social community, and the medical establishment. The extrafamilial support system might serve as a mediator for several reasons. First, child chronic illness might evoke certain reactions (supportive or nonsupportive) from specific members of this extrafamilial system, which in turn the child perceives and which thereby influence the child's own attitude toward his or her illness, feelings of acceptance, confidence, or self-esteem. Second, social support and family characteristics in conjunction might lead to more complicated pathways of the influence through which chronic illness influences child adjustment. For example, extrafamilial supports might affect parental stress and coping abilities, influencing the parent's emotional availability to the child, and ultimately affecting child adjustment. Child illness in a family might cause friends, neighbors and relatives to rally to the family's aid by providing financial support, child care, or simply a shoulder on which to lean. Conversely, friends and relatives might become distant or avoidant in an attempt to respect the family's privacy or as a way of dealing with their own awkwardness, or they might become more actively nonsupportive, perhaps irrationally fearing contagion, such as in the case of pediatric AIDS.

Fox and Feiring (1985) studied the effect of illness and prematurity on the social network responsiveness, both after childbirth and on mother–child interaction 3 months later. Infants were classified as either *healthy preterm, sick preterm* (experiencing severe respiratory distress syndrome), *healthy term,* or *sick term* (experiencing asphyxia during labor and delivery). Overall, in comparison with mothers of sick babies, mothers of healthy babies reported people providing more advice and services, such as help with baby-sitting and household chores. In addition, mothers of healthy babies were found to display more positive affect and greater engagement with their infant in toy play at 3 months. It is unclear from these simple correlations, however, whether mother–child interaction was influenced directly by the response of the mothers' social support systems or whether mothers and members of their social networks both were influenced by a baby's health status. Interestingly, Fox and Feiring reported a different pattern of results with respect to social support in the form of providing goods, such as clothing or baby supplies. In contrast to support in the form of services, which depended on infant health status, support in the form of goods depended on the health and birth status of the infant. Mothers of sick preterm infants reported the least amount of support in the form of goods, perhaps because these infants remained in the hospital for a prolonged period of time, were less visible to family and friends, and perceived as being less likely to live. In contrast, mothers of sick full-term infants reported the most support in the form of receiving goods, perhaps because members of the social support network perceived the infant as more viable than the preterm infant and the families in need of assistance. Sick full-term babies had mothers who were more involved in caregiving but less involved in positive social interaction at 3 months. Interestingly, DeMaso et al. (1991) found that size of the parents' social support network was not associated with adjustment in either healthy children or children with chronic heart disease, suggesting that it is not the number of people with whom the family has contact, but the quality of that contact that is most important. These studies point out the potential complex relations that exist among the the infants's health status, social support provision, maternal interaction and child adjustment.

Kazak (1989) pointed out that not only a family's informal supports but also their formal supports, in particular the medical establishment's response to a chronic illness, might have dramatic effects on the child and the child's family. Research and technological advances that change our treatment of diseases have both short- and long-term implications for families. Moreover, Myer (1988) emphasized the important role of medical personnel, specifically pediatric nurses, who provide emotional support and education to the families of children with CF.

A third potentially important source of support that might affect a chronically ill child's adjustment is the child's own peer group. The peer group's perceptions of an illness is particularly likely to affect child adjustment during the middle childhood and adolescent developmental periods, during which conformity with peers and the need for acceptance and peer approval become prevalent (Perrin & Gerrity, 1984). The child's illness might be a primary identifying characteristic for peers, who see the child as "different." Moreover, well-intending adults might try to help the child by encouraging him or her to be discreet or hide the illness, in effect teaching the child that the illness is something of which to be ashamed (Perrin & Gerrity, 1984).

In conclusion, the onset and course of a chronic illness will likely change both family environments as well as the social network surrounding the family and the child. Changes in these systems might, in turn, influence one another and ultimately child adjustment, serving to mediate the effects of chronic illness on child adjustment and helping to explain the reasons a chronic illness produces quite diverse adjustment outcomes. Such a mediating model might provide some insight into the reasons some children with a chronic illness have serious adjustment problems, whereas others appear resilient and well-adjusted.

IMPLICATIONS FOR FUTURE RESEARCH, INTERVENTION, AND SOCIAL POLICY

The previous two sections highlighted the value of examining factors that moderate and mediate the influence of chronic illness on child adjustment. This section draws attention to the implications of such an approach for future research, intervention efforts, and social policy.

The majority of research examining adjustment of children with chronic illnesses looks only for direct relations (i.e., simple correlations) between psychosocial variables and child outcome. Although identifying such simple correlations is necessary and indeed informative, it is not adequate for addressing the issue of under what circumstances certain outcomes, such as maladjustment, will emerge. This question instead requires researchers to test for moderating influences statistically by examining the interaction between variables of interest, such as illness severity or type and various psychosocial variables. It is very possible, and in many cases probable, that the interaction term of two variables significantly predicts an outcome even though neither variable demonstrates a significant simple relation with the outcome on its own. Thus, we encourage researchers not only to think conceptually about potential moderating influences when designing their studies but also to allow for such influences in their statistical models. Of particular importance is examination of the potential for child gender, age, cognitive level, temperament, illness type, and family characteristics to moderate the impact of chronic illness on child adjustment. For example, some illnesses might place children of particular ages at greater risk for adjustment problems.

As argued previously, identifying significant moderators of predictor–outcome relations might help reconcile disparate findings in the literature regarding adjustment outcomes of chronically ill children. Examining moderating influences also has the potential to shed light on some of the larger, conceptual questions still troubling the field. For example, assessing whether relations between predictors and outcome measures are present and equally strong regardless of the type of illness investigated might help answer the larger question of whether or not chronic illness should be conceptualized as a homogeneous phenomenon, or conversely if the factors influencing adjustment to specific illnesses differ. By looking at the unique combinations of illness, child, and family characteristics, clinicians might target more accurately specific types of prevention and early intervention services for the families that most need them.

Also, the possibility of mediational influences should also be incorporated into our conceptual models and empirical investigations. Examining mediators is the key to moving the state of the literature from the level of description to explanation. Although it is becoming increasingly common in the literature on child adjustment to chronic illness for researchers to discuss factors that "mediate" the impact of illness on adjustment, such mediators have typically not been empirically examined, even in multivariate investigations that simultaneously study illness, child, and environmental parameters. Analytic strategies employed rarely move beyond a concern for how much additional variance in adjustment can be accounted for by adding variable X to a regression model. If the literature on adjustment to chronic illness is to progress to the level of understanding why individual differences in adjustment emerge, and why certain relations among adjustment and its predictors exist, more sophisticated analytic strategies must be employed.

Statistically testing for a mediator involves identifying simple relations among variables of interest (predictor, proposed mediator, and outcome variable), and then examining what happens to those relations when the variables are in statistical models together. As discussed by Baron and Kenny (1986), three regression equations should be estimated to test for mediation; the first examines the relation between the predictor and proposed mediator, the second examines the relation between the predictor and the outcome variable, and the third examines the relation of the predictor and proposed mediator to the outcome variable when placed together in the model. If the relation between a significant predictor and the outcome diminishes in the presence of the proposed mediator, then there is reason to believe that the way in which that predictor exerts its influence on the outcome is via the mediating variable. Examining relations in this way would further our understanding of the process of adjustment to chronic illness over time and the ways it emerges as a function of changes in the parent–child system. In addition, such knowledge would inform clinicians about the potential avenues for intervention.

These suggestions for future research, which are directed at increasing our scientific knowledge of adjustment to chronic childhood illness, also have social policy implications. As our nation's health care system changes dramatically, it is important that appropriate services for chronically ill children and their families be available. The available research suggests, however, that optimizing the adjustment of chronically ill children requires that we attend not only to their specific medical needs but also to the broader needs of the child–family system. Coordination of medical- and family-related services is thus crucial (Perrin & Ireys, 1984). Future research in this area should be helpful in refining the structure of such intervention programs. Moreover, empirical information regarding which chronically ill children are at greatest risk for adjustment problems could be invaluable, particularly in cases when limited monies for intervention programs are available and decisions must be made to provide intervention only to those children most in need. Thus, equally important to utilizing the knowledge that available research efforts have provided is recognizing what future efforts have yet to tell us. This chapter has attempted to point out key gaps in our research practices. Addressing these gaps will require considerable commitment on the part of the scientific community and society. Existing research often falls short of answering important questions (such as under what circumstances maladjustment might occur, or how exactly it emerges). Moreover, it seems evident that because of the developmental nature of adaptation to chronic illness that child adjustment would be best investigated in cohorts spanning large age-ranges and involving a variety of specific diagnostic categories. However, because the number of children with specific illnesses is often quite limited within a particular geographical area, it is difficult to conduct research of the magnitude needed to answer some of our most basic questions. For this reason, the organization and funding of large-scale multisite collaborative projects seems imperative for understanding the variety of factors that influence adjustment among chronically ill children and their families.

REFERENCES

Austin, J. K., & Huberty, T. J. (1993). Development of the child attitude toward illness scale. *Journal of Pediatric Psychology, 18*, 467–480.

Barnett, W. S., & Boyce, G. C. (1995). Effects of children with Down syndrome on parents' activities. *American Journal on Mental Retardation, 100*(2), 115–127.

Baron, R. M., & Kenny, D. A. (1986). The moderator-mediator variable distinction in social psychological research: Conceptual, strategic, and statistical considerations. *Journal of Personality and Social Psychology, 51*, 345–353.

Burbach, D. J., & Peterson, L. (1986). Children's concepts of physical illness: A review and critique of the cognitive-developmental literature. *Health Psychology, 5*, 307–325.

Cadman, D., Boyle, M., Szatmari, P., & Offord, D. R. (1987). Chronic illness, disability, and mental and social well-being: Findings of the Ontario Child Health Study. *Pediatrics, 79*, 805–813.

Crnic, K., & Greenberg, M. (1987). Maternal stress, social support, and coping: Influences on the early mother-infant relationship. In Z. Boukydis (Ed.), *Research on support for parents and infants in the postnatal period.* Norwood, NJ: Ablex.

Crnic, K., Greenberg, M., Ragozin, A., Robinson, N., & Basham, R. (1983). Effects of stress and social support on mothers and premature and full-term infants. *Child Development, 54*, 209–217.

DeMaso, D. R., Campis, L. K., Wypij, D., Bertram, S., Lipshitz, M., & Freed, M. (1991). The impact of maternal perceptions and medical severity on the adjustment of children with congenital heart disease. *Journal of Pediatric Psychology, 16*, 137–149.

Dunn, L. M., & Dunn, L. M. (1981). *Peabody Picture Vocabulary Test–Revised.* Circle Pines, MN: American Guidance Services.

Dyson, L., & Fewell, R. (1986). Stress and adaptation in parents of young handicapped and nonhandicapped children: A comparative study. *Journal of the Division for Early Childhood, 10*, 25–34.

Fox, N. A., & Feiring, C. (1985). High-risk birth: Effects of illness and prematurity on the mother-infant interaction and the mother's social support system. In S. Harel & N. J. Anastasiow (Eds.),

The at-risk infant: Psycho/socio/medical aspects (pp. 19–28). Baltimore, MD: Paul H. Brookes Publishing Co., Inc.

Fritz, G. K., McQuaid, E. L., Spirito, A., & Klein, R. B. (1996). Symptom perception in pediatric asthma: Relationship to functional morbidity and psychological factors. *Journal of the American Academy of Child and Adolescent Psychiatry,* 35, 1033–1041.

Goldberg, S., Simmons, R. J., Newman, J. Campbell, K., & Fowler, R. S. (1991). Congenital heart disease, parental stress, and infant–mother relationships. *The Journal of Pediatrics, 119*(4), 661–666.

Gortmaker, S. L., Walker, D. K., Weitzman, M., & Sobol, A. M. (1990). Chronic conditions, socioeconomic risks, and behavioral problems in children and adolescents. *Pediatrics, 85,* 267–276.

Jennings, K. D., Stagg, V., Connors, R. E., & Ross, S. (1995). Social networks of mothers of physically handicapped and nonhandicapped preschoolers: Group differences and relations to mother-child interaction. *Journal of Applied Developmental Psychology, 16,* 193–209.

Kazak, A. E. (1989). Families of chronically ill children: A systems and social ecological model of adaptation and challenge. *Journal of Consulting and Clinical Psychology, 57,* 25–30.

Klinnert, M. D., Gavin, L. A., Wamboldt, F. S., & Mrazek, D. A. (1992). Marriages with children at medical risk: The transition to parenthood. *Journal of the American Academy of Child and Adolescent Psychiatry, 31*(2), 334–342.

Krusac, K. M., Passo, M., Hovanitz, C., Taylor, J., & Noll, R. B. (1997, April). *Social and emotional functioning of children with juvenile rheumatoid arthritis and matched classroom comparison peers.* Paper presented at the biennial meeting of the Society for Research in Child Development, Washington, DC.

Lavigne, J. V., & Faier-Routman, J. (1992). Psychological adjustment to pediatric physical disorders: A meta-analytic review. *Journal of Pediatric Psychology, 17,* 133–157.

Lavigne, J. V., & Faier-Routman, J. (1993). Correlates of psychological adjustment to pediatric physical disorders: A meta-analytic review and comparison with existing models. *Journal of Developmental and Behavioral Pediatrics, 14,* 117–123.

Lavigne, J. V., Nolan, D., & McLone, D. G. (1988). Temperament, coping, and psychological adjustment in young children with myelomeningocele. *Journal of Pediatric Psychology, 13,* 363–378.

MacLean, W. E., Perrin, J. M., Gortmaker, S., & Pierre, C. B. (1992). Psychological adjustment of children with asthma: Effects of illness severity and recent stressful life events. *Journal of Pediatric Psychology, 17,* 159–172.

Mattsson, A. (1972). Long-term physical illness in childhood: A challenge to psychosocial adaptation. *Pediatrics, 50,* 801–811.

Moos, R. H., & Tsu, U. D. (1977). The crisis of physical illness: An overview. In R. H. Moos (Ed.), *Coping with physical illness* (pp. 3–21). New York: Plenum.

Myer, P. A. (1988). Parental adaptation to cystic fibrosis. *Journal of Pediatric Health Care, 2,* 20–28.

O'Dougherty, M., Wright, F. S., Garmezy, N., Loewenson, R. B., & Torres, F. (1983). Later competence and adaptation in infants who survive severe heart defects. *Child Development, 54,* 1129–1142.

Perrin, E. C., Ayoub, C. C., & Willet, J. B. (1993). In the eyes of the beholder: Family and maternal influences on perceptions of adjustment of children with a chronic illness. *Journal of Developmental and Behavioral Pediatrics, 14,* 94–105.

Perrin, E. C., & Gerrity, S. (1984). Development of children with a chronic illness. *Pediatric Clinics of North America, 31,* 19–31.

Perrin, J. M., & Ireys, H. T. (1984). The organization of services for chronically ill children and their families. *Pediatric Clinics of North America, 31,* 235–257.

Pless, I. B., & Pinkerton, P. (1975). *Chronic childhood disorders: Promoting patterns of adjustment.* Chicago: Year-Book Medical Publishers.

Powell, T. H., & Gallagher, P. A. (1993). *Brothers and sisters: A special part of exceptional families.* Baltimore: Brookes and Company.

Reid, G. J., Dubow, E. F., & Carey, T. C. (1995). Developmental and situational differences in coping among children and adolescents with diabetes. *Journal of Applied Developmental Psychology, 16,* 529–554.

Silver, E. J., Stein, R. E. K., & Dadds, M. R. (1996). Moderating effects of family structure on the relationship between physical and mental health in urban children with chronic illness. *Journal of Pediatric Psychology, 21,* 43–56.

Spaulding, B. R., & Morgan, S. B. (1986). Spina bifida children and their parents: A population prone to family dysfunction? *Journal of Pediatric Psychology, 11,* 359–374.

Speltz, M. L., Endriga, M. C., Fisher, P. A., & Mason, C. A. (1997). Predictors of attachment in infants with cleft lip and or palate. *Child Development, 68,* 12–25.

Thompson, R. J., Gil, K. M., Burbach, D. J., Keith, B. R., & Kinney, T. R. (1993). Role of child and maternal processes in the psychological adjustment of children with sickle cell disease. *Journal of Consulting and Clinical Psychology, 61,* 468–474.

Thompson, R. J., & Gustafson, K. E. (1996). *Adaptation to chronic childhood illness.* Washington, DC: American Psychological Association.

Thompson, R. J., Gustafson, K. E., Hamlett, K. W., & Spock, A. (1992). Psychological adjustment of children with cystic fibrosis: The role of child cognitive processes and maternal adjustment. *Journal of Pediatric Psychology, 17,* 741- 755.

Troster, H., & Brambring, M. (1993). Early motor development in blind infants. *Journal of Applied Developmental Psychology, 14,* 83–106.

Walker, D. K. (1984). Care of chronically ill children in schools. *Pediatric Clinics of North America, 31,* 221–233.

Walker, L. S., Ortiz-Valdes, J. A., & Newbrough, J. R. (1989). The role of maternal employment and depression in the psychological adjustment of chronically ill, mentally retarded, and well children. *Journal of Pediatric Psychology, 14,* 357–370.

Wallander, J. L., Hubert, N. C., & Varni, J. W. (1988). Child and maternal temperament characteristics, goodness of fit, and adjustment in physically handicapped children. *Journal of Clinical Child Psychology, 17,* 336–344.

Wallander, J. L., Varni, J. W., Babani, L., Banis, H. T., & Wilcox, K. T. (1989). Family resources as resistance factors for psychological maladjustment in chronically ill and handicapped children. *Journal of Pediatric Psychology, 14,* 157–173.

Washington, J., Janus, M., & Goldberg, S. (1997, April). *The heart of the matter: Differential effects of chronic illness.* Paper presented at the biennial meeting of the Society for Research in Child Development, Washington, DC.

PART III

Adulthood, Aging, and Health

10

Adulthood and Aging: Transitions in Health and Health Cognition

Thomas V. Merluzzi
Raymond C. Nairn
University of Notre Dame

IN CONTRAST TO the abundant information about the health and development of children and about older adults, relatively little is known about young adulthood and midlife. Perhaps the bias in health and psychology toward the beginning and end of the life span is fostered by the abundance of striking changes that occur during those periods. However, from a life-span perspective there is continuity among all those phases. Genetic predispositions, as well as behaviors and attitudes learned as a child affect health in young adulthood, midlife, and old age. Although there are gaps in the information we have about health across the life span, more is being written about adulthood generally and about midlife in particular (Lachman & James, 1997). This chapter examines health and development during young, middle, and older adulthood.

Because young adults perceive themselves as being healthy and have few peers facing serious illness, they tend to think they are invulnerable to illness. A distinguishing characteristic of this population is a tendency to engage in risky behaviors that often have serious health consequences (e.g., drug and alcohol abuse, unprotected sex, reckless driving, suicide). In addition, negative health behaviors acquired during this time (e.g., smoking, poor diet) may set the stage for illnesses later in life.

The assumption that midlife is a time of little change from a health perspective has been called into question in the popular literature (Sheehy, 1976, 1995) and recently in research literature of health psychology (Resnick & Rozensky, 1996). Whereas youth is often perceived as a time of invulnerability and metabolic activity, and aging might provoke images of vulnerability and catabolic activity, midlife represents an enigmatic transition influenced by the lifestyle of youth and sets the staging for old age. Despite middle age being a time of relatively good health for most people, many serious illnesses begin to emerge and mortality rates begin to accelerate during this period. In addition, there is an increasing consciousness about health that comes about as a result of emerging medical problems and the emphasis that the medical community places on health screening, early detection, and healthy behaviors. Thus, middle age appears to signify a shift in women's and men's cognitive representations of health and a concomitant increase in vulnerability for disease.

Although there are considerable individual differences in the health and longevity of the elderly, disability increases significantly in old age (Verbrugge, 1994). However, many of the common health problems of old age (e.g., cancer, hypertension, heart disease) are conditions that result, in part, from unhealthy lifestyles that were adopted in youth and midlife.

The focus of this chapter is on midlife; however, young adulthood and old age are compared with midlife. Other chapters in this volume cover aspects of old age in more detail (cf. Bergeman & Wallace, chapter 11; Vachon, chapter 12; and McIntosh, chapter 13).

First, the stages of adult life are discussed, highlighting the importance of health in overall life satisfaction. Second, biological, psychosocial, and environmental factors that might account for individual differences in adult health are reviewed. Finally, the health beliefs model is described and its utility as a conceptual tool for understanding the nature of the cognitive shift in health consciousness that occurs in adulthood is examined.

SATISFACTION WITH HEALTH IN EARLY, MIDDLE, AND LATE ADULTHOOD

Determining what early adulthood, midlife, and old age are by some objective standard, such as chronological age, is difficult. Perhaps a better marker of transitions in adulthood would be to determine whether certain events are "on time" or "off time" in the process of development (Neugarten & Hagestad, 1976). An alternative strategy, albeit a subjective one, is to consider midlife as a "time to look back and a time to look ahead, a time to ask how things are going and what is left to do" (Lachman & James, 1997, p. 3). In contrast, young adults are more likely to focus on the future, and elderly adults tend to turn their attention primarily to the past (Lachman & James, 1997). Midlife includes a perspective that "includes both the past and future perspective along with the present focus" (Lachman & James, 1997, p. 4). For the sake of simplicity, and at the same time risking accuracy, we use age ranges to characterize adult development as we discuss health and its relation to life satisfaction. Although these age ranges may help demarcate a stage, there are numerous exceptions to this arbitrary system of dividing adulthood.

Early adulthood (ages 22–34 years) has been characterized as a time of affirmation (Medley, 1980). These adults search for economic stability and attempt to establish themselves as independent adults. Although much has been written about the tendency of children to stay at home longer than in previous generations, the child who does stay at home during this period is considered somewhat aberrant (Neugarten & Hagestad, 1976). For the most part, young adults experience very good health. Medley (1980) found that during this stage of development, *family life* is the most important predictor of life satisfaction; standard of living is the second most important. Satisfaction with health was not a significant predictor of life satisfaction (Medley, 1980).

In general, changes in the social domain characterize this period of development. Early adulthood is marked by role transitions that include completing education, beginning full-time employment, establishing an independent household, marriage, and becoming a parent (Hogan & Astone, 1986). These role transitions do not apply to all persons. Moreover, the actual age at which these transitions occur has changed over the past century. For example, during the 20th century, the number of people attending college has risen dramatically; thus, the average age of finding full-time employment has risen. Most role transitions can be used as markers of adulthood; however, despite the transitions, the initiation of adulthood is not clearly demarcated in our culture (Kail & Cavanaugh, 1996) because most Western cultures have no socially prescribed rituals or rights of passage.

Overall, the health of young adults is very good. About 90% of young adults indicate that their health is good or excellent (U.S. Department of Health and Human Services [USDHHS], 1990). The leading causes of death among young adults are accidents, followed by cancer, cardiovascular disease, and murder (USDHHS, 1994). Despite cancer being the most prevalent cause of death by disease, the rate per 10,000 deaths is fewer than 1 compared to 16 per 10,000 in midlife (ages 45–54 years) and 106 per 10,000 in people older than 65. Thus, relatively speaking, young adulthood is a time of excellent health. However, the seeds of health problems might be growing during this age because young adults tend to downplay or deny certain negative outcomes associated with risky behaviors (e.g., unprotected sex, smoking, excessive alcohol, and poor diet; Fromme, Katz, & Rivet, 1997).

In contrast to early adulthood, early middle age (ages 35–44 years) is dominated by the notion of *attainment*. There is particular emphasis on the material trappings that accompany successes. Frequently, financial demands are created by the need for a larger home to accommodate a larger family. Sheehy (1995) referred to this period as *middlescence* because some experience an identity conflict that may be compared to adolescence. That identity crisis is due to a reluctance to move into middle age, particularly in the baby boomer cohort. That is, acknowledging the transition to middle age is tantamount to admitting that one is aging and that the the phase in life where one can be described as youthful is gone.

Toward the end of this period there is usually some evaluation of one's value orientation. For example, the workaholic may question the value of work style and its impact on marriage and family. Not surprisingly, "standard of living" is the greatest predictor of life satisfaction during middle age, followed by "family life."

In contrast to early adulthood, in which family issues focus on establishing independence from the primary family, for those in early middle age family issues have to do with the quality of their relationships with spouse and children. Similar to early adulthood, satisfaction with health is not a significant predictor of overall life satisfaction (Medley, 1980).

Late middle age (ages 45–64 years) may be characterized by *accommodation*. "Individuals are confronted with a series of crucial situations—each requiring adjustment, adaptation, compliance and reconciliation" (Medley, 1980, p. 204). These adults recognize that there will be more stability in one's personality and financial condition. From a social perspective, families of persons in their 50s are changing. Under normal circumstances children make a transition outside the home, leaving the "empty nest." However, because of the trend in delaying childbearing, there is a new phenomenon termed the *sandwich generation*—those who have children at home and aging dependent parents who need caregiving. In addition, during this time there is a recognition of losses (Baltes, 1993); including a decline in physical stamina and health status.

In late midlife there is typically a transition in thinking about balancing work and relationships as well as an interest in the moral aspects of work and social responsibility. Psychologically, men might become more nurturing, and women might become more assertive (Sheehy, 1995). There is a also a focus on restructuring time to maximize the value of the time left to live. For example, a professional might start working fewer hours to pursue some personal goal or to spend more time at home. In summary, midlife represents a time of reflection on the "bigger picture," which might result in some transition in the concept of self and health.

During this period as in previous stages, "family life" is the most significant predictor of overall life satisfaction followed by "satisfaction with health," which emerges for the first time as a significant predictor of life satisfaction (Medley, 1980). "Standard of living" is the third most significant predictor of life satisfaction. Thus, at this stage good health represents a salient and desired state with the cognitive shift in health consciousness representing attempts to maintain, regain, or grieve the loss of health.

Biologically, late midlife is a time when hormonal changes occur. Decreases in testosterone, growth hormone, and estrogen typically are experienced. Also, vulnerability to disease increases markedly. In particular, the incidence of cancer and heart disease raises precipitously after age 50 (Siegler, 1997). During this phase of life, persons might confront serious illness and death among friends or family. For the first time, the experience of loss of health or a close relationship might provoke conscious concern about one's health and mortality. Also, there is an emphasis on participating in medical screenings for breast, colon, and prostate cancer as well as for heart disease (e.g., blood pressure and cholesterol screenings). The combination of the exposure to illness and death, the existential crisis, and the pressure from health messages in the media invokes a more significant role for health in late middle age.

Despite greater biological vulnerability, about 85% of people in midlife report good health (USDHHS, 1990). Prior to age 35, the leading cause of death is accidents. After age 35 the most frequent causes of death during midlife are heart attack, stroke, and cancer. Moreover, the death rate doubles from 35 to 45 years of age and doubles again from 45 to 55 years of age (Bernard & Krupat, 1994). Thus, lifestyle choices in conjunction with increasing biological vulnerability and genetics facilitate the disease process. The increase in cancer has been quite pronounced over the past two decades as a function of the precipitous rise in lung cancer deaths (Bernard & Krupat, 1994). In contrast, death rates from heart attacks and strokes have actually decreased by about 25% over the past 40 years. These declines might be due both to improvements in medical care and significant lifestyle changes.

Late adulthood (65 years and older) has been characterized as a time of consolidation, of letting go of certain roles, and of reconciling the losses that accompany an aging body (Medley, 1980). According to Baltes (1993), changes and losses are more evident in this stage than in previous stages. For most there is the termination of employment, as well as changes in their relationship with spouse and children. In addition, there are more physical illnesses and psychological adjustments than at any other time of life, and the caregiver role is more common than before. In essence, there is an age-normative expectation of illness at this stage compared to all previous stages.

Compared to young and middle-age adults, older persons have many more chronic health conditions. About 86% of people older than 65 have one or more chronic health conditions. Hospitalization rates for those older than 65 are double compared to that of those younger than 64. However, for the most part, people in their 60s are not severely impaired. About 85% are able to function independently, compared to only 51% of those over 85 (Kail & Cavanaugh, 1996).

Decline in old age is not uniform across individuals. Moreover, there is some indication that health status of older adults as a group is improving (Palmore, 1986). If the decline in smoking as well as the increase in preventive health practices continues (e.g., reducing serum cholesterol, adhering cancer screenings), successive cohorts might enjoy better health than their predecessors. Although overall longevity might not be significantly affected by better health, the onset of chronic and debilitating diseases might be postponed (Crandall, 1991). There also seems to be a relation between subjective evaluation of health and longevity. In a study of older adults, Kaplan, Burell, and Lusky (1988) found that impressions of health status was related to survival even when the researchers controlled for chronic conditions. Thus, the perceptions of health in old age might be a strong determinant of longevity.

During late adulthood, "family life" is again the best predictor of life satisfaction followed by "standard of living." "Satisfaction with health" followed as a significant predictor, albeit less salient than in the late middle-age group (Medley, 1980). It is fascinating that at a stage in life when illness is so prevalent that the significance of health for life satisfaction actually decreases. Perhaps the normative nature of illnesses at this stage, the acceptance of mortality, and a lifetime of coping skills helps to moderate the impact of illness on life satisfaction.

ACCOUNTING FOR INDIVIDUAL DIFFERENCES IN HEALTH IN ADULTHOOD

A myriad of factors may influence health in adulthood and old age. Consistent with the model presented in chapter 1, these influences are categorized into three domains: biological, psychosocial, and environmental. The section of the biological domain discusses briefly the prevalent theories of aging that account for the limitations of longevity and the prevalence of disease in old age. Psychosocial influences include social support, lifestyle choices, and personality. Finally, racism and poverty are discussed as environmental influences on health in adulthood.

Biological Changes

Compared to young adulthood, midlife is when biological decrements begin to become more evident and even more pronounced than they are in old age. However, it is important to distinguish *aging* from *disease*. Normal biological changes are not diseases—but they are losses of function. Thus, menopause, loss of hair, decreased capacity for exercise, and so on, are not midlife disorders that make one more susceptible to death. However, other aspects of aging do increase our vulnerability over the life span. For example, with aging the immune system might lose some of its capacity to recognize foreign cells, DNA replication might falter when errors in DNA are not detected and corrected, cells might lose their capability to replicate (Hayflick, 1994), free radicals might cause damage to chromosomes (Harman, 1992), and levels of hormones (e.g., estrogen) might decrease, resulting in more vulnerability to heart disease (Bernard & Krupat, 1994).

Other physiological changes might contribute to the development of health problems in old age. For example, changes that occur in neurons in that axon fibers might become twisted and form spiral-shaped neurofibrillary tangles. These axon tangles might disrupt the normal functioning of the neurons. In addition, dendrites might atrophy, and neurotransmitter activity might be impaired. These changes in neurons are implicated in the development of Alzheimer's disease.

In addition to changes in neurons, significant changes might occur in the cardiovascular and respiratory systems that might be exacerbated by smoking, poor diet, and sedentary lifestyle, thus making older persons more vulnerable to heart disease and strokes, the leading causes of deaths in the late adulthood population. However, despite the greater prevalence of illness, older people adjust better to illness than their younger counterparts (Merluzzi & Martinez Sanchez, 1997).

Social and Environmental Factors

Social factors may mitigate the aging process and protect against disease. For example, the social context of aging may protect or exacerbate the biological effects of aging and concomitant vulnerability. Perhaps the most well-studied aspect of the social context is social support; literally hundreds of studies support the stress-buffering effects of social support. For example, social support may buffer some of the negative effects of stress that otherwise might compromise the immune system. On another level, large-scale epidemiological studies (e.g., Kaplan, Seeman, Cohen, Knudsen, & Guralnik, 1987) demonstrate the positive influence of social support in lowering the incidence and duration of disease and improving longevity. Either the mechanisms underlying social support provide needed resources to promote health, or those who have an adequate social network are more apt to take better care of themselves.

Another social phenomenon that might affect health in adulthood is the birth cohort. In theory, the experiences that a group of individuals share (e.g., depression era) can have a profound effect on their development. These effects accumulate over a lifetime and may contribute to lifestyle preferences, behaviors, and social norms that affect health and longevity. For example, African Americans born after 1960 have different experiences in American culture from those born before 1940. Although racism might be endemic to our society, the laws enacted and opportunities made available to the younger group probably had a profound effects on their life courses and their health. Other birth cohort effects are evident throughout American society. For example, the image of grandparent has changed dramatically. Grandparents in their 50s and 60s do not resemble the grandparents of previous cohorts; they are younger looking and acting (Sheehy, 1995). Also, the present cohort of grandparents is more concerned about health—they smoke less and are more weight and diet conscious than previous cohorts were at that age (Perlmutter & Hall, 1992).

Lifestyle Factors

The impact of positive health practices seems to emerge in midlife. In a series of longitudinal studies, about 7,000 residents of Alameda County, California were asked how many of the following seven behaviors describe them: sleep 7 to 8 hours each night, eat breakfast every day, never or rarely eat between meals, maintain appropriate weight for height, never smoked, use alcohol moderately, and partake in regular physical activity. Overall, after 10 years those who engaged in more of the healthy behaviors had more positive health than those who engaged in fewer health behaviors (Belloc, 1973). The men who engaged in all seven healthy behaviors had an overall mortality that was only 28% of that for men who engaged in zero to three of those health practices. The overall mortality for women who engaged in all seven was 43% of that of women who engaged in zero to three of the healthy behaviors (Breslow & Enstrom, 1980). The authors noted that there was a great deal of stability in these behaviors over the years that people were followed.

The survival benefit for men who engaged in six or seven of the healthy behaviors was more substantial for those ages 50 to 74 than for those younger than 50 or older than 74. In fact, at about age 75 the death rates for those who engaged in zero to three and those who engaged in six or seven converged to a great extent. Thus, it appears that the maximal benefits of a healthy lifestyle occur in later midlife and early old age. For women, the survival benefit of healthy behaviors tends to emerge about age 60 and continues through age 85. Prior to age 60, estrogen or menses might be a protective factor for all women. In summary, the benefits of healthy behaviors appears to have its largest impact in midlife for men and women. However, the benefits of these health behaviors may be rooted in lifestyle choices that span all of adulthood.

Education and Income

Higher educational level and greater income are strongly correlated with good health (see Bolig, Borkowski, & Brandenberger, chapter 4, this volume). This relation becomes evident at midlife and is even more pronounced at old age (Ross & Wu, 1996). The higher death rates among those elderly who are lower in socioeconomic status (SES) would suggest that the divergence in health as a function of age is understated. That is, those older adults who are poor represent a much more hardy subset of that cohort because they were able to survive the disadvantages of poverty. Thus, although there is a consistent pattern of decline in health over the life span, educational attainment, income, and factors associated with these variables appear to slow that decline.

Psychological Factors: Changes in Health Cognitions

As noted earlier in the chapter, early adulthood is characterized by relatively little disease and little decline in physical reserve capacity. Moreover, in early adulthood there is a cognitive set that has been called the *personal fable*, which is characterized by a perception of personal invulnerability. As noted by Gondoli (chapter 8, this volume) young adults actually might perceive the danger of certain behaviors but, nonetheless, are willing to take rather substantial risks. Middle age represents a transition in the representation of the self with respect to health. There is enough physical reserve capacity lost and enough of life experienced to provoke thoughts of mortality. Moreover, there are enough cases of friends or peers with heart disease, heart attacks, and cancer to reinforce the notion that vulnerability is increasing. This midlife scenario also may be contrasted with an older group's whose reserve capacity is more limited and in whom disease is much more prevalent. The representation of the self in late adulthood includes a substantial vulnerability component (Cavanaugh, 1997).

One of the overriding themes in this transition from perceived invulnerability and risk-taking to substantial vulnerability and frailty is a sense of personal control. This concept has a rich history in health psychology and has been associated with positive health outcomes (Taylor, 1995). The following sections review some of the constructs and empirical findings related to control and interpret that data from a life-span perspective.

Personal and Perceived Control. Personal control and responsibility-taking have been linked to health and health-related behaviors. Ziff, Conrad, and Lachman (1995) found that a sense of control accounted for a significant amount of the variance in the prediction of self-rated health and health-related behaviors. This sense of control or perceived control appears to have a profound impact not only on the health of individuals but also on their adjustment to illness (Taylor & Brown, 1988). It appears that actual control is less important than perceived control or illusion of control (Taylor, 1989).

Although there might be some variation as a function of personality or disease in the need for control, generally the perception of control allows individuals to regulate affect and enhance coping in stressful situations. However, situations in which increasing control is accompanied by a high degree of responsibility that actually might be detrimental (Taylor, 1995). For example, it would be deleterious for someone to assume responsibility for the recurrence of cancer after being in remission for a period of time.

Perhaps the most well-known construct in the literature on control is locus of control (Rotter, 1966). *Internal locus of control* refers to the belief that the outcomes that we experience in life are a result of our own behaviors. In contrast, *external locus of control* refers to the belief that outcomes occur as a result of chance or external forces that are beyond our control. Those who believe in an internal locus of control appear to have an advantage in health over those who believe in an external locus of control. They seek more information about health, engage in more behaviors that would be considered health promoting, are more inclined to exercise, and are much less likely to have heart disease (Quadrel & Lau, 1989; Strickland, 1979; Tinsley & Holtgrave, 1989; Waller & Bates, 1992). Compared to external locus of control, an internal locus of control is associated with significantly less serious illnesses (Brandon & Loftin, 1991).

Self-efficacy is similar to locus of control (Bandura, 1997). Self-efficacy judgments are behavior expectancies or estimations of one's ability to perform certain behaviors. However, one's willingness to perform the behavior generally is related to an expected outcome. Thus, *control* may be defined as having positive efficacy expectations (the notion that you can accomplish the appropriate behaviors) and positive outcome expectancies (the notion that positive outcomes will result). There are health benefits to self-efficacy. High self-efficacy is associated with weight loss

(Stotland & Zuroff, 1991), smoking cessation (Kok et al., 1992), adaptation to serious illness (Merluzzi & Martinez Sanchez, 1997), changing AIDS-related risk behaviors (Bandura, 1990), and adoption of health behaviors (e.g., healthy diet and regular exercise; Schwarzer, 1992). High self-efficacy expectations also are associated with adherence to exercise regimens (Fruin, Pratt, & Owen, 1992), adaptive coping with pain (Litt, 1988), positive stress-immune functioning (Zautra, Okun, Roth, & Emmanual, 1989), relapse prevention (Borland, Owen, Hill, & Schofield, 1991), adjustment to rheumatoid arthritis (O'Leary, Shoor, Lorig, & Holman, 1988), and practice of safe sex (Wulfert & Wan, 1993). However, in a study that examined physical rehabilitation, efficacy expectations did not predict progress as well as the performance feedback that led the authors to suggest that in some instances the impact of the disease or the physical functioning level of the person might be a stronger predictor of outcome than self-efficacy (Toshima, Kaplan, & Reis, 1992).

Perceived control, internal locus of control, and high self-efficacy are associated with the construct of control that, in turn, is associated with more positive states of health. In addition to the notion that control fosters a sense of agency in the health domain, control also has been postulated to moderate the effects of stress on health, which is critical for the adult body. The *stress–diathesis paradigm,* which states certain conditions that exacerbate the effects of stress, may be a particularly useful heuristic in conceptualizing health at midlife compared to young adulthood, when physical resilience may obviate many effects of stress, and older adulthood, when vulnerability is much more evident. We conclude, therefore, that the effects of stress, in the absence of control, are likely to be more devastating in midlife than in youth. For example, blood pressure rises with age, thus many people in their 50s have borderline hypertension (i.e., 140 systolic, 90 diastolic). Unless buffered or moderated by perceived control, extreme stress may push blood pressure up into a range that has more serious consequences for health. Thus, the increased vulnerability the comes with midlife may potentiate the effects of stress; on the other hand, control may moderate the relation between stress and illness.

Control is a multidimensional construct that must be evaluated in the context a particular situation. Moreover, the expectancies for control should be reasonable for a given situation. Some people are characterized by unreasonable expectations that may be detrimental to their health. For example, the Type A behavior pattern, which is characterized by intense competition, impatience, anger, hostility, and aggressiveness, doubles the risk for cardiovascular disease (Bernard & Krupat, 1994). The Type A behavior pattern might represent an extreme need for control, and the failure to acquire it in the long term might lead to devastating consequences. Thus, control, which involves reasonable positive behavior expectancies (self-efficacy) and reasonable positive outcome expectancies usually is the most adaptive pattern of behavior for beneficial adjustment and health.

The development of control beliefs begins in infancy and progresses throughout the life span (Skinner, 1995). During adulthood there is generally an overestimation of controllability; that is, the perception that behaviors and events are more controllable than they really are. Also, throughout adulthood there is the perception that we can control desired personal attributes. In addition, compared to young and middle-aged adults, older persons believe that undesired attributes are more controllable (Heckhausen & Baltes, 1991). Thus, older adults develop a sense of responsibility for negative attributes and believe that they are controllable, which enables them to cope with adversity better. It appears actual experience with the changes that occur in life fosters control beliefs that are not present at earlier stages of life.

Older adults also might foster self-efficacy by making favorable social comparisons despite overall losses in functioning. If older persons perceive themselves as exceeding the capabilities of their age cohort, their self-efficacy might remain relatively high. One extension of this line of thought is that if older persons maintain skills, then the social comparisons with same age peers provide even more support for their self-efficacy expectations. In many instances, performance or skill actually might be declining on some absolute level; however, efficacy and perceptions of control are maintained based on performance or skill evaluations relative to same-age peers (Bandura, 1997). Moreover, there may be a tendency to make social comparisons without knowledge of the norms; thus, the process of making positive social comparisons, rather than making accurate age-related social comparisons, might be critical in maintaining efficacy in old age.

There also appears to be some modification of control beliefs as a consequence of the older adult's life situation (Flammer, 1995). This reconciliation of control beliefs with reality (i.e., becoming more realistic about what can be controlled) does not result in a total loss of control. There may be some compensatory strategy to retain control while also experiencing losses in reserve capacity. Baltes and Baltes (1990) referred to this process as *selective optimization with compensation*. In late middle age, a series of experiences provoke the aging person to think differently about capacity for control. First, activities or behaviors are selected from a previously larger repertoire. Then, they are practiced so that expertise is gained in a narrower range of activities. Finally, losses are compensated for by performing those activities differently from the way they were performed in the past. For example, a once excellent singles tennis player might, in old age, concentrate on excelling in doubles.

In summary, control and self-efficacy are important for maintaining health in midlife and old age. The developmental aspects of control provide a context for the maintenance of control beliefs. In particular, differences develop in the perceptions of control in the progression from midlife to old age. For example, compared to younger cohorts, older persons perceive that negative attributes are more controllable. In addition, the tendency to align expectations more with reality and implement strategies to maintain efficacy, such as the adoption of age-related performance standards, social comparison with same-age peers, and optimization of skills in well-chosen areas increases as the body ages.

Personality Characteristics: Hardiness.   Some social leaning theorists (e.g., Bandura) view control as a learned characteristic and, therefore, alterable. Others, however (e.g., Rotter and Kobasa) view control as a dimension of personality that is not easily changed. Kobasa (1979b) hypothesized that some individuals experience high levels of stress but do not suffer serious deterioration as a consequence because they possess the hardy personality. Stressful events are defined in this context as events that "cause changes in and demands readjustment of an average person's normal routine" (Kobasa, 1979a, p. 2).

There are three components to hardiness: commitment, control, and perception of change as a challenge. Committed individuals have the ability to feel deeply involved in—or committed to—the activities of their lives. They recognize their own particular values, goals, and priorities, have a sense of purpose for their lives, and make decisions appropriate to these purposes. This belief or value system reduces the perceived threat of stressful life events and, therefore, increases the ability of the person to cope successfully. In general, committed individuals approach life with the notion that stressful situations provide an opportunity to implement or clarify one's meaning system (Funk, 1992; Kobasa, Maddi, & Courington, 1981). In addition, committed persons are not alienated from others; therefore, they may turn to others for assistance to help themselves readjust under stressful conditions (Kobasa, 1979a).

Hardy individuals also have a strong sense of control. As noted earlier, personal control allows the individual to view stressors as changeable and to believe in their own ability to control or influence the outcomes in their lives (Funk, 1992; Kobasa et al., 1981). As a result of coping successfully in a variety of situations, they develop a repertoire of coping skills to call on in stressful situations (Kobasa, 1979a).

Third, hardy persons view change as a challenge that provides opportunities to obtain new insights (Funk, 1992; Kobasa et al., 1981). Because they view change as a challenge rather than a nuisance, they are more apt to engage new situations as opposed to avoiding them. In addition, they are predisposed to being cognitively flexible, which means they integrate and appraise information from new situations and unexpected events.

An early study of hardiness investigated the stress resistance of middle-aged male business executives (Kobasa, 1979b). A large sample of participants who were midlevel managers in large corporations were asked to indicate the stressful life events they had experienced and the number of illness episodes they had in the 3 years prior to the study. In addition, they filled out a number of measures that tapped the three main dimensions of hardiness. Participants who had stress scores above the median and who had illness scores below the cohort median were assigned to a high stress–low illness group. Participants whose stress and illness scores were above the median were assigned to a high stress–high illness group. The study revels that those who experienced high levels of stressful life events without becoming ill were more committed, more in control, and more oriented toward viewing change as a challenge than those who experience high degrees of stressful life events and become sick. Thus, hardiness seemed to act as a buffer that moderated the effects of stress on illness.

It is interesting that a similar buffer effect of hardiness was not replicated with younger (college-age) samples (Funk & Huston, 1987; Hull, Van Treuren, & Virnelli, 1987). Perhaps there is something unique about midlife that distinguishes it from earlier stages of life. For example, college students, as compared to middle-aged managers, might not experience serious illnesses because of greater physical reserve capacity and might not encounter stressors as severe as those in the competitive world of business. Because midlife involves more biological vulnerability and more difficult stressors, the role of psychological variables, such as hardiness, might increase as a salient health protective factor. ·

In summary, control and hardiness appear to serve not only as health protective factors, but they also have a developmental pattern. Control beliefs and hardiness appear to develop at a young age, transform as moderator variables in midlife, and transform again in old age to compensate for some loss of reserve capacity.

A CONCEPTUAL FRAMEWORK
FOR HEALTH IN ADULTHOOD

Health in adulthood may be described in terms that are thematic in this book—biological, environmental, and psychological factors that impinge on our health status. In midlife and old age there is increased biological vulnerability to disease, but more pressure from the environment (e.g., physicians and the media) to engage in healthy lifestyles. A number of social and psychological variables might influence health (e.g., SES, race, social support, coping skills, personal control, hardiness). A health consciousness also emerges that gradually appears during midlife in spite of the fact that this population is relatively healthy. That awareness and the actions that follow might have a substantial impact on the individual's health over the remainder of the person's life into old age. For example, mammography and prostate screening during midlife might determine whether serious illnesses are discovered early enough to treat and cure the patient. Moreover, engaging in other healthy behaviors such as weight loss, cholesterol reduction, and controlling blood pressure might have marked effects on one's quality of life and longevity.

Rosenstock (1974) indicated that a "cue to action" may be necessary to prompt health behaviors. Those cues may be internal, external, or a combination of the two. For example, a middle-aged, overweight man who smokes may experience chest pain and immediately have thoughts about the need to quit smoking. His urge to quit may be reinforced as a consequence of a co-worker's heart attack. Thus, the cognitive shift in health consciousness may be characterized as a shift in health beliefs that are informed by external events (e.g., messages from the media, the death of a close friend, support from spouse or friend to consult a physician, etc.) or internal events (e.g., chest pain, shortness of breath, headaches, decreased stamina, impotence, etc.). These events or symptoms may invoke what Prochaska and DiClemente (1992) called *contemplation* and promote a transition from not thinking very much about health (i.e., precontemplation) to a more conscious awareness and consideration of health problems.

This emergence of and focus on health beliefs during midlife is contained in the well-known health beliefs model (HBM; Rosenstock, 1974). The HBM, derived from value-expectancy theory, postulates that certain behaviors will be executed if their outcome is valued and reasonably probable. The HBM was developed by psychologists in the Public Health Service to explain why people would or would not take advantage of certain public health programs, such as tuberculosis screening.

The model consists of several components. The first component is perceived threat, that is, the perceived severity of the illness and the perceived susceptibility of the person to the illness. The second component is the perceived efficacy of engaging in health-oriented behaviors. Included in that component are the perceived benefits of the behaviors and the perceived barriers to executing the behaviors. The latest component to be added to the model is self-efficacy, that is, the confidence an individual has to perform appropriate health-oriented behaviors. A combination of these components leads to some estimation of the likelihood of engaging in a health-protective or health-promoting behavior.

The HBM has been represented by an equation suggested earlier (Seibold & Roper, 1979) with the addition of self efficacy:

$$LA(f)PV_{w1} + PS_{w2} + (PB - PC)_{w3} + SE$$

In other words, the likelihood of a particular health behavior (LA) is a function of perceived vulnerability (PV), plus perceived severity (PS), plus the balance of perceived benefits (PB) minus the barriers (PC) plus self-efficacy (SE). An examination of each of the components helps illuminate the midlife cognitive shift presented in this chapter. For example, a woman who has had several close relatives contract breast cancer may feel that her family history makes her very susceptible to the disease. Also, she may have witnessed the impact of chemotherapy treatments or even the effects of metastatic disease and determined that the severity of the disease is rather extreme. She then may compare the perceived benefits of a health behavior (in this case mammogram screening and clinical breast examination) with the perceived barriers (i.e., financial costs, anticipated pain, anxiety, inconvenience, etc.) to determine if the outcomes are positive relative to the costs.

A critique of the HBM is beyond the scope of this chapter; however, the model provides insight into the cognitive shift in health consciousness that takes place in midlife. Based on the health of young adults and their perceived invulnerability, one would hypothesize that the weight for perceived vulnerability (PV_{w1}) is relatively low in young adulthood, then increase significantly during midlife and old age. The increase may be caused by the attention devoted to salient biological, environmental, social, and psychological cues that appear to increase during middle age. There is some evidence to support the notion that thinking about disease leads to more thoughts about susceptibility (PV) and severity (PS; Millar & Millar, 1995).

The weight for severity (PS_{w2}) should also be relatively low during young adulthood because severe illness is uncommon, then increase during midlife and old age. However, perceptions of severity might be tempered by the efficacy of procedures to detect disease in its early stages. This conclusion is supported in the cancer screening literature in which susceptibility, benefits, and barriers were significant predictors of compliance with screening mammography but not severity (Aiken, West, Woodward, Reno, & Reynolds, 1994). Similarly, in another study of adherence, Champion and Miller (1996) found that severity did not predict adherence and nonadherence.

In a comprehensive review of studies that used the health beliefs model, Janz and Becker (1984) found that barriers were the best overall predictors of compliance. The implication was that barriers outweighed benefits. However, from a life-span perspective we might hypothesize that benefits increase with age, peak during midlife and decrease slightly in old age. Thus, prevention and early detection are major factors in controlling disease in midlife and might decrease somewhat with old age. Therefore, the benefits of being proactive in health are more advantageous in midlife than in youth, when the body is relatively disease-free, or in old age, when disease already might be present.

The difference between benefits and barriers ($PB - PC_{w3}$) should decrease during midlife and then gradually increase in old age. First, if barriers are consistent predictors of health behaviors and some increasing effect of benefits occurs in midlife, then the difference between the two would be less in midlife based on the strength of benefits, the general health of the midlife population, and the resources available to them. Thus, the overall impact of benefits at midlife offsets the barriers, such as physical, economic, and convenience, to a greater extent than it does in younger years, when the benefits are not apparent and the inconvenience is great, and old age when the benefits are not as great and the barriers are very salient.

The HBM provides a conceptual template for understanding the shift in health consciousness in midlife. Internal and external health cues provide impetus for more thought about disease detection, and a feeling of vulnerability begins to emerge in midlife that, in turn, might lead to a greater focus on health behaviors. Finally, the increase in health consciousness varies considerably based on individual differences reviewed earlier in this chapter.

SUMMARY

The intent of this chapter has been to explore in a life-span perspective the unique phenomena that are characteristic of adulthood. Most people in early adulthood report excellent health, with increasing age people become more aware of internal biological cues, external cues such as from the media and the environment in general. Those cues are interpreted with respect to their salience for well-being. This shift in health consciousness might be understood by using the health beliefs model in a life-span perspective, which emphasizes increased perceptions of vulnerability to disease and the evaluation of the benefits of certain health protective behaviors. Whereas the health beliefs model might help set the stage for the cognitive shift in midlife, actual health behaviors also might be determined by a number of individual difference variables, such as education, income, lifestyle, heredity, cohort, locus of control, self-efficacy, and hardiness.

REFERENCES

Aiken, L. S.,West, S. G., Woodward, C. K., Reno, R. R., & Reynolds, K. D. (1994). Increasing screening mammography in asymptomatic women: Evaluation of a second-generation, theory-based program. *Health Psychology, 13*, 526–538.

Baltes, P. B. (1993). The aging mind: Potential and limits. *The Gerontologist, 33*, 580–594.

Baltes, P. B., & Baltes, M. M. (Eds.). (1990). *Successful aging: Perspectives from the behavioral sciences.* Cambridge, England: Cambridge University Press.

Bandura, A. (1990). Perceived self-efficacy in the exercise of control over AIDS infection. *Evaluation and Program Planning, 13*, 9–17.

Bandura, A. (1997). *Self-efficacy: The exercise of control.* New York: Freeman.

Belloc, N. (1973). Relationship of health practices and mortality. *Preventive Medicine, 2*, 67–81.

Bernard, L. C., & Krupat, E. (1994). *Health psychology.* New York: Harcourt Brace.

Borland, R., Owen, N., Hill, D., & Schofields, P. (1991). Predicting attempts and sustained cessation of smoking after the introduction of workplace smoking bans. *Health Psychology, 10*, 336–342.

Brandon, J. E., & Loftin, J. M. (1991). Relationship of fitness to depression, state and trait anxiety, internal health locus of control, and self-control. *Perception and Motor Skills, 73*, 563–568.

Breslow, L., & Enstrom, J. E. (1980). Persistence of health habits and their relationship to mortality. *Preventive Medicine, 9*, 469–483.

Cavanaugh, J. C. (1997). *Adult development and aging.* Pacific Grove, CA: Brooks/Cole.

Champion, V., & Miller A. M. (1996). Recent mammography in women aged 35 and older: Predisposing variables. *Health Care for Women International, 17*, 233–245.

Crandall, R. C. (1991). *Gerontology: A behavioral science approach.* New York: McGraw-Hill.

Flammer, A. (1995). Developmental analysis of control beliefs. In A. Bandura (Ed.), *Self-efficacy and changing societies* (pp. 69–113). New York: Cambridge University Press.

Fromme, K., Katz, E. C., & Rivet, K. (1997). Outcome expectancies and risk-taking behavior. *Cognitive Therapy and Research, 21*, 421–442.

Fruin, D. J., Pratt, C., & Owen, N. (1992). Protection Motivation Theory and adolescents' perceptions of exercise. *Journal of Applied Social Psychology, 22*, 55–69.

Funk, S. (1992). Hardiness: A review of theory and research. *Health Psychology, 11*, 335–345.

Funk, S., & Huston, B. K. (1987). A critical analysis of the Hardiness Scale's validity and utility. *Journal of Personality and Social Psychology, 53*, 572–578.

Harman, D. (1992). Free radical theory of aging. *Mutation Research, 275*, 257–266.

Hayflick, L. (1994). *How and why we age.* New York: Ballantine Books.

Heckhausen, J., & Baltes, P. B. (1991). Perceived controllability of expected psychological change across adulthood and old age. *Journal of Gerontology: Psychological Sciences, 46*, 165–173.

Hogan, D. P., & Astone, N. M. (1986). The transition to adulthood. *Annual Review of Sociology, 12*, 109–130.

Hull, J. G., Van Treuren, R. R., & Virnelli, S. (1987). Hardiness and health: A critique and alternative approach. *Journal of Personality and Social Psychology, 53*, 518–530.

Janz, N. K., & Becker, M. H. (1984). The health belief model: A decade later. *Health Education Quarterly, 11*, 1–47.

Kail, R. V., & Cavanaugh, J. C. (1996). *Human development*. Pacific Grove, CA: Brooks/Cole.

Kaplan, G., Burell, V., & Lusky, A. (1988). Subjective state of health and survival in elderly adults. *Journal of Gerontology, 43*, 5114–5120.

Kaplan, G. A., Seeman, T. E., Cohen, R. D., Knudsen, L. P., & Guralnik, J. (1987). Mortality among the elderly in the Alameda County study: Behavioral and demographic risk factors. *American Journal of Public Health, 77*, 307–312.

Kobasa, S. (1979a). Personality and resistance to illness. *American Journal of Community Psychology, 7*, 413–423.

Kobasa, S. (1979b). Stressful life events, personslity, and health: An inquiry into hardiness. *Journal of Personality and Social Psychology, 37*, 1–11.

Kobasa, S. C., Maddi, S. R., & Courington, S. (1981). Personality and exercise as buffers in the stress-illness relationship. *Journal of Behavioral Medicine, 5*, 391–404.

Kok, G., Den Boer, D. J., De Vries, H., Gerards, F., Hospers, H. J., & Mudde, A. N. (1992). Self-efficacy and attributional theory in health education. In R. Schwarzer (Ed.), *Self-efficacy: Thought control of action* (pp. 245–262). Washington DC: Hemisphere.

Lachman, M. E., & James, J. B. (Eds.). (1997). *Multiple paths of mid-life development*. Chicago: University of Chicago Press.

Medley, M. L. (1980). Life satisfaction across four stages of adult life. *International Journal of Aging and Human Development, 11*, 193–209.

Merluzzi, T. V., & Martinez Sanchez, M. (1997). Assessment of self-efficacy and coping with cancer: Development and validation of the Cancer Behavior Inventory. *Health Psychology, 16*, 163–170.

Millar, M. G., & Millar, K. U. (1995). Spontaneous responses to thinking about disease detection and health promotion behaviors. *Social Behavior and Personality, 23*, 191–198.

Neugarten, B., & Hagestad, G. G. (1976). Age and the life course. In R. H. Binstock & E. Shanas (Eds.), *Handbook of aging and the social sciences* (pp. 35–55). New York: Van Nostrand Reinhold.

O'Leary, A., Shoor, S., Loring, K., & Holman, H. R. (1988) A cognitive-behavioral treatment for rheumatoid arthritis. *Health Psychology, 7*, 527–544.

Palmore, E. B. (1986). Trends in the health of the aged. *The Gerontologist, 16*, 298–302.

Perlmutter, M., & Hall, E. (1992). *Adult development and aging*. New York: Wiley.

Prochaska, J. O., & DiClemente, C. C. (1992). Stages of change in the modification of problem behaviors. In M. Hersen, R. M. Eisler, & P. M. Miller (Eds.), *Progress in behavior modification* (vol. 28, pp. 184–218). Terre Haute: Sycamore.

Quadrel, M. J., & Lau, R. R. (1989). Health promotion, health locus of control, and health behavior: Two field experiments. *Journal of Applied Social Psychology, 19*, 1497–1521.

Resnick, R. J., & Rozensky, R. H. (Eds.). (1996). *Health psychology through the life span*. Washington, DC: American Psychological Association.

Rosenstock, I. (1974). The health beliefs model and preventive health behavior. *Health Education Monographs, 2*, 354–386.

Ross, C. E., & Wu, C. (1996). Education, age, and the cumulative advantage in health. *Journal of Health and Social Behavior, 37*, 104–120.

Rotter, J. B. (1966). Generalized expectancies for internal versus external control of reinforcement. *Psychological monographs, 80*, 1–28.

Schwarzer, R. (1992). Self-efficacy in the adiption and maintenance of health behaviors: Theoretical approaches and a new model. In R. Schwarzer (Ed.), *Self-efficacy: Thought control of action* (pp. 217–243). Washington DC: Hemisphere.

Siebold, D. R., & Roper, R. E. (1979). Psychosocial determinants of health care intentions: Test of the Triandis and Fishbein models. In D. Nimmo (Ed.), *Communications yearbook* (vol 3. pp. 625–643). New Brunswick, NJ: Transaction Books.

Siegler, I. C. (1997). Promoting health and minimizing stress in mid-life. In M. E. Lachman & J. B. James (Eds.), *Multiple paths of mid-life development.* Chicago: University of Chicago Press.

Sheehy, G. (1976). *Passages.* New York: E. P. Dutton & Co.

Sheehy, G. (1995). *New passages.* New York: Ballantine Books.

Skinner, E. A. (1995). *Perceived control, motivation, and coping.* Thousand Oaks, CA: Sage.

Stotland, S., & Zuroff, D. C. (1991). Relations between multiple measures of dieting self-efficacy and weight change in a behavioral weight control program. *Behavior Therapy, 22,* 47–59.

Strickland, B. R. (1979). Internal-external expectancies and health-related behaviors. *Journal of Consulting and Clinical Psychology, 46,* 1192–1211.

Taylor, S. E. (1989). *Positive illusions: Creative self-deception and the healthy mind.* New York: Basic Books.

Taylor, S. E. (1995). *Health psychology* (3rd ed.). New York: McGraw-Hill.

Taylor, S. E., & Brown, J. D. (1988). Illusion and well-being: A social psychological perspective on mental health. *Psychological Bulletin, 103,* 193–210.

Tinsley, B. J., & Holtgrave, D. R. (1989). Maternal health locus of control beliefs, utilization of childhood preventive health services, and infant health. *Journal of Developmental and Behavioral Pediatrics, 10,* 236–241.

Toshima, M. T., Kaplan, R. M., & Ries, A. L. (1992). Self-efficacy expectancies in chronic obstructive pulmonary disease rehabilitation. In R. Schwarzer (Ed.), *Self-efficacy: Thought control of action* (pp. 325–354). London: Hemisphere.

United States Department of Health and Human Services. (1990). *Health United States 1989.* (DHHS Publ. No. PHS 90–1232). Washington, DC: U.S. Government Printing Office.

United State Department of Health and Human Services. (1994). *Vital statistics of the U.S., 1991. Vol. 2: Mortality.* Hyattsville, MD: U.S. Public Health Service.

Verbrugge, L. M. (1994). Disability in late life. In R. P. Abeles, H. C. Gift, & M. G. Ory (Eds.), *Aging and quality of life* (pp. 30–95). New York: Springer.

Waller, K., & Bates, R. C. (1992). Health locus of control and self-efficacy beliefs in a healthy elderly sample. *American Journal of Health Promotion, 6,* 302–309.

Wulfert, S. K., & Wan, C. K. (1993). Condom use: A self-efficacy model. *Health Psychology, 12,* 346–353.

Zautra, A. J., Okun, M. A., Roth, S. H., & Emmanual, J. (1989). Life stress and lymphocyte alterations among patients with rheumatoid arthritis. *Health Psychology, 8,* 1–14.

Ziff, M. A., Conrad, P., & Lachman, M. E. (1995). The relative effects of perceived personal control and responsibility on health and health related behaviors in young and middle-aged adults. *Health Education Quarterly, 22,* 127–142.

II

Resiliency in Later Life

C. S. Bergeman
K. A. Wallace
University of Notre Dame

EARLIER IN this century, acute infectious conditions were the major causes of death. In contrast, conditions such as heart disease, cancer, and stroke are the leading causes of morbidity and mortality in the late 1990s. Accompanying this shift, a new emphasis is being placed on chronic illness and disability and on understanding the complex interactions among social, psychological, and biological factors that contribute to health and well-being in later life (Ory, Abeles, & Lipman, 1992). The decrease in mortality over the latter part of this century has also resulted in an increase in life expectancy and a significant growth in the ageband known as the *oldest old.* Recent predictions indicate that the age group of 75 years and older will increase by 76% in the 1990s alone (U.S. Bureau of the Census, 1991). This rate of increase is expected to continue, with the largest expansion predicted between 2010 and 2030 as the "baby boom" generation reaches age 65 (American Association of Retired Persons, 1987).

Not only has the number of older individuals in the population increased, but research has also indicated that people age differently (Bergeman, 1997). Age-related diseases and physiological changes that we have come to think of as a part of normal aging do not occur in the same way for all people, nor do all individuals necessarily experience identical changes as they reach a given age (Dannefer & Sell, 1988). As a group, older people are more diverse than younger people in health, psychological functioning, and dimensions of social interaction (Nelson & Dannefer, 1992). As a result, the members of a cohort are thought to "fan out" as they age, becoming increasingly dissimilar for any given characteristic (Baltes, 1979).

A review of the behavioral genetic literature indicates that both genetic and environmental influences contribute to this diversity (Bergeman, 1997). There is also a growing consensus that the environmental influences contributing to individual differences in the aging process are related to the experience of life events (Murrell,

Norris, & Grote, 1988). Individuals who experience life events as stressful often have more physical health problems (Adler & Matthews, 1994), higher levels of depression, and lower levels of life satisfaction (George, 1989). Other individuals, however, manage to maintain high self-esteem, good physical health, and a positive outlook on life despite facing the same adversities that lead others to give up, get sick, or lose hope. Why do some people age more optimally than others? Why do some older people thrive in the face of adversity? What are the turning points that change an individual's developmental trajectory and which qualities result in more optimal outcomes? How do these qualities develop and how do they change across the life course?

   This chapter identifies psychosocial attributes that promote stress resistance and resiliency in later life as well as the factors and processes that are important for the development of intervention and prevention strategies targeted at older individuals. This discussion is based on the notion that individuals who overcome the risks and challenges associated with aging and an increased number of life experiences may have important resources of resilience that promote more optimal outcomes in later life. More generally, these resilience factors may influence the way in which one perceives life events (e.g., as stressful or nonstressful), or they may facilitate the coping process used to expedite recovery after the experience of an adverse event. To examine resiliency in later life, this chapter is organized in three sections. First, resiliency is defined from a life-span developmental perspective. Second, potential resilience factors are identified and considered in terms of their relations with physical health and psychological well-being. The discussion of the individual attributes includes speculation on the ways in which each contributes to the underlying process of resiliency and thus produces more optimal health outcomes in later life. The chapter concludes with a model depicting the multidimensional nature of resiliency and a discussion of the etiology and developmental nature of specific protective mechanisms.

LIFE-SPAN DEVELOPMENTAL PERSPECTIVE

The search for the protective mechanisms that underlie resiliency and stress resistance in late adulthood is theoretically based in a life-span developmental perspective. From this perspective, development is viewed as a dynamic and continuous interplay between growth (gain) and decline (loss). Rather than viewing development as a period of growth during young adulthood followed by a decline in the last three quarters of the life span, *development* is defined as any change in the adaptive capacity of an organism, whether positive or negative (Baltes, 1987). This perspective also suggests that there is much intraindividual plasticity (within-person variability); thus, even in later life, individuals have the potential for different developmental trajectories and can improve and modify their adaptive capacity (Baltes, Reese, & Nesselroade, 1988). Because knowledge of the range and limits of intraindividual functioning is a cornerstone of the life-span perspective, this perspective conveys the dynamic and developmental nature of aging, with a primary focus on aging as a process, not just as an outcome at the end of life (Lachman & Baltes, 1994). Using the life-span perspective as a framework, this chapter not only demonstrates the link between various resilience mechanisms and more optimal outcomes, but speculates on the processes that underlie this link.

Plasticity, resiliency, and reserve capacity are important concepts in understanding the antecedents and sequelae that influence the course of adaptation in human behavior. *Plasticity* is an index of the potential for change and an indicator of how flexible or robust an individual might be in dealing with life's challenges and demands (Staudinger, Marsiske, & Baltes, 1993). An individual's degree of plasticity is determined by his or her reserve capacity or resiliency. *Resiliency* refers to latent resources that can be activated in times of stress to aid in returning to a previous state after a stress or trauma. *Reserve capacity* is an expansion of resilience that includes resources that promote growth beyond a previous level of functioning. The ability to activate these existing internal (e.g., attributes of personality) and external (e.g., social support) resources, in turn, serves to protect the individual in times of stress (Rutter, 1987). The next section provides an overview of possible resilience mechanisms and a description of how these mechanisms might produce more optimal outcomes in later life.

PROTECTIVE FACTORS, RESILIENCE, AND OPTIMAL AGING

Previous researchers have suggested that protective factors fall into two broad areas (see Fig. 11.1): individual factors and familial/community support factors (Garmezy, 1985; Rutter, 1987). Individual factors include dispositional attributes of the individual, such as personality. For example, individuals who are open to new experiences are better able to adapt to change; similarly, individuals who exhibit behavioral flexibility are likely to have a greater repertoire of coping mechanisms to deal with stressful or disadvantageous conditions. Although it should be noted that the resilience mechanisms or protective factors in the "individual factors" domain are not necessarily limited to these dimensions, three possible reserve resources are explored in this chapter, including self-concept, control, and hardiness.[1] The second dimension, *familial and community support factors*, refers to affectional ties between family members that provide support in times of stress (e.g., a cohesive family environment), as well as supports that come from outside of the family, including friends, community organizations (e.g., club memberships, church), and socioeconomic factors.

---

[1]The conceptualization of cognitive functioning as a resilience resource has been described in detail elsewhere and is not discussed further here (see Staudinger et al., 1993).

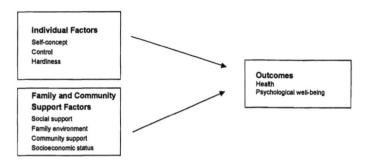

FIG. 11.1. Individual and familial and community support factors that are suggested to work as resilience mechanisms in later life.

Although previous research on resiliency has been focused primarily on earlier
segments of the life span, protective factors are hypothesized to be applicable to developmental processes in later life as well. A brief review of research on each of
these components, including the proposed mechanisms by which each may promote more optimal outcomes in later life, is provided.

Individual Factors

Self-Concept. A review of the literature on self-concept suggests that more
optimal outcomes in later life are positively related to how well one plans and engages in socialization (Carstensen, 1992), selects age-friendly environments (Lawton, 1982), optimizes certain skills, compensates for the loss of others (Baltes &
Baltes, 1990), and engages in a successful life review (Butler, 1963). Each of these
processes, in turn, can be tied to a view of self-concept. *Self-concept* is regarded as a
multifaceted and dynamic entity that integrates an individual's experiences across
time, catalyzes action, and provides continuity and meaning to those experiences
(Markus & Herzog, 1991). As such, it is a primary component of all aspects of psychological experience, including emotion, well-being, motivation, control, efficacy, and competence.

A number of the functions of the self-concept provide potential insights into
the process by which self-concept works as a resilience mechanism (Markus &
Herzog, 1991). Three of these mechanisms—life review, possible selves, and selective social comparison—are discussed here. First, the self-concept provides organization to one's life experiences and a sense of coherence and continuity across diverse life experiences. Often referred to as the *life review,* this complex process of
self-regulation encompasses the reconstruction, explanation, and evaluation of the
past, and as such is a rich resource for the restoration of psychological balance in
the face of life transitions (Butler, 1963). Because the self-concept is an integral
component of emotional control and affect regulation, evaluation of one's life history as well as the various components of one's life can be used to enhance self-

esteem. For example, if the sense of self is threatened in interpersonal relations, a person may focus on career strengths to bolster his or her self-concept.

Second, what has been referred to as *possible selves* refers to what one thinks about oneself in the past, what one knows about oneself in the present, and what one believes is possible for oneself in the future. Self-concept from this perspective may also be viewed as a resource to protect the individual because it serves as a motivational source and is linked to goals that are strived for or are to be avoided (for more detail, see Markus & Nurius, 1986). Third, people can maintain their self-evaluation through *selective social comparison;* that is, as life changes, people find new points of comparison to help them reorganize their standards or values (Paulus & Christie, 1981). For example, an individual who loses a spouse may know others who have experienced the same, or worse. Comparing him or herself to these "others" helps promote and maintain a sense of self. Consequently, the selection of an appropriate comparison group is an important mechanism that empowers an elderly individual to manage the gains and losses of old age.

Although little research has explicitly tested the ways in which self-concept acts as a resilience factor, research does indicate that there are significant relations between a positive self-concept and physical and mental health outcomes in later life (Markus & Herzog, 1991). For example, after a heart attack or other serious illness, an individual might be forced to change aspects of his/her lifestyle. Such changes may invoke new self-schemas, or perceptions of the self, that are relevant to maintaining reasonable health. As a result, an individual may now view him or herself as able to maintain a regular medical regimen. This positive sense of self can result in changes in diet and exercise, and in obtaining routine health examinations. Thus, people with a positive self-concept are motivated to follow health-promoting practices, thereby improving health (Markus & Herzog, 1991).

Control and Self-Efficacy. Control has been defined in a number of ways (see Skinner, 1996), but generally reflects the extent to which individuals think they can take charge of their lives, including the ability to bring about desired outcomes through their own efficacy (Lachman, Ziff, & Spiro, 1994). Many older individuals report a decrease in objective and subjective control (Heckhausen & Schulz, 1995), and this loss has been associated with functional impairment (Duffy & MacDonald, 1990), cardiovascular disease (Engel, 1978), cancer (Schmale & Iker, 1971), deterioration of the immune system (Rodin, 1986), and mortality (Wolinsky & Johnson, 1992). A sense of control, on the other hand, is a robust predictor of psychological well-being (e.g., achievement, optimism, motivation, personal adjustment) and good physical health (Baltes & Baltes, 1986; Skinner, 1996).

Perceptions of control, or feelings of self-efficacy, may function to promote resilience for several reasons. First, control beliefs foster health and well-being (or conversely lead to disease and depression) by influencing whether actions are taken to prevent or remedy health problems. For instance, perceptions of control might affect the extent to which an individual gathers health-related information, engages in self-care behaviors, is active in interactions with medical providers, or shows compliance with medical regimens. More specifically, self-judgments of efficacy determine a person's choice of behaviors, such as a reduction in alcohol consumption or the cessation of cigarette smoking.

Second, control may affect physical and mental health through its impact on physiological functioning. Efforts to link loss of control and physiological processes have indicated that giving up in response to situations of loss may affect changes in the neuroendocrine system, which may lead to the development of illness. For example, research has indicated that catecholamines and corticosteroids increase when individuals are confronted with uncontrollable situations (Rodin, Timko, & Harris, 1985). An increase in these hormones, in turn, has been related to coronary disease (via increased blood pressure and heart rate, elevation of blood lipids, and changes in the regulation of the metabolism of cholesterol) and to the suppression of the immune system.

A third way in which perceptions of control can influence health is their impact on whether an event is appraised as stressful (Rodin et al., 1985). That is, uncontrollable life events are often more stressful than controllable ones. Perceiving an event as controllable increases the predictability of the event, which, in turn, has a positive effect on psychological well-being and health. Related to the effects of control on the appraisal of the stressfulness of an event is the link between control and health through the labeling of symptoms (Rodin & Timko, 1992). In studies using experimental manipulations, participants with perceptions of little or no control over life events reported more physical symptoms than those who felt more in control (Matthews, Scheier, Brunson & Carducci, 1980). As a result of this type of research, it has been suggested that a loss of control caused by situational changes related to aging (e.g., retirement) elicits bodily preoccupation, symptom monitoring, and an entrance into the "sick role" (Rodin & Timko, 1992).

Variability in preference for control also changes with age; that is, people differ in their desire for personal control, and there are some conditions in which perceived control is more likely to induce stress than to have a beneficial impact. In addition, it has been speculated that in situations in which having control produces stress, the negative effects may have a greater impact on older adults (Rodin & Timko, 1992). In their review of research, Rodin and Timko (1992) also indicated that medical patients whose treatments offer options congruent with their control beliefs show the best psychological and physical adjustment. This type of relation is exemplified by research-assessing factors that are important in the recovery from heart attacks (Cromwell, Butterfield, Brayfield, & Curry, 1977).

Similar to the idea of congruency, researchers have posited a theory of person–environment fit, which predicts that the fit or match between the characteristics of an individual and the characteristics of that person's environment, is important for more optimal outcomes in later life (Conway, Vickers, & French, 1992). Thus, a critical issue of control in later life involves the goodness-of-fit between one's perception of control and one's desire for control (Wallace & Bergeman, 1997). In this study, *person* was conceptualized as an individual's desire to have control (i.e., the extent to which an individual is motivated to control the events in his/her life); *environment* was defined in terms of perceptions of actual control (i.e., belief in the ability to bring about certain outcomes). Results indicated that the fit between desired and perceived control was a significant predictor of self-reported health and well-being in later life above and beyond the main effects of desired and perceived control.

Hardiness. Another way to characterize resiliency is through a dispositional characteristic such as hardiness, a trait that has its theoretical basis in existential personality theory (Kobasa & Maddi, 1977). Researchers have identified three main dimensions underlying the hardy personality style, including commitment, control, and challenge. *Commitment* refers to a belief in oneself and the value of one's activities (Kobasa, 1982), which helps prevent alienation from the self and the outside world. *Control*, as described previously, is the extent to which one sees oneself as influential in bringing about certain outcomes, whereas *challenge* involves an openness to experience that is characterized by the acceptance of change as a normal part of life and as necessary for growth (Kobasa, Maddi, & Kahn, 1982). Although the majority of hardiness researchers have focused on young and middle-aged samples, the concept of the hardy personality may be especially relevant in later life. In particular, the idea of the hardy personality style as a dispositional resilience (Bartone, Ursano, Wright, & Ingraham, 1989) may begin to explain the reasons some individuals age more optimally than others (Magnani, 1990).

Although main effects for the importance of hardiness on physical health have been extensively reported (Kobasa, 1982), hardiness was first conceptualized to buffer the negative effects of stress on health (Kobasa, 1979). As a buffer or moderator, the effect of hardiness (i.e., hardy vs. nonhardy) was expected to be different depending on the levels of stress (i.e., high stress vs. low stress); specifically, the difference between hardy and nonhardy individuals should be greater in high, rather than low, stress situations. Despite the original moderator conceptualization, the empirical support for such an effect has been inconclusive. A concurrent moderation effect on reported physical health was found for male executives (Kahn, 1987) and for women with higher education (Rhodewalt & Zone, 1989). Similarly, a prospective moderation effect on reported physical health was found for managers (Kobasa, Maddi, & Kahn, 1982). In contrast, no support for the buffer hypothesis was found for female undergraduates, although a possible ceiling effect was noted in this sample (Schlosser, 1986). No research to date has tested the buffer hypothesis using a sample of older adults.

Because the importance of hardiness has not been rigorously investigated in an older population, an important first step is to determine whether the theoretical conceptualization of hardiness (including the proposed components of commitment, challenge, and control) is commensurate in a sample of elderly individuals and to assess whether hardiness plays a similar role in directly promoting more positive outcomes in later life. A recent study suggests that the theoretical components deemed essential in samples of young and middle-aged adults (commitment, control, and challenge) were also necessary in a sample of older adults. In addition, hardiness was significantly related to self-reported physical health and psychological well-being, and as such may be an important component of stress resistance in later life (Wallace & Bergeman, 1997).

Hardiness may work to promote health and well-being in a number of ways. Most simply, dispositional resilience may affect the way in which individuals appraise their physical and psychological health. Aspects of hardiness also may influence the interpretation of an event (e.g., as stressful or nonstressful), and the imaginative ways the individual confronts or copes with events appraised as stressful (Kobasa, Maddi, Puccetti, & Zola, 1985). Another question is whether hardy people experience fewer life events or appraise their events differently than individuals who are low in hardiness (Orr & Westman, 1990). The research, although limited, appears to support the latter (Kobasa et al., 1982). Furthermore, Kobasa and colleagues theorized that hardiness affects stress via transformational coping, including the process of stress appraisal and problem-solving strategies: Hardy people use coping mechanisms to decrease emotional strain; emotional well-being then decreases physiological strain, which in turn decreases the impact on physical health (Kobasa et al., 1985). Finally, researchers have looked for physiological differences (blood pressure, finger pulse amplitude, heart rate, and skin conductance) between hardy and nonhardy individuals during a stressful situation (Allred & Smith, 1989). Compelling evidence surfaced that hardy individuals have lower levels of these physical indicators of stress (e.g., blood pressure, and heart rate) after or during recovery than during the actual stress-inducing task. This finding suggests that hardy individuals may recover more quickly from stressful situations and as a result may have fewer negative outcomes.

Not only are there differences in the appraisal of life events as stressful, but hardy people may also be better able to mobilize resources that decrease the negative effects of stress on physical, psychological, or social health. Hardiness has been associated with a variety of coping strategies. For example, recruiting social support (a resistance resource) may be one way hardy people transform a negative event. Also, the quality of the support network is more closely related to hardiness than is the size of the support network, but research has not addressed how this relation relates to health and well-being in later life (Orr & Westman, 1990). Consequently, the amount of support is not important, but what is important is whether it is viewed as beneficial. This is discussed in detail in the next section.

Familial and Community Support Factors

Social Support.   Many attributes associated with resiliency and aging (e.g., self-concept, hardiness) involve mobilizing social resources in times of stress; thus it is not surprising that strong relations have been found between aspects of social support and physical and mental health. *Social support* refers to the provision and receipt of tangible (e.g., help when ill) and intangible (e.g., advice, companionship, and emotional support) goods, services, and benefits. Objective reports of social support reflect the frequency of a specific supportive transaction, whereas measures of subjective support portray the perceived adequacy or satisfaction with the quality or amount of support. A review of the research on the social support–health outcome relation indicates that there is a consistent positive relation between social support from family, friends, and neighbors and physical health, mental health, and mortality, even when the effects of socioeconomic status (SES), initial health status, and health practices are statistically controlled (for a review, see George, 1989; Schulz & Rau, 1985; Shumaker & Czajkowski, 1994). Research also indicates a direct effect of social ties (including both the quantity and quality of social support) on neuroendocrine function, although the relation is stronger for males than for females (Seeman, Berkman, Blazer, & Rowe, 1994).

The influence of social support on health can be direct (e.g., support members provide transportation to doctor appointments) or indirect (e.g., family or friends provide emotional support that mitigates the influence of a stressful life event). This latter type of influence has been a primary focus of social support research and has been called the *buffer hypothesis*. Proponents of the buffer hypothesis have suggested that social support serves a protective role, primarily during times of stress, through an enhancement of adaptive coping strategies. More specifically, Cohen (1988) suggested that social support can buffer the adverse effects of stress in four ways: First, friends and neighbors can provide older individuals with information (the network provides stress-buffering information that results in a benign appraisal of events or in an increased ability to cope with stress); second, support networks can enhance older individual's sense of identity or self-esteem (increasing feelings of self-worth and control can influence both appraisal and coping abilities); third, pressure by a social network can catalyze the adoption of normative coping behaviors; and finally, support providers can make tangible resources available or can provide aid that facilitates coping behaviors.

Unfortunately, not all support is beneficial; both benefits and liabilities are associated with a strong support network. Excessive support can sometimes lower autonomy, self-reliance, or feelings of control, and may result in feelings of helplessness (Krause, 1990). Moreover, helping behaviors may be effective only if they satisfy the needs created by a particular stressor (Cutrona, Russell, & Rose, 1986; Krause, 1990). Thus, for a support network to provide adequate support, members of the support group must have the ability, knowledge, and motivation to meet a person's support needs (Schulz & Rau, 1985).

Additionally, providing support to others might be as important as receiving social support. The inability to reciprocate may lead to feelings of dependence, which, in turn, might diminish feelings of well-being among older adults. One way that older individuals use social resources optimally is to have a support "reserve" they can draw on in times of need (Antonucci & Jackson, 1987). The ability of older people to provide support to others may allow them to ask for support in return. That is, elderly individuals may feel that providing support to others enables them to accumulate "credit" toward receiving future support for themselves.

Family Environment. Contrary to the notion that Americans are abandoning their elders, network size and frequency of contact with close kin remains relatively stable across the life span (Schulz & Rau, 1985). A review of the literature in this area leads to the inescapable conclusion that family support can facilitate the effective functioning and health of older adults (Antonucci & Jackson, 1987; Carstensen, 1993). Generally, older people turn first to family members for emotional and social support and for crisis intervention because they are more likely than anyone else to help in times of need (Carstensen, 1993). For example, the availability of support from a spouse or from children is the most important factor keeping older individuals out of institutions (Hanson & Sauer, 1985). In addition, older siblings may experience a renewed emotional closeness with one another (Cicirelli, 1989), oftentimes as a result of the normative losses associated with aging (e.g., death of a spouse), which in turn enhances their own self-esteem. Although little research has addressed the significance of a cohesive family environment beyond the importance of the supportive relationships just described, the characteristics of the family environment also may be meaningful in later life. Researchers have found that family interactions marked by warmth and cohesion promote resiliency in children (Masten & Garmezy, 1985). In addition to a supportive family milieu, an extended community support system is also an important protective factor for helping children become stress-resilient (Rutter, 1987).

Community Support. Researchers often overlook the importance of formal (e.g., home health care agencies) and community support networks (e.g., church groups; club memberships) for promoting more optimal outcomes in later life (Krause, 1990). Formal support may be important in later life because many elderly individuals do not want to receive support from family and friends unless they can provide support in return (Lee, 1985). That is, the failure or inability to reciprocate when support is provided may lead to feelings of dependency and a loss of autonomy. As a result, aging individuals may prefer to receive aid from a formal (versus more informal) support network, which tends not to be bound by the issue of reciprocity (e.g., when services are purchased).

Consequently, formal support networks do not necessarily replace informal ones, but rather they complement them; older individuals who have support from a variety of sources may have more resources with which to deal with life's adverse circumstances. Therefore, assessments of community involvement are very important. Measures of these interactions not only provide information concerning the potential for supportive interactions but also reflect level of activity and embeddedness in the larger community. Because social integration results in enhanced coping skills and thus provides an increase in social relationships outside the family, social integration through involvement in voluntary organizations or church attendance may result in better health outcomes. Conversely, a lack of social integration can result in role loss, which may affect feelings of self-worth. Additional research in this area is needed to explicate the relations between formal support, informal support, and community involvement and to assess how these influences relate to health outcomes in later life.

Financial Assets and SES. One final dimension associated with better physical health and psychological well-being is SES. Social status in general, and financial resources in particular, are important to perceptions of well-being, either because they contribute directly to quality of life, or because their effects are indirect, via social activities or health (George, 1990). Additionally, SES, especially indicators such as education and income, are strongly related to physical health (George, 1996). Social status may be associated with health due to related exposure to stress, access to quality health care, or associated coping resources.

THE MULTIDIMENSIONAL NATURE OF RESILIENCE

The first step in understanding the resilience process in later life is to move beyond the identification of broadly based protective factors to focus on the developmental and situational mechanisms involved in developing these protective processes (Rutter, 1987). In pursuit of this goal, the previous discussion of each of the individual and familial or community support factors included possible mechanisms and processes through which each attribute may contribute to more optimal health outcomes. In brief, the self-concept serves an overarching function that evaluates and synthesizes the gains and losses of old age. Evidence suggests that having a well-established feeling of one's own self-worth, as well as the confidence and conviction of being able to cope successfully with life's challenges is protective. These perceptions form another dimension of personality called *control* or *self-efficacy.*

The process by which control affects health is thought to occur in at least three ways. First, feelings of control or self-efficacy are related to whether individuals engage in health-promoting behaviors, including actions to prevent disease (e.g., smoking cessation) and promote health (e.g., exercising). Second, feelings of control, and, more specifically, a lack of control, can affect health through physiological mechanisms, such as the immunological or neuroendocrine systems. Finally, control can affect health through cognitive factors (the appraisal process), which, in turn, bias a person's awareness and reporting of stressful events and aspects of health. Hardiness is a multidimensional personality trait that in many ways incorporates aspects of both self-concept (commitment) and self-efficacy (control). An additional characteristic (challenge) adds a component of openness to experience and behavioral flexibility that may be especially important to resiliency in later life.

Hardiness, like control, is thought to affect the appraisal of stress and to be an important dimension in the mobilization of coping resources, such as social support.

Not suprisingly, a plethora of research indicates that social resources from family and friends can affect health directly through tangible aid (e.g., a ride to a doctor's appointment; the management of medications) or indirectly via emotional support. Additionally, a supportive family environment or being embedded in the larger community (e.g., church, voluntary organizations, or home health networks) can provide elders with many reserve resources with which to deal with life's ups and downs.

Assimilating the research in these broad domains reveals many similarities in how the individual resources of self-concept, control, and hardiness, for example, are thought to affect health-related behaviors, and ultimately health outcomes. In other words, it may be through the confluence of the individual and familial and community support factors just described that resiliency is achieved. The ways these factors interrelate is less clear, however. Do these dimensions have a cumulative influence, or is there an underlying attribute of the individual that is being indirectly assessed by these different measures? Do these factors produce better health outcomes through similar pathways, or are the mechanisms different? Research designed to test the interrelation among these factors, assessing their impact both individually and in harmony, is an important next step in the process of understanding resiliency in later life.

Figure 11.2 depicts one theoretical representation of the multidimensional nature of the resilience factors, and portrays several avenues through which the fac-

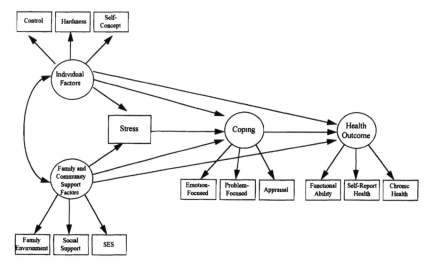

FIG. 11.2.   A theoretical model depicting the multidimensional nature of the resilience factors, the relations among these factors, and the possible avenues through which they contribute to more optimal health outcomes.

tors might produce optimal health outcomes in later life. In this model, resiliency factors are represented by the correlated latent variables of *individual resources,* which include personality dimensions such as hardiness, control, and self-concept, and *Familial and community support factors,* which refer to important influences associated with the family environment, with social support provided by friends and family, and with socioeconomic factors. Based on the research reviewed, this schematic is designed to depict the direct influence of these individual and support factors on stress (or perceived stress), coping behaviors (e.g., problem-focused, emotion-focused, and/or appraisal), and health outcomes (e.g., functional ability, self-reported health, and chronic health). The figure also illustrates an indirect effect of these resilience resources on coping through the intervening variable of stress and on outcome through stress and coping.

From this general model, a variety of hypotheses can be generated to test the influence of individual and social resources on health-related behaviors, physiological mechanisms, and, ultimately, health outcomes in later life. For instance, examples of research questions that this model might generate include the following: How do personality factors influence perceptions of stress, and how does this relation change depending on social support factors? What is the nature of these relations, taking into account the coping strategies that individuals use? How do each of these components contribute individually and in concert with other factors to promote positive health outcomes? Although a model of the type illustrated in Fig. 11.2 has not been tested explicitly, the evidence available from research using older populations suggests that protective processes include those that promote self-esteem or self-efficacy through the availability of secure and supportive personal relationships or successful task accomplishment. These dimensions, in turn, are likely to play key roles in the processes involved in people's response to stressful circumstances.

Although discussion of the multidimensional nature of the relations among the various resilience attributes is important, additional research is needed to explicate the developmental processes underlying these relations. That is, it is unlikely that successful or optimal aging begins in later life. Thus, to understand more fully how these factors work as resilience mechanisms, future research is needed to address questions such as the following: What permits some individuals to have social supports that they can use effectively in times of crisis? Why do some individuals perceive that they have control over their lives, and others do not? Is "hardiness" innate, or is it a personality characteristic that is learned from a lifetime of environmental interaction? Is it the "spin of the roulette wheel," inherent predispositions, or did prior circumstances or actions bring about this desirable state? The longitudinal assessment of resilience attributes (i.e., individual and social resources) will begin to answer questions about the *process* of aging, not just the *outcome* in later life. Empirical work is needed to assess how attributes such as a strong social network, feelings of self-efficacy and self-esteem, and personality attributes, such as hardiness, develop not only in later life but also across the entire life span.

THE ETIOLOGY OF RESILIENCE MECHANISMS

Although little research is available on the etiology of the resilience mechanisms proposed in this review, behavioral genetic studies have included these or related concepts. A brief overview of this research provides a foundation for understanding individual differences in resiliency factors. In the Individual Factors domain, research has assessed self-concept (McGue, Hirsch, & Lykken, 1993), control (Pedersen, Gatz, Plomin, Nesselroade, & McClearn, 1989), and aspects of personality related to hardiness (Bergeman et al., 1993). In the familial and community support area, behavioral genetic research has assessed the etiology of social support (Bergeman, Plomin, Pedersen, McClearn, & Nesselroade, 1990; Kessler, Kendler, Heath, Neale, & Eaves, 1992), family environment (Plomin, McClearn, Pedersen, Nesselroade, & Bergeman, 1988, 1989; Schaie & Willis, 1995), and SES (Lichtenstein, Hershberger, & Pedersen, 1995; Lichtenstein, Pedersen, & McClearn, 1992). In general, the results indicate that the resilience attributes discussed in this chapter are influenced by both genetic and environmental factors (for a review, see Bergeman, 1997). Interestingly, the experience of life events themselves also might reflect an inherent predisposition (Plomin, Lichtenstein, Pedersen, McClearn, & Nesselroade, 1990).

Consideration of genetic contributions to measures of environmental risks and protective factors suggests new ways of thinking about individual differences in later life. If environmental risks and protective factors show genetic influence, as do outcome measures, such as physical or mental health, then hereditary factors are likely to contribute to the correlations among them. For example, multivariate genetic analyses have been used to explore the etiology of the association between measures of social support and physical health (Lichtenstein & Pedersen, 1995) and psychological well-being in later life (Bergeman, Plomin, Pedersen, & McClearn, 1991; Kessler et al., 1992). Results consistently indicate that both genetic and nonshared environmental influences are important in the etiology of this relation. That is, the genetic influences that contribute to the perceived adequacy of the support network also contribute to the assessment of overall health, depressive symptoms, and life satisfaction.

That nonshared environmental influences also mediate the social support–physical health relation is not surprising. This result indicates that elements of the environment that are specific to an individual (and not to a twin pair) influence both the perception of the social support system and physical health. Schulz and Rau (1985) reviewed social support across the life span and provided examples of life course events that are related to aspects of social support. For example, life events, such as the death of a family member or close friend or a move to a new location, can reduce the number of individuals available for support; these same events are also likely to affect (or be affected by) overall health status (Bergeman et al., 1991). In summary, although much research is still needed in this area, the work to date indicates that individual differences for many of the protective mechanisms thought to produce more optimal outcomes in later life are due to both inherent and experiential factors. Research of this type affects the ways in which resilience factors are conceptualized in relation to outcomes and how prevention and intervention strategies are directed.

THE ROLE OF RESILIENCY IN PREVENTION AND INTERVENTION STRATEGIES

The purpose of the search for resilience mechanisms in later life is not to find qualities that make people feel good but to identify processes that protect individuals from adverse situations (Rutter, 1987). From the perspective of prevention, a favorable circumstance for promoting stress resistance is not necessarily a life without adversity, but more likely it is a life with graduated challenges that enhance the mastery of skills, flexible coping strategies, positive self-concept, and feelings of efficacy. Specifically, physiological studies suggest that inoculation against stress might be provided best by controlled exposure to stress in circumstances that are favorable to coping or adaptation. Because life involves unavoidable encounters with all types of stressors, it is unrealistic to assume that individuals who age "successfully" have led a life without adversity. Rather, protection probably lies in the safeguarding qualities that accrue from successful coping with life's stressors when the exposure is of a type and degree that is manageable in the context of the individual's capacities and social situation (Rutter, 1987).

The process by which resilience mechanisms promote more optimal outcomes in later life is important for intervention strategies as well. Some risk factors for disease are preventable (e.g., cigarette smoking) or modifiable (e.g., through diet or exercise), but others might not be (e.g., stressful life events). Because people age differently, however, not all intervention strategies will work for all people. Rather than trying to change specific behaviors, enhancing feelings of self-concept through strategies aimed at a life review or selecting an appropriate comparison group might be more advantageous. For some individuals, providing support from a variety of sources (e.g., family, friend, or community) might be important; for others, however, encouraging reciprocity of support may be the key to a successful intervention. It is important to identify target groups for intervention and to know who is at greatest risk or who can benefit most from specific interventions. Optimal health outcomes may result from the goodness-of-fit among the attributes of the individual (e.g., their individual factors, such as personality) and the aspects of the environment (familial and community support factors). Knowing how to best promote change requires knowledge of the developmental process linking risk and protective factors with optimal versus pathological aging (Masten & Garmezy, 1985).

REFERENCES

Adler, N., & Matthews, K. (1994). Health psychology: Why do some people get sick and some stay well? *Annual Review of Psychology, 45,* 229–259.

Allred, K. D., & Smith, T. W. (1989). The hardy personality: Cognitive and physiological responses to evaluative threat. *Journal of Personality and Social Psychology, 56,* 257–266.

American Association of Retired Persons. (1987). *A profile of older Americans.* Long Beach, CA: Author.

Antonucci, T. C., & Jackson, J. S. (1987). Social support, interpersonal efficacy, and health: A life course perspective. In L. L. Carstensen & B. A. Edelstein (Eds.), *Handbook of clinical gerontology* (pp. 291–311). New York: Pergamon.

Baltes, M. M., & Baltes, P. B. (1986). *The psychology of control and aging,* Hillsdale, NJ: Lawrence Erlbaum Associates.

Baltes, P. B. (1979). Life-span developmental psychology: Some converging observations on history and theory. In P. B. Baltes & O. G. Brim, Jr. (Eds.), *Life-span development and behavior* (vol. 2, pp. 256–279). New York: Academic Press.

Baltes, P. B. (1987). Theoretical propositions of life-span developmental psychology: On the dynamics between growth and decline. *Developmental Psychology, 23,* 611–626.

Baltes, P. B., & Baltes, M. M. (1990). Psychological perspectives on successful aging: The model of selective optimization with compensation. In P. B. Baltes & M. M. Baltes (Eds.), *Successful aging: Perspectives from the behavioral sciences,* (pp. 1–34). New York: Cambridge University Press.

Baltes, P. B., Reese, H. W., & Nesselroade, J. R. (1988). *Life-span developmental psychology: Introduction to research methods,* Hillsdale, NJ: Lawrence Erlbaum Associates.

Bartone, R. T., Ursano, R. J., Wright, K. M., & Ingraham, L. H. (1989). The impact of a military air disaster on the health of assistance workers: A prospective study. *The Journal of Nervous and Mental Disease, 177,* 317–328.

Bergeman, C. S. (1997). *Aging: Genetic and environmental influences.* Thousand Oaks, CA: Sage.

Bergeman, C. S., Chipuer, H. M., Plomin, R., Pedersen, N. L., McClearn, G. E., Nesselroade, J. R., Costa, Jr., P. T., & McCrae, R. R. (1993). Genetic and environmental effects on openness to experience, agreeableness, and conscientiousness: An adoption/twin study. *Journal of Personality, 61,* 159–179.

Bergeman, C. S., Plomin, R., Pedersen, N., & McClearn, G. E. (1991). Genetic and environmental etiologies of the relationship between social support and psychological well-being. *Psychology and Aging, 6,* 640–646.

Bergeman, C. S., Plomin, R., Pedersen, N., McClearn, G. E., & Nesselroade, J. R. (1990). Genetic and environmental influences on social support: The Swedish Adoption/Twin Study of Aging (SATSA). *Journal of Gerontology, 45,* 101–106.

Butler, R. (1963). The life review: An interpretation of reminiscence in the aged. *Psychiatry, 26,* 65–76.

Carstensen, L. L. (1992). Motivation for social contact across the life span: A theory of socioemotional selectivity. In R. Dienstbier & J. E. Jacobs (Eds.), *Developmental perspectives on motivation: Nebraska symposium on motivation* (pp. 209–254), Lincoln, NB: University of Nebraska Press.

Carstensen, L. L. (1993). Perspectives on research with older families: Contributions of older adults to families and family theory. In P. A. Cowan, D. Field, D. A. Hansen, A. Solinick, & G. E., Swanson (Eds.), *Family, self and society: Toward a new agenda for family research* (pp. 353–360). Hillsdale, NJ: Lawrence Erlbaum Associates.

Cicirelli, V. G. (1989). Feelings of attachment to siblings and well-being in later life. *Psychology and Aging, 4,* 211–216.

Cohen, S. (1988). Psychosocial models of the sole of social support in the etiology of physical disease. *Health Psychology, 7,* 269–297.

Conway, T. L., Vickers, R. R., & French, J. R. (1992). An application of person-environment fit theory: Perceived versus desired control. *Journal of Social Issues, 48,* 95–107.

Cromwell, R. L., Butterfield, D. C., Brayfield, F. M., & Curry, J. J. (1977). *Acute myocardial infarction: Reaction and recovery.* St. Louis, MO: Mosby.

Cutrona, C., Russell, D., & Rose, J. (1986). Social support and adaptation to stress by the elderly. *Psychology and Aging, 1,* 47–54.

Dannefer, D., & Sell, R. R. (1988). Age structure, the life course and "aged heterogeneity": Prospects for research and theory. *Comprehensive Gerontology—B, 2,* 1–10.

Duffy, M. E., & McDonald, E. (1990). Determinants of functional health of older persons. *The Gerontologist, 30,* 503–509.

Engel, G. L. (1978). Psychological stress vasodepressor, (vasobasal) syncope, and sudden death. *Annals of Internal Medicine, 89,* 403–412.

Garmezy, N. (1985). Stress resistant children: The search for protective factors. In J. Stevensen (Ed.), *Recent research in developmental psychopathology* (pp. 213–233). Oxford, England: Pergamon.

George, L. K. (1989). Stress, social support, and depression over the life-course. In K. S. Markides & C. Cooper (Eds.), *Aging, stress, social support, and health.* Chester, England: Wiley.

George, L. K. (1990). Social structure, social processes and social-psychological states. In R. H. Binstock & L. K. George (Eds.), *Handbook of aging and the social sciences* (3rd ed., pp. 186–204). New York: Academic Press.

George, L. K. (1996). Social factors and illness. In H. Binstock & L. K. George (Eds.), *Handbook of aging and the social sciences* (4th ed., pp. 229–252). San Diego: Academic Press.

Hanson, S. H., & Sauer, W. G. (1985). Children and their elderly parents. In W. J. Sauer & R. T. Coward (Eds.), *Social support networks and the care of the elderly: Theory, research and practice* (pp. 41–66). New York: Springer.

Heckhausen, J., & Schulz, R. A. (1995). Life span theory of control. *Psychological Review, 102,* 284–304.

Kahn, S. (1987, August). *Descriptive statistics and alpha coefficients for third-generation hardiness scale and subscales.* Paper presented at the Hardiness Conference, City University of New York, New York.

Kessler, R. C., Kendler, K., Heath, A., Neale, M., & Eaves, L. (1992). Social support, depressed mood, and adjustment to stress: A genetic epidemiologic investigation. *Journal of Personality and Social Psychology, 62,* 257–272.

Kobasa, S. C. (1979). Stressful life events, personality, and health: An inquiry into hardiness. *Journal of Personality and Social Psychology, 37,* 1–11.

Kobasa, S. C. (1982). The personality: Toward a social psychology of stress and health. In G. S. Sanders & J. Suls (Eds.), *Social psychology of health and illness* (pp. 3–32). Hillsdale, NJ: Lawrence Erlbaum Associates.

Kobasa, S. C., & Maddi, S. R. (1977). Existential personality theory. In R. Corsini (Ed.), *Current personality theories* (pp. 243–276). Itasca, IL: T. F. Peacock.

Kobasa, S. C., Maddi, S. R., & Kahn, S. (1982). Hardiness and health: A prospective study. *Journal of Personality and Social Psychology, 42,* 168–177.

Kobasa, S. C., Maddi, S. R., Puccetti, M. C., & Zola, M. A. (1985). Effectiveness of hardiness, exercise, and social support as resources against illness. *Journal of Psychosomatic Resources, 29,* 525–533.

Krause, N. (1990). Perceived health problems, formal/informal support, and life satisfaction among older adults. *Journal of Gerontology, 45,* S193–205.

Lachman, M. E., & Baltes, P. B. (1994). Psychological ageing in lifespan perspective. In M. Rutter & D. F. Hay (Eds.), *Development through life: A handbook for clinicians* (pp. 583–606). Oxford: Blackwell.

Lachman, M. E., Ziff, M. A., & Spiro, A., III (1994). Maintaining a sense of control in later life. In R. P. Abeles, H. C. Gift, & M. G. Ory (Eds.), *Aging and quality of life* (pp. 216–232). New York: Springer.

Lawton, M. P. (1982). Environments and living arrangements. In R. H. Binstock, W. S. Chow, & J. H. Schulz (Eds.), *International perspectives on aging* (pp.159–192). New York: United Nations Fund for Population Activities.

Lee, G. (1985). Kinship and social support among the elderly: The case of the United States. *Aging and Society, 5,* 19–38.

Lichtenstein, P., Hershberger, S. L., & Pedersen, N. L. (1995). Dimensions of occupations: Genetic and environmental influences, *Journal of Biosocial Science, 27,* 193–206.

Lichtenstein, P., & Pedersen, N. L. (1995). Social relationships, stressful life events, and self-reported physical health: Genetic and environmental influences. *Psychology and Health, 10,* 295–319.

Lichtenstein, P., Pedersen, N. L., & McClearn, G. E. (1992). The origins of individual differences in occupational status and educational level: A study of twins reared apart and together. *Acta Sociologica, 35,* 13–31.

Magnani, L. E. (1990). Hardiness, self-perceived health, and activity among independently functioning older adults. *Scholarly Inquiry for Nursing Practice: An International Journal, 4,* 171–184.

Markus, H. R., & Herzog, A. R. (1991). The role of the self-concept in aging. *Annual Review of Gerontology and Geriatrics, 11,* 111–143.

Markus, H. R., & Nurius, P. (1986). Possible selves. *American Psychologist, 41,* 954–969.

Masten, A. S., & Garmezy, N. (1985). Risk, vulnerability and protective factors in developmental psychopathology. In B. B. Lahey & A. E. Kazdin (Eds.), *Advances in child psychology* (vol. 8, pp. 1–52). New York: Plenum.

Matthews, K., Scheier, M. F., Brunson, B. I., & Carducci, B. (1980). Attention, unpredictability and reports of physical symptoms. *Journal of Personality and Social Psychology, 38,* 535–537.

McGue, M., Hirsch, B., & Lykken, D. T. (1993). Age and the self-perception of ability: A twin analysis. *Psychology and Aging, 8,* 72–80.

Murrell, S. A., Norris, F. H., & Grote, C. (1988). Life events in older adults. In L. H. Cohen (Ed.), *Life events and psychological functioning* (pp. 96–122). Newbury Park, CA: Sage.

Nelson, E. A., & Dannefer, D. (1992). Aged heterogeneity: Fact or fiction? The fate of diversity in gerontological research. *Gerontologist, 32,* 17–23.

Orr, E., & Westman, M. (1990). Does hardiness moderate stress, and how?: A review. In M. Rosenbaum (Ed.), *Learned resourcefulness: On coping skills, self-control, and adaptive behavior* (pp. 64–94). New York: Springer.

Ory, M. G., Abeles, R. P., & Lipman, P. D. (1992). Introduction: An overview of research on aging, health, and behavior. In M. G. Ory, R. P. Abeles, & P. D. Lipman (Eds.), *Aging, health, and behavior* (pp. 1–23). Newbury Park, CA: Sage.

Paulus, D., & Christie, R. (1981). Spheres of control: An interactionist approach to assessment of perceived control. In H. M. Lefcourt (Ed.), *Research with the locus of control construct. Vol. 1: Assessment Methods* (pp. 161–188). New York: Academic Press.

Pedersen, N. L., Gatz, M., Plomin, R., Nesselroade, J. R., & McClearn, G. E. (1989). Individual differences on locus of control during the second half of the life span of identical and fraternal twins reared apart and reared together. *Journal of Gerontology, 44,* P100–P105.

Plomin, R., Lichtenstein, P., Pedersen, N. L., McClearn, G. E., & Nesselroade, J. R. (1990). Genetic influences on life events during the last half of the life span. *Psychology and Aging, 5,* 25–30.

Plomin, R., McClearn, G. E., Pedersen, N., Nesselroade, J. R., & Bergeman, C. S. (1988). Genetic influences on childhood family environment perceived retrospectively from the last half of the lifespan. *Developmental Psychology, 24,* 738–745.

Plomin, R., McClearn, G. E., Pedersen, N., Nesselroade, J. R., & Bergeman, C. S. (1989). Genetic influence on adults' ratings of their current family environment. *Journal of Marriage and the Family, 51,* 791–803.

Rhodewalt, F., & Zone, J. B. (1989). Appraisal of life change, depression, and illness in hardy and nonhardy women. *Journal of Personality and Social Psychology, 56,* 81–88.

Rodin, J. (1986). Aging and health: Effects of sense of control. *Science, 233,* 1271–1276.

Rodin, J., & Timko, C. (1992). Sense of control, aging and health. In M. G. Ory, R. P. Abeles, & P. D. Lipman (Eds.), *Aging, health and behavior* (pp. 174–206). Newbury Park, CA: Sage.

Rodin, J., Timko, C. & Harris, S. (1985). The construct of control: Biological and psychosocial correlates. In C. Eisdorfer, M. P. Lawton, & G. L. Maddox (Eds.), *Annual review of gerontology and geriatrics* (vol. 5, pp. 3–55). New York: Springer.

Rutter, M. (1987). Psychosocial resilience and protective mechanisms. *American Journal of Orthopsychiatry, 57,* 316–331.

Schaie, K. W., & Willis, S. L. (1995). Family environments across generations. In V. L. Bengston, K. W. Schaie, & L. Burton (Eds.), *Adult intergenerational relations: Effects of societal change* (pp. 174–209). New York: Springer.

Schlosser, M. B. (1986, August). *Anger, crying, and health among females.* Paper presented at the 94th annual convention of the American Psychological Association. Washington, DC.

Schmale, A., & Iker, H. (1971). Hopelessness as a prediction of cervical cancer. *Social Science Medicine, 5,* 95–100.

Schulz, R., & Rau, M. T. (1985). Social support through the life course. In S. Cohen & S. L. Syme (Eds.), *Social support and health* (pp. 129–149). Orlando, FL: Wiley.

Seeman, T. E., Berkman, L. F., Blazer, D., & Rowe, J. W. (1994). Social ties and support and neuroendocrine function: The MacArthur Studies of Successful Aging. *Annals of Behavioral Medicine, 16,* 95–106.

Shumaker, S. A., & Czajkowski, S. M. (1994). *Social support and cardiovascular disease.* New York: Plenum.

Skinner, E. A. (1996). A guide to constructs of control. *Journal of Personality and Social Psychology, 71,* 549–570.

Staudinger, U. M., Marsiske, M., & Baltes, P. B. (1993). Resilience and levels of reserve capacity in later adulthood: Perspectives from life-span theory. *Developmental Psychopathology, 5,* 541–566.

U.S. Bureau of the Census (1991). *Statistical abstract of the United States: 1991 (111th Ed.).* Washington, DC: Author.

Wallace, K., & Bergeman, C. S. (1997). *Hardiness in the elderly: Maximizing reserve potential.* Poster presented to the Midwest Psychological Association, Chicago, IL.

Wallace, K., & Bergeman, C. S. (1997). Control and the elderly: "Goodness of Fit." *International Journal of Aging and Human Development, 45,* 323–339.

Wolinsky, F. D., & Johnson, R. J. (1992). Perceived health status and mortality among older men and women. *Journal of Gerontology: Social Sciences, 47,* S304–S312.

12

The Health Effects of Caregiving for Adults in Later Life

Dominic O. Vachon
University of Notre Dame

As ADULTS AGE, the likelihood increases that they will experience temporary or chronic illnesses or disabling conditions requiring a dependence on others for assistance. Caregiving is most often associated with assisting the frail elderly, especially those with chronic medical conditions or dementias. Conditions that might require caregiving include stroke, coronary problems, cancer, accidents involving physical injury such as traumatic brain injuries, AIDS, and severe mental disorders.

Caregiving is generally defined as the provision of nonordinary help to persons who are unable to take complete care of themselves due to a mental illness, physical illness, disability, or a condition such as frailty due to aging (Marks, 1996). Most often, family members such as spouses, adult children, siblings, and other relatives provide caregiving, but friends of the ill or disabled person also may be involved in caregiving.

Typically, primary caregivers provide most of the care to, and have most of the responsibility for the care of, the person suffering from a disabling condition; secondary caregivers are those who provide at least some significant services for the ill or disabled person and may also provide support to the primary caregiver. Caregivers are motivated by a sense of attachment or affection for the ill or disabled person, as well as guilt, a sense of duty, or a sense of being forced to become a caregiver. It is well documented in the popular media as well as in the clinical and research literature that extended caregiving might affect the caregiver negatively, including psychological problems (e.g., depression), physical illnesses, social isolation, financial burden, interference with career or childrearing, and disruptions of routine and preexisting roles (e.g., inability to work). Caregiver burden and strain has been researched extensively with regard to caring for individuals with dementia, especially Alzheimer's disease (AD). However, more recently, there has been a move toward examining the positive effects of caregiving on various aspects of the caregiver's life (Miller & Lawton, 1997).

Part of the difficulty for those who become caregivers is that the need to care for an ill or disabled relative, partner, or friend is often unexpected and experienced as an interruption in their lives. In U.S. culture, which emphasizes independence and the meeting of individual needs, caregiving is often thought of as an infrequent occurrence (Vachon, 1996). However, it is actually common. In a sample of 13,017 adults living in the continental United States aged 19 years and older (National Survey of Families and Households), Marks (1996) calculated population estimates of in- and out-of-household caregiving from persons of all ages. In this cross-sectional study, Marks concluded that caregiving is not rare in a person's life. In fact, during young adulthood (ages 19–34), approximately 15% of women and 11% of men were giving in- or out-of-household care to dependent relatives or friends. Moreover, a significant number of care recipients were children or other relatives who were not elderly. In early middle age (ages 35–49), one in five women and almost one in seven men were engaged in some type of caregiving. By later middle age (ages 50–64) and early older age (65–74), approximately one in five adults (men and women) were caregivers. In the older age group, caregiving tended to be for elderly family members and friends. A significant number (16.4%) of caregivers at all ages were providing care for more than one ill or disabled person.

In terms of in-household care, Marks found that 1 in 20 adults were caregivers for a disabled person (most likely a child or younger adult) during early adulthood (ages 19–34) and early middle age (ages 35–49). About 1 in 10 adults in later middle age (ages 50–64) and young old age (ages 65–74) provide in-household care. Most of the care recipients for the later middle age group are younger than age 65; but for the young old (ages 65–74) and the older old (ages 75 and older), in-household caregiving was typically for persons over 65 years old. However, most of out-of-household caregiving was for persons who are 65 or older. About 10% of all adults provided some type of out-of-household caregiving in the year prior to the study. Approximately 15% of all middle-aged women (35–64) were involved in out-of-household caregiving (Marks, 1996).

The caregiving experience is a frequent one and often has negative consequences for the caregiver's mental and physical health. This chapter examines the caregiving process as well as the effects of caregiving on the caregiver followed by a review of factors that place caregivers at risk for or protect them from adverse health outcomes. The dynamics of the negative as well as positive aspects of caregiving are explored. Also, the impact of caregiving on the health of the care recipient is discussed. Finally, types of interventions for improving the health and well-being of caregivers is reviewed.

PHASES IN THE JOURNEY OF THE CAREGIVER

Being a caregiver for an ill or disabled person is a continuous and a complex process. The caregiving process is affected by the care recipient's type of illness or disability. If the illness or disability is progressive, the demands on the caregiver will
change and increase. Initially, the individual must decide to become a caregiver
and then decide how to enact that role. In conceptualizing the caregiver experiences, some researchers have called it a *career*. Consistent with that perspective,
Aneshensel, Pearlin, Mullan, Zarit, and Whitlatch (1995) identified three stages of
caregiving, each with its own sources of stress; these are "preparation for and acquisition of the caregiver role; enactment of care-related tasks and responsibilities
within the home and possibly within a formal institution; and disengagement
from caregiving, which often entails bereavement, recovery, and social reintegra-
tion" (p. 17).

In my own workshops and clinical work, I have found it useful to describe
phases in the journey of the caregiver, which helps caregivers articulate their own
experiences of the caregiving process and provides validation of their personal reactions as typical parts of the caregiver's journey (Vachon, 1996). The *Antecedent*
phase comes first. In this phase, preexisting family dynamics and personal history
set the stage for the type of response a potential caregiver may have to someone in
need of care. Phase 2, the *Crisis* phase, is when either sudden or gradual caregiving
is needed because of a medical or psychiatric diagnosis. Decisions about what is to
be done in the short term are required and, if caregiving is needed, family members
or acquaintances work out who will help provide it. In this phase, these individuals
decide whether to act as caregivers and the extent of their involvement. A number
of factors influence the making of these decisions: the family's relationships, personal resources of the potential caregivers and the care recipients, situational factors such as distance from the ill person or the occupation of the caregiver, and the
extent of caregiving required by an illness or disabling condition.

Assuming that individuals have decided to be caregivers, the third phase is the
Despairing/Exhaustion phase. At this point, the condition requires an increasing
amount of the caregiver's energy, and the caregiver might experience negative feelings about the personal, physical, and social costs of the task. The fourth phase is
"Hitting the Wall"/Acceptance. As caregivers fully realize the long-term nature of
the role and possible costs, they may shift their perception of the situation; at times
they may even decide to pass caregiving responsibilities to someone else or to use a
long-term care institution or agency. In the fifth phase, the *Long Haul*, the caregiver is coping satisfactorily with caring for a person whose illness or disabling
condition is stable, worsening, or improving. This phase is characterized by having
good personal and social resources as well as a reliance on a transcendent spirituality or philosophy of life.

In the sixth phase, the *End of Caregiving*, caregiving has ended or shifted in some way (e.g., death, recovery, institutionalization) and the caregiver must adjust to a new way of living. The caregiver often experiences a mixture of grief, relief, guilt, and even a sense of purposelessness. Finally, in the seventh phase, *Readjustment*, the person's life is changed (positively or negatively) by the caregiving experience. Readjustment is complete but a number of dimensions might be changed, such as enduring negative feelings, physical effects, or attitudinal changes related to the caregiving experience. The phases in this model should not be thought of as proceeding linearly necessarily but at times in circular fashion; for example, cycling through the crisis phase and "hitting the wall"/exhaustion each time there is a worsening condition for the patient.

As Aneshensel et al. (1995) and others have argued, the process of caregiving is ongoing and dynamic. Each caregiving phase can place specific types of demands on caregivers that in turn can in some way affect health. In terms of this review, a biopsychoenvironmental model is used to discuss the impact of caregiving on the caregiver's mental and physical health with medical, psychological, and environmental factors all interacting to influence caregiver outcomes.

THE EFFECTS OF CAREGIVING ON THE CAREGIVER

Psychological Effects

A number of psychological effects associated with caregiving have been documented. Some caregivers have been found to have higher levels of psychological or emotional distress as well as increased psychiatric disorders (Russo, Vitaliano, Brewer, Katon, & Becker, 1995; Schulz, Visintainer, & Williamson, 1990). A higher percentage of caregivers use psychotropic drugs than does the general population (Clipp & George, 1990). In a review of caregivers of stroke survivors, Tyman (1994) found that caregivers do suffer from more psychological health problems such as depression, anxiety, and fatigue. Also, increased depression has been found among caregivers for spouses and parents with dementias as well as other medical problems (Gallagher, Rose, Rivera, Lovett, & Thompson, 1989; Schulz et al., 1990).

McNaughton, Patterson, Smith, and Grant (1995) found a sample of caregivers of AD patients to be mildly depressed in comparison with a control group. Becker and Morrissey (1988) also found that caregivers tend to have disturbed sleep, worries about the future, and feelings of helplessness, but they suggested that these symptoms might be related to the caregiving situation and not indicative of clinical depression. Finally, Schulz, Newsom, Mittlemark, Burton, Hirsch, and Jackson (1997) found in a large population-based sample comparing caregivers to a matched control group that caregivers have more depressive symptoms and higher levels of anxiety and report not having enough time for sleep, self-care, and other health-related activities.

Research has also focused on the positive practical and emotional benefits of caregiving (Miller & Lawton, 1997). Referring to these benefits, Kramer (1997) used the term *gain*, defined "as the extent to which the caregiving role is appraised to enhance an individual's life space and be enriching" (p. 219). Based on the review of 29 studies, Kramer found a number of measurement problems and a lack of theory in assessing beneficial outcomes of caregiving. Nonetheless, she found evidence that the positive appraisals of caregiving appear to contribute to caregiver adaptation and to positive well-being. Moreover, positive feelings about caregiving (e.g., feelings of mutuality, self-satisfaction, rewards) has been related to lower caregiver stress (Given & Given, 1991).

Physical Effects

Research examining the physical health of caregivers is limited, but the intensity of the demands of caring for a seriously ill or disabled person is associated with negative effects on subjective ratings of physical health (Marks, 1996; Schulz et al., 1990; Schulz et al., 1997). Employing objective health ratings, Kiecolt-Glaser, Dura, Speicher, Trask, and Glaser (1991) found negative immunological changes in caregivers of persons with dementia. Although these caregivers did not manifest a greater number of illnesses than did a control group, their illnesses tended to last longer and required more medical attention. Caregiving has also been found to be associated with deficits in virus-specific immune response (Glaser & Kiecolt-Glaser, 1997), slower wound healing (Kiecolt-Glaser, Marucha, Malarkey, Mercado, & Glaser, 1995), and poor influenza vaccine responses (Kiecolt-Glaser, Glaser, Gravenstein, Malarkey, & Sheridan, 1996). In comparison with a control group, Schulz et al. (1997) found that psychiatric and physical health effects occur the most for caregivers who reported strain in providing care. Of their sample, 40% felt little distress and difficulty and did not have significant negative health effects. Yet, several reviews have not found this effect on physical health (Baumgarten, 1989; Connell & Gibson, 1997). Overall, the link between caregiving and negative physical health effects has limited support at this time. In general, it appears that caregivers are at risk for negative health effects particularly when the demands of care are high and the caregiver experiences strain (Schulz et al., 1997).

Social Effects

The time demands of caregiving, the requirements of caregiving tasks, and emotional energy also affect dimensions of the caregiver's social, family, and work life. Donaldson, Tarrier, and Burns (1997) reported that many studies find that the care recipient's dementia symptoms do affect the caregiver's social and recreational activities negatively. Specifically, restrictions in caregivers' social activities are related to dementia symptoms in the care recipient that require a great deal of caregiver supervision (e.g., because of disturbed behavior) or that are labor-intensive (e.g., problems in activities of daily living [ADL]). In a longitudinal study of caregivers of spouses with dementia, caregivers reported less social support than did controls and a decline in social support 13 months later (Kiecolt-Glaser et al., 1991).

The addition of caregiving de facto affects other roles in a caregiver's life. Energy given to caregiving for an ill or disabled parent, sibling, partner, or friend negatively affects the amount of energy available for significant others, such as children. Also, family members who are secondary caregivers likewise experience changes in their life not only from the additional work but also from the psychological effects of witnessing a relative's suffering. A number of studies indicate that caregiving restricts the social lives of family members as well as their interactions with each other (Given & Given, 1991).

Another social effect is a possible change in the relationship with the ill or disabled care recipient, such as the role reversal of an adult child caring for a parent. Negative feelings such as resentment or guilt may also enter into the relationship. For caregivers of persons with dementia, feelings toward the care recipient typically became more negative with the emergence of disturbed behaviors such as mood changes, aggression, and withdrawal (Donaldson et al., 1997). On the other hand, positive changes in the family are also possible as family members encounter a very stressful situation. Beach (1997) studied the positive caregiving experiences of adolescents whose families were caring for a relative with AD. She found that those adolescents experienced increased sibling activity, sharing, and bonding; developed increased empathy for older adults; experienced greater mother–adolescent bonding and increased their selection and maintenance of relationships with empathic friends.

The increased demands of caregiving often affects work. In a sense, caregiving becomes an additional job with periods of crisis that can affect employment productivity. In a review of the literature, Given and Given (1991) found that caregivers reported disruption, inhibition, and withdrawal from their work roles. Caregiving also conflicts with parenting, marital relationships, or other responsibilities. Although some studies find increased burden with multiple roles, others find that caregiver well-being may depend on having outside employment and other roles (Given & Given, 1991). Moreover, negative work effects are not always found. For example, Neal, Chapman, Ingersoll-Dayton, Emlen, and Boise (1990) found that although caregivers may experience more work interruptions than noncaregivers, there were no differences in terms of absenteeism, late arrival, or leaving work early.

RISK FACTORS AND CAREGIVING

A number of factors have been associated with mental and physical health outcomes in caregivers. First, the major theoretical models used in this research are briefly described. Second, the research on the characteristics of care recipients that relate to caregiver burden as well as mental and physical health effects are discussed. Third, the personal factors relating to these effects are presented; these include psychological factors, gender effects, health status, and spirituality and philosophy of life factors. Fourth, the social factors of social support, racial or ethnic background, and the quality or type of caregiving relationship are summarized. Finally, the limitations of the current research are mentioned.

Theoretical Models

The transactional model of stress appraisal proposed by Lazarus and Folkman (1984) has been used commonly in caregiver research. This model incorporates environmental, person, and situation factors to explain how the caregiving process affects the caregiver. In terms of how appraisal and coping affect physical health, Lazarus and Folkman pointed out three possibilities. First, the frequency, duration, intensity, and patterning of neurochemical stress reactions may be influenced by coping. Second, coping can affect health in terms of the habits and activities in which a person engages such as drug abuse, smoking, or high-risk activities. Third, the use of emotion-focused coping, such as denial or avoidance of a psychological or physical problem, can interfere with adaptive health- or illness-related behavior. As they explained, "Appraisal processes provide a common pathway through which person and environment variables modify psychological responses, and hence emotions and their biological concomitants" (p. 224). In a more specified theory of appraisal by caregivers, Lawton, Moss, Kleban, Glicksman, and Rovine (1991) argued for a two-factor model that they called the *parallel channel hypothesis*, in which positive and negative emotional states are partially independent and have different antecedents. Partial support for this theory has been found in which the objective stressors, the subjective appraisal (measured by caregiving satisfaction and burden), and the caregiver resources relate differently to positive affect and depression (Lawton et al., 1991; Pruchno, Peters, & Burant, 1995). For example, in spouse caregivers of persons with AD, caregiving satisfaction was more strongly associated with positive affect than it was with lessening depression; and caregiving burden was more strongly associated with increasing depression than it was with decreasing positive affect (Lawton et al., 1991).

Haley and Pardo (1987) proposed three models of ways in which caregiver health is affected. The first is the wear-and-tear hypothesis, in which caregivers become more overwhelmed and deteriorate in their functioning as the care recipient's condition worsens. The second is the adaptation model, in which the caregiver adapts to the situation even if the patient's condition worsens; the caregiver either maintains or improves functioning in response. Third, the trait hypothesis model proposes that caregivers maintain a level of functioning because of preexisting levels of resources, coping skills, and social support.

Characteristics of Care-Recipient Factors

A number of factors relate to the care recipient that may affect caregiver health. For example, the type of illness of the care recipient has been investigated as an objective stressor that affects health. Aspects of the illness or disability such as severity, types of symptoms, and assistance in ADL have been studied to determine if there are links to caregiver stress and burden, physical health, and mental health. Highlights of this research are presented here.

With respect to the effect of care-recipient factors on caregiver stress, burden, and psychological symptoms, the research findings have been inconsistent and complex. In general, Hooker, Monahan, Shifren, and Hutchinson (1992) concluded that caregiver stress or burden appears to relate more to caregiver characteristics such as coping skills and social support than to care-recipient factors. That is, caregiver stress or burden is not related to the functional impairment in the care recipient (Hooker et al., 1992). However, Schulz et al. (1990) found that depressive symptoms were worse when a patient was more severely impaired, and females tend to be more depressed than males. They are cautious about these findings because the selection strategies for caregiver studies are biased toward the most distressed caregivers.

Donaldson et al. (1997) reviewed 17 well-designed studies conducted between 1980 and 1995 regarding the relation between types of dementia symptoms and the negative impact on caregivers. They found that most studies did not find a significant relation between caregiver burden and ADL (e.g., bathing, toileting, feeding, using transportation, and everyday instrumental activities). Increased burden or caregiver strain and depression was related in most studies to the noncognitive features of dementia (i.e., psychotic symptoms, depressive features, and behavioral disturbances). They argued that the key factor in caregiver distress was psychopathology in the dementia patient. In terms of the effect of dementia symptoms on caregiver anxiety and stress, the relation appears to be similar to the results just noted. That is, the association between caregiver anxiety and stress has been found with demanding, disturbed, and dependent behaviors in patients (Donaldson et al. 1997).

Because most of the research on caregiving has been done with dementia patients, an important issue is whether these findings apply to other types of illnesses. Rabins, Fitting, Eastham, and Fetting (1990) compared AD patient caregivers to cancer patient caregivers and found no significant differences in negative or positive emotional states between the two groups. Similar levels of psychological distress also have been found for caregivers of stroke victims (Silliman, Fletcher, Earp, & Wagner, 1986).

Pruchno and Resch (1989) hypothesized that the complex relation between caregiver stressors and outcomes might be partially resolved by focusing on the course of a disease like AD in which particular stressors change as the disease progresses. They found some evidence supporting a wear-and-tear hypothesis: A social and disoriented behaviors in care recipients were related in linear fashion to perceived burden, negative consequences of caring, and decrease in social activities. However, indicating an adaptation pattern, the increase of forgetful behaviors at first is related to increased caregiver stress, but then reverses at high levels of forgetful behaviors. The authors argued that forgetful behaviors, at first, is more stressful because the mild impairment does not meet family norms, but when the care recipient has more severe impairment, the expectations change and the shift is to care for more basic needs. Zarit, Todd, and Zarit (1986) also found support for the adaptation hypothesis; caregivers whose spouses had dementia developed the ability to tolerate problem behaviors better even if the disease worsened. They either developed skills to manage the situation better or did not let the behaviors bother them as much.

The relation between dementia symptoms and caregiver physical health has been less clear than the relation between dementia symptoms and psychological health (Donaldson et al., 1997). Some studies report no significant relations. However, Deimling and Bass (1986) found that physical health in caregivers was most affected by ADL limitations followed by patient disruptive behavior and deficits in social functioning (e.g., withdrawal, poor cooperation). Shaw, Patterson, Sempe, Ho, et al. (1997) found in a sample of AD caregivers that there was a physical health decline in the caregiver when ADL caregiving demands were great, but this was not related to problem behaviors of the care recipient. In another study that controlled for caregiver gender, familial generation, and living arrangement, Cattanach and Tebes (1991) tested the health effects of caring for three types of elderly care recipients in the home: cognitively impaired, functionally impaired, and nonimpaired. Among the negative psychosocial and health effects found in all three types of caregivers, no differences were found in the severity of the health effects due to the type of care-recipient impairment. The authors argued that other aspects of the caregiving context, such as gender, familial generation, and living arrangement must lead to differential effects on psychological and physical health.

At this time there are contradictory findings regarding how care-recipient factors relate to caregiver health. What does seem clear is that caregiver health is affected more by the caregiver's stress appraisal, coping skills, situational factors, as well as social support than by care-recipient characteristics. Care-recipient factors appear to negatively affect caregiver health in particular phases in caregiving such as when the caregiver is adapting to severe impairment in the care recipient or when there are high ADL caregiving demands. Future research will continue clarifying how this occurs.

Personal Factors

Psychological Factors. Cognitive appraisal, coping styles, and personality factors have been the psychological variables most often related to caregiver health. Caregiver perception of stress appears to determine the caregiver's psychological well-being, burden, psychological symptoms, and physiological reactions. That is, the caregiver's feelings of burden, not the severity of the patient's symptoms, relates to the decision to institutionalize spouses with dementia (Zarit et al., 1986) In a sample of AD caregivers and matched noncaregiver controls, caregivers were found to be significantly more depressed, but there was no difference in health status. For both groups, depressive symptoms and health were related to irrational beliefs, the degree of life adversity in general, and external locus of control (McNaughton et al., 1995). Interestingly, the subjective ratings of health over 6 months, not the objective health ratings, were most influenced by cognitive appraisal and social support. In another study, subjective perception of lower burden and higher perceived control have been found to be related to greater psychological well-being, better life satisfaction, and less depression in a sample of patients with spinal cord injuries (Schulz, Tompkins, Woods, & Decker, 1987).

A number of studies find physiological changes related to various aspects of the appraisal of caregiver stress. In a longitudinal study of AD caregivers, psychological distress (i.e., more depression, hassles, burden, and lower uplifts) contributed to higher insulin and glucose levels (Vitaliano, Scanlan, Krenz, Schwartz, & Marcovina, 1996). In another study, caregivers who reported significantly more distress regarding their spouses' dementia had more decrements in immune function (Kiecolt-Glaser et al., 1991). Finally, Vitaliano, Russo, and Niaura (1995) found that a sample of AD spouse caregivers compared to matched controls had higher lipid levels (associated with cardiovascular disease).

In addition to appraisal, coping style has been related to perceived stress and psychological outcomes. In a study of spouse caregivers of persons with dementia (Neundorfer, 1991), greater depression was related to the severity of patient problems, higher caregiver stress, and a wishing–emotive coping style. A wishing–emotive coping style is characterized by wishful thinking, tendency to escape, not accepting one's responsibility in the problem and the solution, and a lack of aggressive efforts to change the situation. Higher levels of anxiety were predicted by higher caregiver stress and wishing–emotive coping style. However, health was not predicted by coping style. Neundorfer (1991) noted in her study of spouse caregivers that most of the caregivers were using adaptive coping strategies. Many used positive reappraisal, which focuses on personal growth, turning to prayer, and seeing the benefits of caregiving. Moreover, this coping style was not related to depression and anxiety levels. Similarly, other researchers found that coping methods such as reframing the problem, existential growth, and spiritual support were beneficial to caregivers (Pratt, Schmall, Wright, & Cleland, 1985; Quayhagen & Quayhagen, 1988).

Personality traits affect the coping process by influencing how a situation is appraised and by influencing a person's coping capacities and strategies (Lazarus, 1966). Preexisting negative traits increase the risk for negative caregiving outcomes and positive traits provide more beneficial results. Caregivers with a higher degree of personality hardiness (i.e., control, challenge, and commitment) were found to have less depression and dissatisfaction (Clark & Hartman, 1996). Commitment was especially predictive of decreased psychological distress, pointing to the important role of the belief in the importance and meaning of a person's activities and goals despite the negative aspects of any situation. Hardy appraisals of various caregiving situations were also related to less psychological distress. In terms of physical health, however, only commitment related to fewer physical symptoms; no other relations with medical diagnoses and symptoms were found.

In a study of caregivers of cancer and AD patients, positive emotional experiences were associated with lower neuroticism and higher extraversion (Rabins et al., 1990). Hooker et al. (1992) found that neuroticism is related to higher perceived stress, more depressive symptoms, lower psychological well-being, poorer self-reported physical health, and more chronic health conditions diagnosed by a doctor in a sample of dementia caregivers. They also found that optimism had an indirect effect on psychological health, mainly through the path of perceived stress; decreased optimism is related to increased perceived stress, which, in turn, is related to poorer psychological health.

In short, stress appraisal, coping style, and personality traits underlying appraisal and coping do significantly influence perceived stress and psychological health. Although significant physical health effects are less often found and problems exist in the sole reliance on subjective self-report measures of physical health, there is still substantial evidence that these psychological factors have physical health consequences.

Gender Effects.   Marks (1996) found that in the population as a whole, 9.4% of adults were female caregivers and 6.5% of adults were male caregivers. Women were more likely to be caregivers across the life span, but men who are 75 or older are more likely to be caregivers than the comparable age group of women. Marks concluded "that women caregivers are more likely to be bearing the burden of being squeezed by multiple burdens of responsibilities for care of dependent children and caregiving and/or an intensive workload and caregiving than are men caregivers and, thereby, may need more formal service consideration in handling their loads" (p. 34). Given and Given (1991), in their review of the caregiving literature, reported inconsistent findings regarding the role of gender in response to caregiving. In studies controlling for differences in cognitive or physical functioning of the care recipient, few differences have emerged in caregiver burden based on gender. Yet, others have found poorer physical and mental health among wife caregivers than husband caregivers, with wives and daughters reporting more caregiver burden than husband caregivers (Given & Given, 1991)

Cantor (1983) concluded that gender and type of relationship to the care recipient affect the adaptation, commitment, and involvement in caregiving. For example, in a 2-year longitudinal study of caregivers of spouses who had dementia, Zarit et al. (1986) found that initially wife caregivers reported more subjective burden than did husband caregivers. However, 2 years later, no significant differences were found. The authors speculated that wives changed their coping style to a more instrumental approach that the men adopted from the beginning.

The gender differences in burden initially can be explained by other factors as well. Zarit et al. (1986) speculated that in the early stages of the spouse's illness, wives might have experienced resentment at being put again into a caregiving role or that they had more conflicting demands on them. In another attempt to explain gender differences, Lutzky and Knight (1994) indicated that male and female caregivers tend to report their distressed feelings differently, with men being less attentive to their actual feelings. Also, they found that women are socialized to use coping styles that are less effective in dealing with distress (i.e., greater use of escape-avoidance coping). In general, Kriseman and Claes (1997) concluded from their review that caregiving is a more negative experience for women than for men and that women report greater burden and depression.

Health Factors. There is evidence that mental and physical health have reciprocal effects under caregiver stress. On one hand, caregiver health is associated with better life satisfaction, better psychological well-being, and lower levels of depression. Combined with other factors, such as social support, satisfaction with social contacts, and perceived control, psychological well-being and lower depression is most predicted by health status (Schulz et al., 1987). Pruchno et al. (1995) found that poorer physical health and more negative appraisals were associated with greater depression. But physical health did not predict positive affect. On the other hand, mental health influences physical health as well. Pruchno, Kleban, Michaels, and Dempsey (1990) found that over a 6-month period, depression in wife caregivers predicted declines in physical health. Finally, the psychological health of a person entering the caregiving experience is also important in what occurs during caregiving in terms of mental and physical health effects. Russo et al. (1995) found evidence for a stress–diathesis model of psychopathology in AD caregivers; caregivers who had a psychiatric history of an anxiety or depressive disorder prior to the onset of AD in the care recipient tended to have a mental disorder after onset compared to caregivers without previous disorders.

Spiritual and Philosophy of Life Factors. Although there is little research at this time, there is initial evidence that caregiver well-being can be enhanced by factors such as a sense of finding meaning, spirituality, and religiosity. Farran and Keane-Hagerty (1991) noted there have been no theoretical frameworks devoted only to family caregiving and that usually the research has tended to focus on the negative aspects of caregiving. They found that caregivers try to find meaning in their difficult experiences or else experience an absence of meaning or good from caregiving that leads to despair and hopelessness. Caregiver feelings of being supported and comforted by their religious faith are strongly related to positive emotional experiences and are associated with less emotional distress; however, the number of religious services was not associated with these emotional outcomes

(Rabins et al., 1990). A number of studies have highlighted how much certain caregivers rely on faith, prayer, and religion (Picot, Debanne, Namazi, & Wykle, 1997; Valle, Gook-Gait, & Tazbaz, 1993).

Social Factors

Social Support. Greater social support is a major variable that predicts lower psychological distress, lower burden, higher well-being, improved immune function, lower levels of depression, and lower likelihood of institutionalizing the care recipient (Kiecolt-Glaser et al., 1991; Schulz et al., 1987). In a sample of caregivers of cancer and AD patients, positive emotional experiences were associated with the number of social contacts and the degree of family cohesiveness caregivers have (Rabins et al., 1990). However, the perception of support is most related to reduced caregiver burden or distress rather than the amount of instrumental assistance given by others in caregiving tasks (Given & Given, 1991; Lawton et al., 1991). Furthermore, Li, Seltzer, and Greenberg (1997) found that type of social support, type of stressor, and the individual context interact to result in a particular effect of support; for example, they found that increased social participation was related to lower depressive symptoms for daughters but not for wives; and emotional support differentially buffered different sets of stressful care-recipient characteristics for wives and daughters.

Racial and Ethnic Background Factors. A caregiver's racial or ethnic background also appears to influence psychological and physical health outcomes. Although most of the research on caregiving has been with Euro-American participants, more research is now examining cultural and racial factors. Compared to African-American caregivers, Euro-American caregivers tend to experience higher levels of caregiver stress, burden, and depression; they also report less caregiving mastery and satisfaction and see caregiving as more of an intrusion than do African-American caregivers (Aranda & Knight, 1997; Connell & Gibson, 1997). Factors possibly explaining these differences include African Americans' espousing a more traditional caregiving ideology, having more strongly held beliefs about family support, perceiving more rewards in caregiving, and having higher levels of religiosity than have Euro-Americans.

In a review of the literature focusing on Latino caregivers, Aranda and Knight (1997) reported that Latino caregivers tended to perceive greater burden than African Americans and tended to react more negatively to the overall caregiving situation, the caregiving tasks, and the care recipient's "problem" behaviors than Anglos. Latino caregivers generally appear to have poorer health than Anglos and at least similar or higher levels of burden and depression than Anglos; however, the research on mental and physical effects is limited and inconclusive. In a study comparing caregivers of persons with dementia in Shanghai and San Diego, coping strategies were found to be similar, but caregivers from Shanghai reported less depression and anxiety than San Diego caregivers (Shaw, Patterson, Semple, Grant, et al., 1997). The authors speculated that Chinese cultural ideals of interdependence among family members, veneration of older adults, and passive acceptance of traditional family role might lessen the psychological impact of caregiving for them. Overall, research is emerging with other racial and ethnic groups as well and continue to demonstrate the influence of culture on health through mechanisms like stress appraisal, social support, attitudes toward caregiving, and so on.

Quality and Type of Relationship. Both the premorbid and current quality of the caregiver's relationship to the care receiver is associated with a number of psychological health variables. In a sample of elderly persons with depression or dementia, caregiver psychological distress was associated with rating the premorbid relationship as unsatisfactory (Wijeratne & Lovestone, 1996). Similarly, in a study of caregivers of persons with spinal cord injury, caregivers had better life satisfaction and felt less burden if they were happy with their individual relationships with the care recipients. Also, the more a caregiver considered the disability of the care recipient to be a limitation, the more burden the caregiver felt; in fact, this relation was stronger than the relation between actual time spent assisting the care recipient and perceived burden (Schulz et al., 1987). A very interesting study reported a tendency for some caregivers of spinal cord injured persons not to be accurate in predicting their partners' levels of depression. In fact, they tended to appraise their partners' level of depression by their own feeling state: Caregivers who overestimated their partners' depression tended to feel more burden, felt less control, were less satisfied with their relationship to the care recipient and with social contacts, and were more depressed than the good estimators and underestimators (Schulz et al., 1987). According to the authors, the level of objective needs might influence the level of depression, burden, and so on; or, the tendency to appraise the situation positively or negatively might have colored the self-reports on various measures.

Types of relationships can also be factors that influence caregiver effects. For example, Lawton et al. (1991) found different dynamics between spouse caregivers and adult child caregivers. For spouse caregivers, caregiver satisfaction was not related to giving more help while for adult child caregivers, greater caregiver satisfaction was related to giving more care. Moreover, giving more help was related to less depression for adult children but was unrelated to depression for spouse caregivers. Perhaps for spouse caregivers, providing help is assumed to be part of the marital commitment and is not a source of satisfaction. For spouses, caregiving is a full commitment to their marital relationship, whereas for adult children it is added to other roles in their lives that are more central.

Limitations of the Current Research

Although the research on the impact of caregiving on health is promising and improving, clearly there exists a number of limitations. The first is the difficulty of making causal claims regarding the influence on health of the biopsychoenvironmental factors. This causal argument is complicated by the fact that health status also has a reciprocal influence on the other factors. For example, Schulz et al. (1990) pointed out that negative impact might be counteracted by the benefits of caregiving. In addition, most caregiving research has been cross-sectional. More longitudinal research is needed to help establish causal interactions among stress exposure (e.g., care-receiver characteristics), caregiver vulnerabilities (e.g., age, gender, race, and health history), caregiver resources (e.g., income, social support, and coping), and health effects (Vitaliano, Schulz, Kiecolt-Glaser, & Grant, 1997).

Another major problem with the research on caregiving concerns measurement. Schulz et al. (1990) argued that the areas having inconsistent results suggest validity problems with measurement instruments. They also pointed out that self-report data on health status can be affected by such factors as personality and, thus, more objective health data are needed. In addition, health measures are not always sensitive to the long-term physiological impact of caregiving. Schulz et al. pointed out that some health effects might be detected better after caregiving has ended. In addition to improving the measurement and timing of health data, Schulz et al. proposed that observing changes in preclinical diseases, such as hypertension, cardiac functioning, and blood chemistries, might be useful in that caregiving might aggravate preexisting vulnerabilities rather than precipitate an illness. McNaughton et al. (1995) indicated the need for measures that can distinguish chronic stress responses in caregiving from clinical depression. According to Kramer (1997), positive gain from caregiving is still not measured well and past research has tended to lack a comprehensive theoretical base.

Schulz et al. (1990) also pointed out that sampling problems exist with the current research. Caregiving samples are biased toward selecting more distressed caregivers. Also, there is always a need to have matched noncaregiving control groups or health norms by age and gender to assist making claims about impact on health (Schulz et al., 1990). Finally, although some research is sensitive to the phase of caregiving (Aneshensel et al., 1995), more work is needed on how particular phases of the caregiving journey have unique stressors and risks (e.g., crisis phase and bereavement).

HEALTH EFFECTS OF CAREGIVING ON THE CARE RECIPIENT

Up to this point we have focused on the biopsychoenvironmental model and its relation to health status for caregivers. It is important, however, to discuss elements of this model for the health status of care recipients. This issue is commonly overlooked because the care recipient is chronically ill or deteriorating, and it is just assumed that caregiving has physical benefits to the care recipient. Yet, it is important to determine how the caregiving quality affects the care recipient.

There a number of domains on which to evaluate caregiving quality. Gillis and Belza (1992) identified four types of caregiver work: (a) functional work, which concerns elements such as housecleaning and meals; (b) monitoring work, which concerns supervising elements such as patient diet, medications, and exercise; (c) comfort work, which focuses on the physical needs; and (d) support work, which concerns tending to the care receiver's psychological needs. Vachon and Merluzzi (1997) investigated domains of caregiver self-efficacy involving such skills as attending to the care receiver's physical needs, getting medical information, facilitating medical care, dealing with negative feelings from the care receiver, dealing with personal negative feelings toward the care receiver, and dealing with issues of death and dying. Outcomes for the care receiver range from facilitating recovery from certain illnesses, such as strokes and hip surgery, to promoting optimum quality of life for a chronically ill, terminally ill, or disabled person.

Elder mistreatment is the most dramatic example of how poor caregiving negatively affects the ill or disabled person. Mistreatment, in the form of physical abuse, neglect of physical needs, not providing emotional support, and poor relationships with the ill or disabled person, results in negative health outcomes. Caregiver burden has been associated with elder mistreatment (Fulmer, 1991). Also, caregiver depression and living arrangement are associated with caregiver violence (Paveza et al., 1992). Caregivers who have mental disorders, drug dependencies, or who are impaired in other ways are often prone to abusive or neglectful behavior (Fulmer, 1991). In short, failure of the caregiver to provide good quality care in the various domains of caregiving negatively affects the care receiver's psychological and physical health.

A growing research literature has documented how good caregiving promotes health in the care receiver. Gillis and Belza (1992) discussed the important role family caregivers play in maximizing the emotional and physical recovery of a person following cardiac surgery. With regard to implementing lifestyle changes after an acute cardiac episode, Creasia (1992) noted that it is the informal caregiver who provides encouragement and guidance; a support network that is available and perceived to be helpful was associated with following a risk-reduction lifestyle. For older heart surgery patients, perceived adequacy of support 1 month after surgery was associated with less depression and less ADL impairment 6 months after surgery (Oxman & Hull, 1997). In recovery from hip fracture surgery, poor social support and depression were related to less improvement in walking ability 2 months after surgery (Mutran, Reitzes, Mossey, & Fernandez, 1995). At 6 months, the causal direction reversed with poor improvement in walking leading to greater depression. In older adult populations, increases in depressive symptoms and decreased life satisfaction were predicted by low reported social support (Newsom & Schulz, 1996). Similarly, Hyduk (1996) found in a sample of older adults that an older person's social contact decreases, and if caregivers do not address this decrease in social support, the older person is more at risk for poorer quality of life and institutionalization.

Whereas most research has found that positive psychological and physical outcomes are associated with supportive caregiving relationships, Thompson and Pitts (1992) reported that some studies report negative effects in those who were cared for by a spouse. In reviewing the literature on how caregivers give help with spouses who have cancer, strokes, rheumatoid arthritis, and heart attacks, they found that overprotective and complaining or critical styles of helping were related to negative effects in the care recipient. Overprotective styles were related to being less likely to return to work, experiencing greater depression, being less motivated for physical therapy, and feeling less in control of their lives compared to individuals whose caregivers were not overprotective. Complaining or critical styles of helping characterized by expressed emotion (i.e., hostility toward the patient and emotional overinvolvement) were related to relapse in persons with schizophrenia and even for women who are trying to maintain successful weight loss. In a series of studies with spouses who suffered strokes, those who felt overprotected were significantly more depressed than spouses who did not feel overprotected, and they also perceived less control over their health outcomes. Unrealistic expectations and critical blame by family members also was related to more depression (Thompson & Pitts, 1992).

Thompson and Pitts (1992) theorized three interaction styles that would not increase dependency or reduce perceived control in care recipients: (a) an interaction style characterized by reciprocity and flexibility in helper and help-seeker roles; (b) an interaction style in which it is made "clear that the help is given because of caring and love for the recipient" (p. 142); and (c) an interaction style in which the couple finds ways to handle or avoid some of the resentment either by venting with others or by open communication.

Caregiving quality has important health effects for the care recipient. The caregiver who maintains good psychological and physical health, who does not feel excessively burdened by caregiving, and who has a sense of efficacy in all the domains of caregiving likely will provide better care than one who has deficits in any of these areas. Furthermore, to the degree that caregiving is supportive to the care recipient without promoting dependency or being critical and complaining, there will be an optimum environment providing positive health effects for the care recipient.

INTERVENTIONS TO HELP CAREGIVERS

Given the impact of caregiving on adults by environmental, situational, personal, and social factors, interventions can be geared to improving health status and satisfaction in caregiving by conducting good assessments of the caregiver and the care receiver and then tailoring interventions to meet their needs. From a medical perspective, the caregiver needs information about the illness or disabling condition and needs to learn specific skills to provide quality care. From a psychological perspective, the caregiver's well-being can be enhanced by interventions that deal with central issues already discussed in this chapter. For example, to relieve caregiver burden, support groups, personal counseling, and respite care are useful. Psychosocial interventions to change cognitive appraisals of stress might improve well-being and health for caregivers (McNaughton et al., 1995). Knight, Lutzky, and Macofsky-Urban (1993) conducted a meta-analytic review of interventions for caregiver distress and found that individual psychosocial interventions and respite care programs had moderately strong effects on reducing caregiver burden and distress. Group psychosocial interventions had a small positive effect on distress. Other social and community health services showed no consistent impact on caregiver distress.

Given and Given (1991) found that although respite programs and formal support improved caregiver physical health, they did not always reduce caregiver burden, possibly because caregivers do not use them soon enough or they experience problems in accessing formal services. In a New Zealand study, social relief admissions to hospital-based services available to caregivers did not lower stress but did decrease psychological symptoms, especially depression (Caradoc-Davies & Harvey, 1995).

Buss, Noelker, and Rechlin (1996) examined the stress-buffering effects of interventions that focus on services to the care recipient (e.g., community services in the areas of personal care, household service, escort or transportation, and health care). In a sample of 401 older adults and their caregivers, the use of personal care services (e.g., formal help with eating, toileting, or supervision) buffered the negative effects of care recipients' problem behaviors; and health care services (e.g., formal assistance in getting medications and medical supplies, catheter or colostomy care, giving injections or intravenous treatments, etc.) buffered the effects the recipient's symptoms of cognitive impairment. The result of these interventions was less caregiver depression, less health deterioration, and less social isolation. Household services were related to less caregiver depression by moderating the negative effect of problem behaviors.

Knowing others who have gone through similar experiences is beneficial. Caregivers who knew others who had gone through caregiving for a relative with AD tended to have less depression than those with fewer contacts. These social contacts also tended to act as buffers against stress, especially in the more difficult situations (Pillemer & Suitor, 1996).

In terms of physical health, a good case has been made for how environmental, personal, and social factors might be related, although much more work needs to be done on the causal pathways. Interventions such as those discussed may contribute to health. But the causal pathway from health to psychological well-being, how the caregiving is appraised, and the amount of burden or gain experienced appears also to be supported. Therefore, personal physical care as well as psychological care are appropriate goals for interventions. Good nutrition, rest, exercise, and engaging in health-promoting behaviors would not only affect physical health but would also spill over to feeling less burden, more gain, less depressed and stressed, and to a greater ability to give care.

CONCLUSION

Caregiving for ill or disabled adults is linked with negative mental and physical health outcomes. However, it is being increasingly recognized that caregiving also benefits caregivers and that caregivers are able to manage the stresses of this work. Characteristics of the environment or situation; personal, psychological, and biological characteristics; and social factors influence health status, although much work is still needed on the mediating factors and causal pathways. Attending to these factors in the caregiver promotes health not only for the caregiver but also for the care receiver. Finally, attending to the caregiver's health status itself has reciprocal effects on the quality of the caregiving and the appraisal of the caregiving.

REFERENCES

Aneshensel, C. S., Pearlin, L. I., Mullan, J. T., Zarit, S. H., & Whitlatch, C. J. (1995). *Profiles in caregiving: The unexpected career.* San Diego: Academic Press.

Aranda, M. P., & Knight, B. G. (1997). The influence of ethnicity and culture on the caregiver stress and coping process: A sociocultural review and analysis. *The Gerontologist, 37*(3), 342–354.

Baumgarten, M. (1989). The health of persons giving care to the demented elderly: A critical review of the literature. *Journal of Clinical Epidemiology, 42,* 1137–1148.

Beach, D. L. (1997). Family caregiving: The *positive* impact on adolescent relationships. *The Gerontologist, 37,* 233–238.

Becker, J., & Morrissey, E. (1988). Difficulties in assessing depressive-like reactions to chronic severe external stress as exemplified by spouse caregivers of Alzheimer patients. *Psychology of Aging, 3*(3), 300–306.

Buss, D. M., Noelker, L. S., & Rechlin, L. R. (1996). The moderating influence of service use on negative caregiving consequences. *Journal of Gerontology: Social Sciences, 51B,* S121–S131.

Cantor, M. H. (1983). Strain among caregivers: A study of experience in the United States. *The Gerontologist, 23*(6), 597–604.

Cattanach, L., & Tebes, J. K. (1991). The nature of elder impairment and its impact on family caregivers' health and psychosocial functioning. *The Gerontologist, 31,* 246–255.

Caradoc-Davies, T. H., & Harvey, J. M. (1995). Do "social relief" admissions have any effect on patients or their care-givers? *Disability and Rehabilitation, 17*(5), 247–251.

Clark, L. M., & Hartman, M. (1996). Effects of hardiness and appraisal on the psychological distress and physical health of caregivers to elderly relatives. *Research on Aging, 18,* 379–401.

Clipp, E. C., & George, L. K. (1990). Psychotropic drug use among caregivers of patients with dementia. *Journal of the American Geriatrics Society, 38,* 227–235.

Connell, C. M., & Gibson, G. D. (1997). Racial, ethnic, and cultural differences in dementia caregiving: Review and analysis. *The Gerontologist, 37*(3), 355–364.

Creasia, J. L. (1992). Outcomes of cardiac patients and perceptions of caregiver support. *Family and Community Health, 15,* 31–40.

Deimling, G. T., & Bass, D. M. (1986). Symptoms of mental impairment among elderly adults and their effects on family caregivers. *Journal of Gerontology, 41,* 778–784.

Donaldson, C., Tarrier, N., & Burns, A. (1997). The impact of the symptoms of dementia on caregivers. *The British Journal of Psychiatry, 170,* 62–68

Farran, C. J., & Keane-Hagerty, E. (1991). An interactive model for finding meaning through caregiving. In P. L. Chinn (Ed.), *Anthology on caring* (pp. 225–237). New York: National League for Nursing Press.

Fulmer, T. (1991). Elder mistreatment: Progress in community detection and intervention. *Family and Community Health, 14,* 26–34.

Gallagher, D., Rose, J., Rivera, P., Lovett, S., & Thompson, L. W. (1989). Prevalence of depression in family caregivers. *The Gerontologist, 29,* 449–456.

Gillis, C. L., & Belza, B. L. (1992). A framework for understanding family caregivers' recovery work after cardiac surgery. *Family and Community Health, 15,* 41–48.

Given, B. A., & Given, C. W. (1991). Family caregiving for the elderly. In J. J. Fitzpatrick, R. L. Taunton, & A. K. Jacox (Eds.), *Annual review of nursing research* (pp. 77–101). New York: Springer.

Glaser, R., & Kiecolt-Glaser, J. K. (1997). Chronic stress modulates the virus-specific immune response to latent Herpes Simplex Virus Type 1. *Annals of Behavioral Medicine, 19*(2), 78–82.

Haley, W. E., & Pardo, K. M. (1987, August). *Relationship of stage of dementia to caregiver stress and coping.* Paper presented at the 95th annual meeting of the American Psychological Association, New York.

Hooker, K., Monahan, D., Shifren, K., & Hutchinson, C. (1992). Mental and physical health of spouse caregivers: The role of personality. *Psychology and Aging, 7,* 367–375.

Hyduk, C. A. (1996). The dynamic relationship between social support and health in older adults: Assessment implications. *Journal of Gerontological Social Work, 27,* 149–165.

Kiecolt-Glaser, J. K., Dura, J. R., Speicher, C. E., Trask, O. J., & Glaser, R. (1991). Spousal caregivers of dementia victims: Longitudinal changes in immunity and health. *Psychosomatic Medicine, 53,* 345–362.

Kiecolt-Glaser, J. K., Glaser, R., Gravenstein, S., Malarkey, W. B., & Sheridan, J. (1996). Chronic stress alters the immune response to influenza virus vaccine in older adults. *Proceedings of the National Academy of Sciences, 93,* 3043–3047.

Kiecolt-Glaser, J. K., Marucha, P. T., Malarkey, W. B., Mercado, A. M., & Glaser, R., (1995). Slowing of wound healing by psychological stress. *The Lancet, 346,* 1194–1196.

Kriseman, N. L., & Claes, J. A. (1997). Gender issues and elder care (pp. 199–208). In T. D. Hargrave & S. M. Hanna (Eds.), *The aging family: New visions in theory, practice and reality.* New York: Bruner/ Mazel.

Knight, B. G., Lutzky, S. M., & Macofsky-Urban, F. (1993). A meta-analytic review of interventions for caregiver distress: Recommendations for future research. *The Gerontologist, 33*(2), 240–248.

Kramer, B. J. (1997). Gain in the caregiving experience: Where are we? What next? *The Gerontologist, 37,* 218–232.

Lawton, M. P., Moss, M., Kleban, M. H., Glicksman, A., & Rovine, M. (1991). A two-factor model of caregiving appraisal and psychological well-being. *Journal of Gerontology: Psychological Sciences, 46,* P181–189.

Lazarus, R. S. (1966). *Psychological stress and the coping process.* New York: McGraw-Hill.

Lazarus, R. S., & Folkman, S. (1984). *Stress, appraisal, and coping.* New York: Springer.

Li, L. W., Seltzer, M. M., & Greenberg, J. S. (1997). Social support and depressive symptoms: Differential patterns in wife and daughter caregivers. *Journal of Gerontology: Social Sciences, 52B*(4), S200–211.

Lutzky, S. M., & Knight, B. G. (1994). Explaining gender differences in caregiver distress: The roles of emotional attentiveness and coping styles. *Psychology and Aging, 9*(4), 513–519.

Marks, N. F. (1996). Caregiving across the lifespan: National prevalence and predictors. *Family Relations, 45,* 27–36.

McNaughton, M. E., Patterson, T. L., Smith, T. L., & Grant, I. (1995). The relationship among stress, depression, locus of control, irrational beliefs, social support, and health in Alzheimer's disease caregivers. *The Journal of Nervous and Mental Disease, 183,* 78–85.

Miller, B., & Lawton, M. P. (1997). Positive aspects of caregiving: Introduction: Finding balance in caregiver research. *The Gerontologist, 37,* 216–217.

Mutran, E. J., Reitzes, D. C., Mossey, J., & Fernandez, M. E. (1995). Social support, depression, and recovery of walking ability following hip fracture surgery. *Journal of Gerontology: Social Sciences, 50B,* S354–S361.

Neal, M. B., Chapman, N. J., Ingersoll-Dayton, B., Emlen, A. C., & Boise, L. (1990). In D. E. Biegel & A. Blum (Eds.), *Aging and caregiving: Theory, research, and policy* (pp. 160–183). Newbury Park, CA: Sage.

Neundorfer, M. M. (1991). Coping and health outcomes in spouse caregivers of persons with dementia. *Nursing Research, 40,* 260–265.

Newsom, J. T., & Schulz, R. (1996). Social support as a mediator in the relation between functional status and quality of life in older adults. *Psychology and Aging, 11,* 34–44.

Oxman, T. E., & Hull, J. G. (1997). Social Support, depression, and activities of daily living in older heart surgery patients. *Journal of Gerontology: Psychological Sciences, 52B,* P1–P14.

Paveza, G. J., Cohen, D., Eisdorfer, C., Freels, S., Semla, T., Ashford, J. W., Gorelick, P., Hirschman, R., Luchins, D. and Levy, P. (1992). Severe family violence and Alzheimer's disease: Prevalence and risk factors. *The Gerontologist, 32,* 493–497.

Picot, S. J., Debanne, S. M., Namazi, K. H., & Wykle, M. L. (1997). Religiosity and perceived rewards of black and white caregivers. *The Gerontologist, 37,* 89–101.

Pillemer, K., & Suitor, J. J. (1996). "It takes one to help one": Effects of similar others on the well-being of caregivers. *Journal of Gerontology: Social Sciences, 51B*(5), S250–S257.

Pratt, C. C., Schmall, V. L., Wright, S., & Cleland, M. (1985). Burden and coping strategies of caregivers to Alzheimer's patients. *Family Relations, 34,* 27–33.

Pruchno, R. A., Kleban, M. H., Michaels, J. E., & Dempsey, N. P. (1990). Mental and physical health of caregiving spouses: Development of a causal model. *Journal of Gerontology, 45,* 192–199.

Pruchno, R. A., Peters, N. D., & Burant, C. J. (1995). Mental health of coresident family caregivers: Examination of a two-factor model. *Journal of Gerontology: Psychological Sciences, 50B,* P247–P256.

Pruchno, R. A., & Resch, N. L. (1989). Aberrant behaviors and Alzheimer's Disease: Mental health effects on spouse caregivers. *Journal of Gerontology: Social Sciences, 44*(5), S177–182.

Quayhagen, M. P., & Quayhagen, M. (1988). Alzheimer's stress: Coping with the caregiving role. *The Gerontologist, 28,* 391–396.

Rabins, P. V., Fitting, M. D., Eastham, J., & Fetting, J. (1990). The emotional impact of caring for the chronically ill. *Psychosomatics, 31,* 331–336.

Russo, J., Vitaliáno, P. P., Brewer, D. D., Katon, W., & Becker, J. (1995). Psychiatric disorders in spouse caregivers of care recipients with Alzheimer's disease and matched controls: A diathesis-stress model of psychopathology. *Journal of Abnormal Psychology, 104,* 197–204.

Schulz, R., Newsom, J., Mittlemark, M., Burton, L., Hirsch, C., & Jackson, S. (1997). Health effects of caregiving: The caregiver health effects study: An ancillary study of the cardiovascular health study. *Annals of Behavioral Medicine, 19*(2), 110–116.

Schulz, R., Tompkins, C. A., Wood, D., & Decker, S. (1987). The social psychology of caregiving: Physical and psychological costs of providing support to the disabled. *Journal of Applied Social Psychology, 17,* 401–428.

Schulz, R., Visintainer, P., & Williamson, G. M. (1990). Psychiatric and physical morbidity effects of caregiving. *Journal of Gerontology: Psychological Sciences, 45*(5), P181–191.

Shaw, W. S., Patterson, T. L., Semple, S. J., Grant, I., Yu, E. S. H., Zhang, M. Y., He, Y., & Wu, W. Y. (1997). A cross-cultural validation of coping strategies and their associations with caregiving distress. *The Gerontologist, 37*(4), 490–504.

Shaw, W. S., Patterson, T. L., Semple, S. J., Ho, S., Irwin, M. R., Hauger, R. L., & Grant, I. (1997). Longitudinal analysis of multiple indicators of health decline among spousal caregivers. *Annals of Behavioral Medicine, 19*(2), 101–109.

Silliman, S. A., Fletcher, R. H., Earp, J. L., & Wagner, E. H. (1986). Family of elderly stroke patients: effects of home care. *Journal of the American Geriatrics Society, 34,* 643–668.

Thompson, S. C., & Pitts, J. S. (1992). In sickness and in health: Chronic illness, marriage, and spousal caregiving. In S. Spacapan & S. Oskamp (Eds.), *Helping and being helped: Naturalistic studies* (pp. 115–151). Newbury Park, CA: Sage.

Tyman, R. V. (1994). The stress experienced by caregivers of stroke survivors: Is it all in the mind, or is it also in the body? *Clinical Rehabilitation, 8,* 341–345.

Vachon, D. O. (1996). *The journey of the caregiver: Cultural, psychological, and spiritual perspectives.* Workshop presented to the Caregiver Resource Center, South Bend, IN.

Vachon, D. O., & Merluzzi, T. (1997). *Development of a measure of caregiver self-efficacy.* Unpublished manuscript.

Valle, R., Gook-Gait, H., & Tazbaz, D. (1993, November). *The cross-cultural Alzheimer/dementia caregiver comparison study.* Paper presented at the 46th Scientific Meeting of the Gerontological Society of America, New Orleans, LA.

Vitaliano, P. P., Russo, J., & Niaura, R. (1995). Plasma lipids and their relationships with psychosocial factors in older adults. *Journal of Gerontology: Psychological Sciences, 50B,* P18–P24.

Vitaliano, P. P., Scanlan, J. M., Krenz, C., Schwartz, R. S., & Marcovina, S. M. (1996). Psychological distress, caregiving, and metabolic variables. *Journal of Gerontology: Psychological Sciences, 51B,* P290–P299.

Vitaliano, P. P., Schulz, R., Kiecolt-Glaser, J., & Grant, I. (1997). Research on physiological and physical concomitants of caregiving: Where do we go from here? *Annals of Behavioral Medicine, 19,* 117–123.

Wijeratne, C., & Lovestone, S. (1996). A pilot study comparing psychological and physical morbidity in carers of elderly people with dementia and those with depression. *International Journal of Geriatric Psychiatry, 11,* 741–744.

Zarit, S. H., Todd, P. A., & Zarit, J. M. (1986). Subjective burden of husbands and wives as caregivers: A longitudinal study. *The Gerontologist, 26,* 260–266.

13

Death and Dying Across the Life Span

John L. McIntosh
Indiana University South Bend

BY DEFINITION, the life span involves a beginning (conception and birth) and end (death and dying). Death is a natural part of the life span, despite its denial in the United States (e.g., Kastenbaum & Aisenberg, 1972). Death, often conceptualized as a biological event, is preceded by a period of psychological, social, and biological processes called dying. As is discussed, these factors interact with one another to influence the course and qualities of the process of dying, and the event of death itself, as well as its probability. Although death is commonly associated with late life, it can occur at any age throughout the life span and any number of biopsychosocial forces and their interactions may bring on death and the events that surround the dying process. In addition to multiple factors, many subtopics relate to death across the various life stages. This chapter discusses patterns of death, understanding of death as well as feelings of anxiety and fear surrounding it, and the grief and bereavement that occur following the death of a loved one.

WHEN WE DIE

Although mortality data are available for many countries through the World Health Organization (e.g., 1991), this chapter focuses on official death statistics from the United States. More specifically, figures compiled from death certificates and other death records are provided by each state to the National Center for Health Statistics (NCHS), forming the basis for official statistics in its various publications (such as the annual *Vital Statistics of the United States*). In 1995 (Anderson, Kochanek, & Murphy, 1997), the most recent year available, there were 262.76 million Americans and 2.3 million deaths were recorded (a record number of deaths, reflecting the increasing national population). Most people associate dying with late life, and indeed, 1.7 million of the 2.3 million deaths were among those 65 years of age and older (73.3% of all deaths among only 12.8% of the population, or 33.5 million). By contrast, those 15 to 24 years of age numbered 35.9 million in 1995 (13.7%) but represented a scant 1.5% (34,244) of all U.S. deaths (Anderson et al., 1997). Therefore, although death may occur at any age, Americans usually die in old age.

The maximum length of human life (life span) over time has changed little, being approximately 120 years. The average length of human lives (life expectancy) has increased dramatically over time. That is, more people are living longer lives (the fastest growing age grouping in the population are those 85 years of age and older), but the upper limit of human life has remained essentially constant. Under prevailing death rates, an American born in 1992 could expect to die at 75.8 years of age (this can be compared to a life expectancy at birth of only 62.9 years in 1940; NCHS, 1996, sect. 6). This average, however, masks important differences for demographic groups. Women, on average, die nearly 7 years later than men (79.1 compared to 72.3 years for those born in 1992). Racial differences indicate that Whites live longer than Blacks (76.5 years compared to 69.5), with the influence of gender present across groups. White women (79.8 years) are the longest lived, followed by Black women (73.9 years), White men (73.2 years), and Black men (65 years). Similar figures are seen in the percentage of those who are still alive at age 65. National figures showed that 80.1% of Americans survived from birth to age 65 in 1992. These percentages show that White women are most often still alive at age 65 (86.8%), followed by White men (76.7%), Black women (75.5%), and Black men (58.2%).

HOW WE DIE

Related to the increasing trends for death in late life, people usually die in institutional settings, particularly hospitals and institutions for the aged. This trend represents a dramatic change from earlier patterns of dying (Cook & Oltjenbruns, 1989; Kastenbaum & Aisenberg, 1972; Leming & Dickinson, 1990), in which individuals most often died at home (and instead of institutionalizing death via the funeral industry, family were present and integral in funeral aspects; see Preston, 1977). In the late 1990s, the likelihood that a person will die in the community is less than one in five (Cook & Oltjenbruns, 1989; Kastenbaum, 1978).

The factors are multifaceted that produce any particular death and contribute to the patterns of death, life span, and life expectancy in a culture. Although death itself is associated with and produced biologically, involving organ systems, other nonbiological forces play primary roles. These other factors involve psychological, social, and environmental forces and their interactions in addition to any biological forces operating. It should be noted that global factors such as culture, ethnicity, and race influence all aspects of death, dying, bereavement, as well as concepts and fears about death. Space does not permit presentation of these factors in other than cursory fashion. More information is available in Jackson (1981), Leming and Dickinson (1990), and Parkes, Laungani, and Young (1997). In most deaths it is likely that no single factor can be identified that produced the death and the majority of deaths are undoubtedly the result of interactions of these various factors. However, some extreme examples in clinical literature may help demonstrate the possible effects of nonbiological forces on humans.

Parkes (1973/1980) identified the "broken heart" syndrome to describe the deaths of spouses who had experienced the recent death of their husbands or wives. Clinical research by Parkes and others are presented as evidence for highly elevated death risk following grief, with deaths far above the number expected in the same population in general or those who had not been bereaved. Although several factors may contribute, the first 6 months to 1 year of bereavement have long been established as a period of particularly high risk for mortality (e.g., Epstein, Weitz, Roback, & McKee, 1975/1979; Stroebe & Stroebe, 1983). These findings about the widowed are similar to those for the other end of the life span. Research has indicated elevated risk of negative outcomes and even increased mortality risk later in life among those who were emotionally deprived of their mothers in childhood through death or other reasons (e.g., Critelli, 1983; Tucker et al., 1997). Prior to the 1950s, Spitz (cited in Kastenbaum & Aisenberg, 1972) found that children deprived of their mothers failed to thrive, became demanding, cried a great deal, lost weight, and by 3 months of age refused human contact and assumed a prone position in their cribs. In studies of children in foundling homes, the same responses were often noted and 37% of these children died by the end of 2 years. Spitz referred to this as *anaclitic depression.* Such extreme examples suggest that the loss of significant others and other stressors has profound effects on some individuals, including possible ramifications that influence life itself. The biological event of death must be placed in the entire biopsychosocial context of the process of dying to be fully understood in its often complicated and multifaceted nature.

Taylor (1991) observed that "in the past 90 years, patterns of disease in the United States of such acute infectious disorders as tuberculosis, influenza, measles, and polio-myelitis have declined because of treatment innovations and changes in public health standards" (p. 53). At the same time, however, Taylor noted increases over time in "preventable disorders" such as cardiovascular disease, lung cancer, automobile accidents, and alcohol and drug abuse. Many of these declining disorders are more often associated with youth, whereas cardiovascular disease, as noted later, is more common in old age. The decline in infectious diseases and the concomitant decline in mortality rates at young ages has been contributing factors to the increase in those surviving to late life (McIntosh, 1993).

A close examination of the specific causes of those deaths in Table 13.1 reveals that the primary killers are heart disease, cancers (malignant neoplasms), and strokes (cerebrovascular diseases), in that order. These three causes combined rep-

TABLE 13.1

Deaths, Death Rates, and Rankings for the 10 Leading Causes of Death by Age Groups: United States, 1995

Rank	<1 yr	1–4 yrs	5–14 yrs	15–24 yrs	25–44 yrs	45–64 yrs	65+ yrs	Total
1	Congenital anomalies	Accidents	Accidents	Accidents	HIV	Malignant neoplasms	Heart disease	Heart disease
	6,554	2,280	3,544	13,842	30,754	132,084	615,426	737,563
	168.1	14.5	9.3	38.5	36.9	253.0	1835.3	280.7
2	Short gestation	Congenital anomalies	Malignant neoplasms	Homicide	Accidents	Heart disease	Malignant neoplasms	Malignant neoplasms
	3,933	695	1,026	7,284	27,660	102,738	381,142	538,455
	100.9	4.4	2.7	20.3	33.2	196.8	1136.6	204.9
3	SIDS	Malignant neoplasms	Homicide	Suicide	Malignant neoplasms	Accidents	Cerebrovascular disease	Cerebrovascular disease
	3,397	488	562	4,784	21,985	16,004	138,762	157,991
	87.1	3.1	1.5	13.3	26.4	30.7	413.8	60.1
4	Respiratory distress syndrome	Homicide	Congenital anomalies	Malignant neoplasms	Heart disease	Cerebrovascular disease	Pulmonary disease[a]	Pulmonary disease[a]
	1,454	452	449	1,642	17,064	15,208	88,478	102,899
	37.3	2.9	1.2	4.6	20.5	29.1	263.9	39.2
5	Maternal complications	Heart disease	Suicide	Heart disease	Suicide	Pulmonary disease[a]	Pneumonia and influenza	Accidents
	1,309	251	337	1,039	12,759	12,744	74,297	93,320
	33.6	1.6	0.9	2.9	15.3	24.4	221.6	35.5
6	Placenta, cord, membrane	HIV	Heart disease	HIV	Homicide	Diabetes	Diabetes and influenza	Pneumonia
	962	210	294	629	10,280	12,184	44,452	82,923
	24.7	1.3	0.8	1.7	12.3	23.3	132.6	31.6

Continued

TABLE 13.1 (*Continued*)

Rank	<1 yr	1–4 yrs	5–14 yrs	15–24 yrs	25–44 yrs	45–64 yrs	65+ yrs	Total
7	Perinatal infections	Pneumonia and influenza	HIV	Congenital anomalies	Liver disease	Liver disease	Accidents	Diabetes
	788	156	189	452	4,309	10,603	29,099	59,254
	20.2	1.0	0.5	1.3	5.2	20.3	86.8	22.6
8	Accidents	Conditions of perinatal period	Pulmonary disease[a]	Pulmonary disease[a]	Cerebrovascular disease	HIV	Alzheimer's disease	HIV
	787	87	143	246	3,492	10,499	20,230	43,115
	20.2	0.6	0.4	0.7	4.2	20.1	60.3	16.4
9	Pneumonia and influenza	Septicemia	Pneumonia and influenza	Pneumonia and influenza	Diabetes	Suicide	Nephritis	Suicide
	492	80	128	207	2,458	7,336	20,182	31,284
	12.6	0.5	0.3	0.6	2.9	14.1	60.2	11.9
10	Intrauterine hypoxia	Cerebrovascular disease	Benign neoplasms	Cerebrovascular disease	Pneumonia and influenza	Pneumonia and influenza	Septicemia disease	Liver
	475	57	105	172	2,102	5,537	16,899	25,222
	12.2	0.4	0.3	0.5	2.5	10.6	50.4	9.6

Note: Data from Anderson et al. (1997), pp. 23–24, p. 69.
Rates are per 100,000.
[a]Includes bronchitis, emphysema, and asthma.

253

resent more than 1.4 million (62%) deaths. For the elderly 65 and older, these same three account for 1.1 million (67%) deaths. It is predominantly, in fact, the large number and proportion of deaths among the old as compared to other age groups that result in the high ranking of these three causes. These three become the highest ranking cause of deaths for the group aged 45 to 64 years; younger groups have different primary causes of death.

Although causes of death predominantly characterized as disease-based prevail in middle age and older adulthood, the young die primarily due to their or others' carelessness or actions. That is, those under the age of 45 die mostly in accidents, with homicide and suicide being conspicuous causes of death as well. For the young aged 5 to 14 years these three external causes of death (i.e., accidents, suicide, and homicide) combine to account for more than half (51.7%) of their deaths. By adolescence and young adulthood (15 to 24 years of age) this proportion increases to 3 of every 4 deaths (75.7%). Many of these deaths in recent years are firearm-related. Firearm deaths accounted for 28.6% of all deaths for those aged 15 to 24 years in 1995 (Anderson et al., 1997; see also O'Donnell, 1995). In another recent trend, the rise of deaths related to AIDS has made this disease the top-ranking cause among those aged 25 to 44 in the United States. Although less so than for the young, among those 25 to 44, external causes still represent nearly one of every three deaths (31.7%), falling with each age grouping until they account for only 2.1% of deaths among those 65 and older.

Mortality rates for violent causes of death have increased among the young. One explanation for these trends, and its extension to the future when the present young eventually become older adults, is of particular interest here. Presenting official data, Holinger (1987) documented strong correlations between population changes and violent deaths (accidents, homicides, suicides, and their aggregation) consistent with what has been called the Easterlin hypothesis (Easterlin, 1987). Easterlin suggested that large birth cohorts are particularly associated with high rates of violent death due to increased stress and competition produced by the large number of individuals moving together through the life span and its societal institutions. Holinger (1987) found this hypothesis had strong predictive potential for the changes from 1933 to 1982 for young adult populations. This relation was particularly true for the period between the 1950s and the 1970s when violent deaths increased dramatically among the young. This distressing pattern coincided with the movement of the large "baby boom" cohort through the target ages of 15 to 24 years.

The Easterlin hypothesis suggests that stability and even decline in violent deaths will occur in the near future as smaller, succeeding cohorts of young people reach the target age. Also based on Easterlin's hypothesis, some authors (e.g., Manton, Blazer, & Woodbury, 1987; Pollinger-Haas & Hendin, 1983) have predicted that suicide rates, which are highest in late life (see McIntosh, Santos, Hubbard, & Overholser, 1994), will be markedly higher than at present when the high-risk baby boomer cohort reaches older adulthood in the next century. On the other hand,

predictions of lower rates among future elders have also been advanced. Emphasizing the multifactorial nature of mortality risk, McIntosh (1992) argued that economic factors (e.g., pensions, Social Security benefits, retirement preparation,
etc.), societal and individual attitudes and beliefs (toward aging, old age, and retirement), the nature of late life in the future as it influences an individual's experience, the health of the older adult population, and medical advances might predict
lower suicide rates for aged boomers than for today's elderly.

Returning now to general mortality figures, in addition to age, race and gender
differences in mortality are also prominent. Although the ranking of the leading
causes of death are primarily the same, White mortality rates are generally higher
than those for non-Whites. In addition, there are a number of specific racial differences (as well as ethnic differences, see, e.g., Jackson, 1981). For example, Table
13.2 provides racial differences in mortality and shows that homicide ranks higher
and suicide lower for non-Whites compared to Whites. In addition, higher ranking
of HIV and the causes of death originating in the perinatal period among non-
Whites are other differences, as are higher rates for accidents, particularly among
non-White males (Anderson et al., 1997; Jackson, 1981). The data in Table 13.2
clearly show the reason that mortality rates and not the actual number of deaths
should be compared—different demographic groups often represent quite disparate population sizes. In addition to racial differences in mortality, men have
higher overall mortality rates than women at all ages regardless of race, and the
gender differences increase with advancing age (Anderson et al., 1997). For the
highest ranking causes of death, particularly heart disease and cancer, men's rates
exceed those for women (see Table 13.2).

Explanations for these various differences in mortality by sex have been advanced, and emphasize further the multifactorial nature of influences on death. As
McIntosh (1993) discussed, for instance, the generally higher male mortality rate
has been explained by biogenetic, environmental, and psychosocial forces. Biogenetic explanations include lower susceptibility to disease by women. This may
result from chromosomal differences, higher metabolic rates among males that
could contribute to some diseases, and dietary preferences for men that might combine with metabolic rates to increase vulnerability to cancer or other disorders. Environmental factors proposed to account for gender differences in death risks include the type of work in which men and women engage as well as differential experiences with stress, cigarette smoking, and exercise. Major potential psychosocial
factors that influence gender differences in mortality involve differential societal
roles, expectations, and demands made on males and females (see Stillion, 1985,
for further discussion of these factors).

Turning to the implications of these detailed data for mortality trends, and particularly for prevention and intervention, a multidimensional perspective on the
causes of death becomes useful. As McIntosh (1993) noted, death is inevitable, and
therefore the intervention emphasis is not on death prevention but on intervention in premature death. Intervention that lessens or eliminates problematic be-

TABLE 13.2

Deaths, Death Rates, and Rankings for the 10 Leading Causes of Death by Gender and Race: United States, 1995

Rank	Men	Women	White	Black	White Men	White Women	Black Men	Black Women
1	Heart disease 362,714 282.7	Heart disease 374,849 278.8	Heart disease 649,089 297.6	Heart disease 78,643 237.3	Heart disease 318,751 297.9	Heart disease 330,338 297.4	Heart disease 38,389 244.2	Heart disease 40,254 231.1
2	Malignant neoplasms 281,611 219.5	Malignant neoplasms 256,844 191.0	Malignant neoplasms 468,897 215.0	Malignant neoplasms 60,603 182.9	Malignant neoplasms 244,000 228.1	Malignant neoplasms 224,897 202.4	Malignant neopl asms 32,880 209.1	Malignant neoplasms 27,723 159.1
3	Cerebrovascular disease 61,563 48.0	Cerebrovascular disease 96,428 71.7	Cerebrovascular disease 136,481 62.6	Cerebrovascular disease 18,537 55.9	Cerebrovascular disease 52,045 48.6	Cerebrovascular disease 84,436 76.0	HIV 12,875 81.9	Cerebrovascular disease 10,526 60.4
4	Accidents 61,401 47.9	Pulmonary disease[a] 48,961 36.4	Pulmonary disease[a] 95,077 43.6	HIV 17,139 51.7	Accidents 50,670 47.4	Pulmonary disease[a] 45,757 41.2	Homicide 8,847 56.3	Diabetes 6,292 36.1
5	Pulmonary disease[a] 53,938 42.0	Pneumonia and influenza 45,136 33.6	Accidents 77,748 35.7	Accidents 12,748 38.5	Pulmonary disease[a] 49,320 46.1	Pneumonia and influenza 40,693 36.6	Accidents 8,834 56.2	HIV 4,264 24.5
6	Pneumonia and influenza 37,787 29.4	Diabetes 33,130 24.6	Pneumonia and influenza 73,641 33.8	Homicide 10,783 32.5	Pneumonia and influenza 32,948 30.8	Accidents 27,078 24.4	Cerebrovascular disease 8,011 51.0	Accidents 3,914 22.5

Continued

TABLE 13.2 (Continued)

Rank	Men	Women	White	Black	White Men	White Women	Black Men	Black Women
7	HIV	Accidents	Diabetes	Diabetes	Suicide	Diabetes	Diabetes	Pneumonia and influenza
	35,950	31,919	47,475	10,482	22,853	26,068	4,110	3,784
	28.0	23.7	21.8	31.4	21.4	23.5	26.1	21.7
8	Diabetes	Alzheimer's disease	Suicide	Pneumonia and influenza	HIV	Alzheimer's disease	Pneumonia and influenza	Pulmonary disease[a]
	26,124	13,607	28,187	7,803	22,670	12,826	4,019	2,750
	20.4	10.1	12.9	23.5	21.2	11.5	25.6	15.8
9	Suicide	Pulmonary disease[a]	HIV	Pulmonary disease[a]	Diabetes	Nephritis	Pulmonary disease[a]	Nephritis
	25,369	12,287	25,509	6,667	21,407	9,829	3,917	2,243
	19.8	9.1	11.7	20.1	20.0	8.8	24.9	12.9
10	Homicide	Septicemia	Liver disease	Conditions of perinatal period	Liver disease	Septicemia	Conditions of perinatal period	Conditions of perinatal period
	17,740	11,974	21,432	4,952	14,100	9,744	2,731	2,221
	13.8	8.9	9.8	14.9	13.2	8.8	17.4	12.7

Note: Data from Anderson et al. (1997), pp. 24–32.
Rates are per 100,000 population.
[a]Includes bronchitis, emphysema, and asthma.

257

havior, lifestyles, and environmental risk factors, such as pollution or secondhand smoke, might extend life nearer or to its maximum potential length. In this regard, the Centers for Disease Control and Prevention have estimated that "50% of all deaths from the ten leading causes of death in this country are due to modifiable lifestyle factors" (Taylor, 1991, p. 53).

Thus, examining the threats to life expectancy Woodruff (1984) raised this question: "Can you live to be 100?" In addressing this question, Woodruff pointed out that biological factors, such as genetic endowment or inheritance, family history of diseases such as cancer and diabetes, and gender interact with lifestyle habits (e.g., eating, exercise, and sleeping behaviors), personal characteristics (intelligence, sexual activity, education, socioeconomic status, income, marital status, and social support), and personality traits (e.g., depression or anxiety level) to predict longevity. Although some of these variables are unchangeable and most do not affect life expectancy alone, their joint modification might have a significant impact. In a review of this literature, McIntosh (1993) suggested that prominent among the modifiable behaviors that compromise health are smoking, alcoholism, and problem drinking. Smoking is associated not only with premature death by lung cancer but also with heart disease, respiratory disorders, and even the effects of secondhand smoke on others. Alcohol abuse and alcoholism contribute to premature deaths through their association with liver cirrhosis, some forms of cancer, auto accidents, and deaths from falls and fires.

CONCEPTIONS AND ATTITUDES TOWARD DEATH ACROSS THE LIFESPAN

Long before death becomes imminent, individuals have undergone processes that shape future cognitions and thoughts during the dying process. At the beginning of life, children and adolescents develop conceptions of personal and universal death. Thereafter, throughout life, individuals at various times confront their own mortality and fears about dying. Therefore, although many factors influence personal experiences of death and the dying process, important among them are cognitions that influence behavior at the end of life.

Death Concept

The individual's understanding of the concept of death in general, the possibility of personal death, and attitudes toward death and dying are important lifelong influences that might affect many of his or her behaviors and choices. An extensive literature exists on the development of the conception of death among children and adolescents (e.g., Kastenbaum, 1991, 1992; Kastenbaum & Aisenberg, 1972; Lonetto, 1980). Not surprisingly, children do not have the same conception of death found among adults. Among the primary factors influencing and limiting this developmental progression is cognitive development (e.g., Jenkins & Cavanaugh, 1985/1986). However, cognitive development alone does not explain children's ideas about death (see e.g., Stambrook & Parker, 1987). Hostler (1978) reminded us of the importance of individual differences in his assertion that "The preschool child will respond to encounters with death based on his own experiences, his family's religious and cultural heritage, his own attachment with the dead person, and his developmental level" (p. 9). In addition, such factors as intelligence, mass media, and social class also might influence the development of ideas about death (Stambrook & Parker, 1987).

One of the early and most often cited studies of children's conception of death was conducted in the 1930s by Nagy (1948/1959) who studied more than 300 Hungarian children aged 3 to 10 years. Utilizing drawings, compositions, and discussions whenever appropriate, Nagy found three major stages in the development of the meaning of death to children. Nagy suggested that children younger than age 5 have no concept of death as final or irreversible. Death is denied by conceiving of the dead as having life and awareness just like living individuals (reminiscent of and an extension of animism in early cognitive development). Sometimes this conception of death is like sleep, whereas in other cases death is seen as either gradual or temporary in nature. For these young children death is no different from a departure (and similar to the cognitive idea of object permanence). These children think that we no longer can see the person who dies, but they remain alive although constricted in their ability to experience. Other investigations (e.g., Hoffman & Strauss, 1985) reported children's ideas that the dead continue with internal events, such as thinking, after they have ceased external events, such as moving.

Although Nagy's findings indicated that death for the preschool child is not permanent, Pattison (1977) noted that it is real to the child. That is, people can and do die; it is not pretend. Death has a magical and impermanent nature, but at the same time death is real. Pattison further suggests that whereas death cannot be understood by the youngest children (younger than age 3), who lack the cognitive development to understand concepts and the permanence of objects, death does represent separation, and this aspect is also present in the child aged 3 to 6. The child needs a sense of continuity in her or his life, and death, in a child's short time perspective, means separation and aloneness from parents and others.

As the second stage, for children aged 5 to 9, Nagy (1948/1959) found a personification of death. For most of these children, death is conceptualized as an actual, invisible person. Nagy considered this a move forward, as the child accepts death as a fact. This attribution of death to the actions of a person are similar to the concept of animism, the aliveness of almost everything, in cognitive development. But children attempt to obtain distance from death by conceptualizing it as not relevant to themselves and not necessarily inevitable so long as one can avoid the death-man. However, research with American children (e.g., Koocher, 1974; see also Cook & Oltjenbruns, 1989; Stillion & Wass, 1979/1984) has not supported this stage in the conception of death. It was suggested that Hungarian culture, with its art and literature, reinforced this personification, and such elements are not a part of the U.S. cultural experience.

Nagy (1948/1959) indicated by the age of 9 or 10 that children understand that death represents "the cessation of corporeal life" (p. 96); it is universal, and it is operating inside us. Children finally comprehend that they and everyone else will die (the ability to think abstractly permitting such speculation), and that death is permanent, internal, and inevitable.

Pattison (1977) elaborated further on the conceptualization of death as final in grade-school children. Although children can appreciate the general idea of death, and of their own death on an intellectual plane, death remains distant and still seems impersonal. Death happens, but it happens to others. This point reminds us of the cognitive research on egocentrism in particular. Young children can only appreciate their own perceptual viewpoint and subjective world. With advancing cognitive development, however, egocentrism diminishes. Older children and adolescents evidence beliefs in seemingly personal invulnerability and immortality even when they understand the general concept of death as final, inevitable, and applying to themselves and everyone else. This "personal fable" (Elkind, 1967), therefore, is a seeming paradox with respect to the child and adolescent's conception of death. Other egocentric aspects of intellectual functioning combine with the personal fable in interesting ways. For instance, Pattison (1977) suggested that young people might "make brave soldiers" either because they do not fear that their own death will occur when chances are taken and danger exists, or they are more concerned with appearing courageous and brave to others in a romantic fashion. Looking good in the eyes of others, that is, the quality of one's appearance to this "imaginary audience," is more important. In summarizing the development of the concept of death and their own immortality, Gordon (1986, p. 28) argued that "the early adolescent becomes aware of death, and the late adolescent attempts to impart a meaning to death (as well as to life) that transcends everyday events and infuses the future with hope," with the "cloak of immortality" serving protective purposes during childhood but being set aside by the end of adolescence.

Given normal development, cognitive impediments can be expected to all but disappear and the finality, inevitability, and universality of adult death conceptualization operate. A recent investigation (Noppe & Noppe, 1997) of middle school, high school, and college students suggested a progression of death conceptualization during adolescence and into young adulthood reflecting experience and knowledge of death. These young people became increasingly aware of and concerned about the personal inevitability of death and were more likely to discuss death openly with others. Particularly different from younger ages, the high school and especially the college students ponder issues of an afterlife and their personal legacy. Little research or writing address the timing and final transitions to complete death concept of young adulthood and beyond. Instead, the focus of attention, particularly in adulthood, is not on death concept but rather on attitudes and possible fears about death.

Death Attitudes and Fears

U.S. society has often been characterized as a death-denying society and one that has distanced itself from death, both emotionally and physically (e.g., Rando, 1984). Several writers (e.g., Firestone, 1994; Kastenbaum, 1991; Kastenbaum & Aisenberg, 1972) have discussed at length the defenses and coping methods humans use to deal with their death fears. These methods include denial, living for the moment, religious beliefs, belief in an afterlife, and leaving a personal legacy through future generations.

Often, contradictory findings have emerged for the many demographic and personality variables studied. However, results by gender consistently either show women to have higher death anxiety than men or find no gender differences (see also Kastenbaum, 1992; Stillion, 1985). In a review of the literature, Pollak (1979–80) also noted that "it appears that death anxiety and concern are greater in people lacking in a personal sense of effectiveness, mastery, and power and are markedly diminished in persons who possess high self-esteem, and who experience a high degree of meaning and purpose in their lives" (p. 116). Schulz (1978/1985) concluded that health status was not related to death anxiety among the terminally ill or those close to death. However, Schulz's review provided evidence that high religiosity as measured by beliefs was associated with low levels of death anxiety. On the other hand, extrinsic measures of religiosity such as church attendance were unrelated to death anxiety (see Leming & Dickinson, 1990, for a consideration of various religions and death). The personal experience of loss of significant others, whether in early life or in recent experience, has been found to be related to higher personal fear of death (e.g., Florian & Mikulincer, 1997), perhaps by raising awareness of personal mortality. Interestingly, although higher levels of general education are associated with low levels of death anxiety (e.g., Kastenbaum, 1992), some death education programs actually seem to produce increased death anxiety (Maglio & Robinson, 1994).

With respect to the life span, research has consistently found that death anxiety, as typically measured by self-report instruments, does not increase with age in adulthood (e.g., Kastenbaum, 1992; Pollak, 1979–80). The most intriguing aspect of this finding is the lack of high death anxiety among the group closest to and most often exposed to death, older adults. Most studies report high levels of death anxiety among only a small proportion of the group. Several authors suggested that the general lack of anxiety may be due to denial processes and general lack of readiness to confront the troubling issue of death. Alternatively, the low levels of death anxiety among the elderly might be due to acceptance of death, more exposure to death and dying, physical changes associated with aging, the fact that death represents no threat to an elder's life plans around such issues as career and family (unlike the young and middle aged), and a perception of already living on "borrowed time" (Kalish, 1976; Kastenbaum, 1992). Research to date has not examined the relative importance of these correlates of death anxiety in late life. However, on a clinical note, Kastenbaum (1992) suggested that high levels or surges in death anxiety might be cause for concern and signal the existence of a problem that demands attention.

The transition from midlife to older adulthood might have special significance for death thoughts and possibly anxiety. In a study of more than 400 Los Angeles residents from four ethnic groups, Kalish and Reynolds (1976) found highest fears of personal death among the young and lowest for the elderly, with the middle aged reporting intermediate levels. Munnich (cited in Kastenbaum, 1992) studied death anxiety among 100 older adults in the Netherlands, employing accounts of their lives as told by the participants themselves. Although moving from the last years of midlife and into the early years of late life (what has often been called the young-old), individuals are actively involved in grappling with their own mortality. By the period of old-old age, however, the very old have arrived at an acceptance or resolution of the topic and do not expend much further thought to the issue. Munnich suggested that the oldest old, in fact, seem to largely prefer to avoid or ignore the issue of the end of life, giving little significance to it. This mid- to late-life progression is consistent with late life theories on processes of life evaluation and its implications for death preparedness (e.g., Erikson's, 1963, ego integrity vs. despair; Butler's, 1963, life review). Kastenbaum and Costa (1977) concluded in their review of research findings that "Most studies of death attitudes in old age indicate the ability of well integrated people to accommodate themselves to finitude. Distress at the prospect of death usually has been related to general agitation or to environmental stress or deprivation" (p. 233).

THE DYING PROCESS

Although several "types" and definitions of death have been described (e.g., psychological death, social death, biological death, brain death, see, e.g., Rando, 1984), dying is less an event than a process over time. Research and clinical evidence suggest a variety of factors as potentially affecting the experience of dying, including the nature of the disease, the amount and perception of pain, the course of the dying process, mobility and social isolation, the treatment regimen, expectations regarding the length and course of the illness, gender, ethnicity, culture, personality, cognitive style, coping styles, history, religiosity and spiritual values, social supports and the number and quality of interpersonal relationships, previous experience with death and dying and loss, mental health, financial and economic resources, education, and intelligence (e.g., Kastenbaum, 1991; Rando, 1984). Finally, the age or developmental period of the individual also influences the dying process.

Dying and Life Periods

Reactions to death by the dying individual vary considerably over the life span (see, e.g., Cook & Oltjenbruns, 1989). Pattison (1977) suggested, however, that dying persons of all ages need to be able to express their feelings surrounding their impending death, feel a sense of security and maintenance of self-control, and have the support and continuation of their social relationships, perhaps because they have common concerns, fears of the unknown, loneliness, sorrow, loss of body, suffering, pain, and loss of identity.

The central issue for the youngest children (under age 3 and from 3 to 6) is a fear of separation from parents. Thus, interventions at this age involve maintaining the stability and closeness of the parents or an adult substitute to the dying child to provide love and emotional support (e.g., Pattison, 1977; Rando, 1984). Young children need an environment in which they can develop trust in those around them and normalization of their lives in circumstances of change and stress (Cook & Oltjenbruns, 1989). Even young children seem to realize they are dying and the consensus is that the fact of their dying should be explained to them in terms they can understand. Open discussion should be permitted (e.g., Leming & Dickinson, 1990). Adults often act with paternalistic concerns toward dying children of all ages, wishing to protect them by either not telling them they are dying or lying to them. Not only should the child be told about the fatal nature of their condition, but, more importantly, adults need to help them avoid the loneliness and isolation associated with dying (e.g., Waechter, 1971).

Among grade-school children (6 to 11 years of age), who are beginning to understand the finality of death, the body-related issues of pain and the medical procedures to be endured are causes of concern. There is agreement that dying children need to continue where possible normal living patterns (e.g., play, attending school, contact with peers). Explanations about their condition and treatment is critical (the information in this and the following life periods are derived from Cook & Oltjenbruns, 1989; Leming & Dickinson, 1990; Pattison, 1977; Rando, 1984).

Dying adolescents often express anger and anxiety about death because of its non-normative nature. Death comes just as the young person has begun to gain a sense of self and being. Recognition of their individuality and developing sense of identity are central aspects of assisting with the dying process in this life period. Adolescents also require attention to their normative needs for privacy, independence, control, and peer contacts (see also Adams & Deveau, 1986).

Similarly, young adults who are dying experience disappointment, frustration, and anger. Death at this time, the threshold of adult life, seems unfair, cheating the young adult of his or her fair experience and promise of life. The goals and tasks of life will now be unfulfilled. Assistance in this life period should center on permitting the expression of such feelings of injustice and rage and helping them to cope with impending losses.

In an acceleration of Erikson's (1963) mid- and late-life crises, knowledge that one is dying in midlife might trigger a sense of urgency to evaluate one's life and its accomplishments and failures. Evaluation of one's legacy and contribution to society and other people (and possibly feelings of unfilled obligations and responsibilities, especially in interpersonal relationships) might take on special significance in the context of impending death. Part of this evaluation process also might include assessing one's values and priorities in life.

As already described, older adults generally prepare for the end of their lives by evaluating them. This process is directed at helping them achieve personal affirmation, integration, and preparation for death. On the other hand, a negative evaluation might produce anxiety for some dying older adults. Primary concerns of dying older adults often center on their body. That is, the older adult in particular might worry about the loss of control and decision making in their life and death, dependence on their children, as well as issues of pain and suffering.

Dying and Family Members

Although a voluminous literature exists on grief and bereavement following the death of a loved one, a relatively small literature is devoted to the family and significant others of the dying individual during their terminal phase. Most of their reactions are similar to those they experience after the death of their loved ones. Families in which a member is dying experience high levels of stress and relationships between members might become strained (although in other cases they actually might become closer). Processes of anticipatory grief and "decathection" toward the dying family member begin. While saying goodbye to the dying person, family members simultaneously continue their relationship and provision of emotional support to the dying individual and attempt to attend to the necessary tasks of their lives. Family members often feel anxiety, sorrow for their impending loss, and perhaps even depression. They also might experience feelings of helplessness and even guilt and like the dying person, might have anger and other hostile emotions as well. Rando (1984) suggested a number of interventions for the family members, including the use of support groups to cope with the loss (see also Lipton, 1978). A variety of issues revolving around the interrelationships of those surrounding the dying person need to be confronted. For example, in a family with a dying child, siblings might be excluded from participating in their brother's or sister's case and not allowed to deal with their own concerns (Stillion & Wass, 1979/ 1984). Parents whose child is dying might feel intense guilt and helplessness because society expects parents to protect and care for their children (Kamerman, 1988). Parents also experience frustration and anger at the injustice and perceived inappropriateness of a child's death. In the case of children whose parents are dying, common reactions include guilt and feelings that somehow they caused the parent's death.

Dying "Stages"

Moving to the subjective experiences of individual death, regardless of life period, perhaps the best known characterization of the process of dying with its feelings and emotional experiences resulted from Kübler-Ross' (1969) extensive clinical work with dying patients. She suggested a number of stages with associated coping mechanisms that terminal patients experience following learning of their terminal condition. Although she never intended that the "stages" be taken literally as an immutable sequence or as anything except a set of feelings that came and went among individuals with terminal illness, they have often been portrayed in this manner. The set of stages Kübler-Ross observed in these individuals are as follows: (a) after a period of shock and numbness, *denial* of the information by the person that she or he is dying regardless of the evidence ("It can't be true. I am not dying."); (b) feelings of *anger,* not actually directed at others but rather at the fact that others have what they soon will not—life ("Why me?"); (c) *bargaining,* usually with a higher power, to continue to live ("If you'll just allow me to live until this event . . ."); (d) when denial is no longer possible, reactive *depression,* not to death itself so much as the loss of everything and everyone; and (e) *acceptance* of death, which although most often is expressed as quiet expectation without emotion, does not mean the person desires to die. Despite the criticisms of Kübler-Ross' stage theory of dying (e.g., Kastenbaum, 1991), few can deny that her work brought much-needed public attention to the topic of death and dying and care of the dying individual. One pioneer in death and dying (Feifel, 1990) placed Kübler-Ross' stage theory (and others related to grief and bereavement) in perspective.

> the hard data do not support the existence of any procrustean stages or schedules that characterize terminal illness or mourning. This does not mean that [such theories] . . . cannot provide us with implications and insights into the dynamics and process of dying and grief, but they are very far from being inexorable hoops through which most terminally ill individuals and mourners inevitably pass. We should beware of promulgating a coercive orthodoxy of how to die or mourn. (p. 540)

Current End-of-Life Issues

No contemporary discussion of death and dying would be complete without at least a brief mention of physician-assisted suicide. Although most often viewed as an issue of late life, cases of assisted suicide have been reported among patients representing nearly the entire range of the life span. This issue has produced massive public, professional, and legal debate, with tremendous fervor among both advocates and opponents. Few topics have the potential to change many of the aspects of death already discussed, including the mode of death, the timing of death, as well as subjective feelings and attitudes about dying and death. Detailed discussion of this topic exceeds the scope of this chapter (see, e.g., American Association of Suicidology, 1996; Diekstra, 1995), but contributing factors to patient contemplation of physician-assisted suicide include loss of control, pain, suffering, and so on that concern and frighten both the dying and the rest of the population. The U.S. Supreme Court recently left decisions about assisted suicide to states. The topic has been brought to the foreground because of the deaths assisted by Jack

Kevorkian (1991), a retired Michigan pathologist who at this writing has assisted at least 100 individuals with their suicides, and Timothy Quill (1991), a New York family physician who assisted one of his patients in her suicide and wrote about it in a leading medical journal), as well as the publication of the controversial argument and prescription for rational suicide, *Final Exit* (Humphry, 1991). Arguments favoring as well as opposing assisted suicide have been advanced, as have guidelines to determine appropriate candidates (e.g., Quill, Cassel, & Meier, 1992). Many organizations (e.g., the American Psychological Association, see Farberman, 1997) have presented their viewpoints on physician-assisted suicide as well as the related and broader topics of hastened death, euthanasia, and other end-of-life issues, such as advance directives and living wills. The debate on these issues could well continue for many years and how they are resolved will most certainly influence death and dying in America.

Dying and Hospices

At any life period, an option often suggested to assisting individuals in ending their lives is the hospice movement and its humane approach to the dying process and individual. Because hospice patients are dying, the emphasis is not on curing them as in traditional hospital settings but rather is on caring for their needs. Hospices operate under a philosophy based on providing total care to meet the medical, psychological, emotional, social, spiritual, and other needs of the dying individual of any age. Hospice emphasizes quality and humane treatment of the dying patient. Its goal is to maintain comfort care and pain management along with social and emotional support. Control of care and respect for the wishes of the dying person are keystones. Family members are involved throughout treatment and receive staff support as well, continuing through provision of bereavement care. The staff establishes personal relationships with hospice patients and the families, something often not encouraged in traditional hospital settings, where individuals may feel depersonalized. The care may take place in either a hospital-type setting or in the individual's home (Kastenbaum, 1991; Leming & Dickinson, 1990; Osterweis & Champagne, 1979). There are more than 1,700 hospices in the United States providing an option in care at the end of life.

THE AFTERMATH OF DEATH:
GRIEF AND BEREAVEMENT

It would be impossible in a short space to do justice to the large literature on grief and bereavement (see e.g., Osterweis, Solomon, & Green, 1984; Rando, 1984; Stroebe, Stroebe, & Hansson, 1993; Zisook, 1987). So, following a short general review, grieving at various ages is examined. The reactions of family members and others to someone's death are affected by many of the same and similar biopsychosocial factors already observed for the dying person, as well as issues such as the mode of death, whether the death was anticipated or unexpected, the suddenness of the death, the emotional closeness of the relationship to the deceased, and the specific kinship relation to the deceased (see, e.g., Rando, 1984).

Many who have investigated grieving individuals have suggested stages or phases of normal or uncomplicated bereavement through which the survivors "work" following the loss of a significant other (see, e.g., Leming & Dickinson, 1990; Rando, 1984). Although each of these characterizations involve some unique steps, Rando (1984) summarized them with three broad categories.

Each of the conceptualizations include first an *avoidance phase* in which bereaved individuals experience such reactions as denial, shock, and disbelief about the death that might function as a protective mechanism, providing some time for the person to begin to deal with the death. The second general phase can be labeled the *confrontation phase*, when what is often portrayed as "grief work" is initiated and the death faced after the numbness lessens. During this phase various investigators have observed displays of extremes in emotions such as panic, anxiety, anger, guilt, yearning and longing for the lost loved one, loneliness, sadness and depression, identification and preoccupation with the deceased, concerns about their own sanity, and even relief (which can lead to even more guilt). Other responses such as physical symptoms (e.g., muscle weakness, fatigue, shortness of breath, tightness in the chest and throat), confusion, absentmindedness, sleep and appetite disturbances, social withdrawal, crying and sighing, and memorializing the deceased's objects and memory are all commonly observed in the bereaved. Rando called the final step the *reestablishment phase*. During this phase the grief gradually declines. This represents the start of learning to live again, not only living with the loss, but reestablishing one's involvement and life in the world. People often experience guilt in this phase as well, as they might feel they are somehow dishonoring the deceased loved one with their less active grieving and the return of "normal" life with its everyday activities and experiences. Although many of these stage characterizations seem to imply that recovery or resolution is the end result of the bereavement process, it is apparent that there are tremendous individual differences in all these stages, with the time involved varying widely. In addition, not everyone reaches recovery, and resolution represents not so much an end to grief or a coming to terms as it does getting accustomed to the loss (see Stroebe, van den Bout, & Schut, 1994). This individuality in responses during bereavement is a consistent research finding (e.g., Gilbert, 1996).

In addition to these characterizations of normal or uncomplicated grief, much attention has been given to grief and bereavement that is pathological, complicated, or unresolved. Reviewing the research and clinical literature on risk factors in the outcome of bereavement, Sanders (1993) found that individuals who generally have the most bereavement difficulties include widowers (compared to widows), mothers (compared to fathers), those without solid financial resources, those who had an ambivalent relationship with or were excessively dependent on the deceased, those whose loved one died from sudden and unexpected (e.g., death by suicide, homicide, catastrophes) or stigmatized causes (such as AIDS or again, suicide), cases where the deceased was a child (including deaths by sudden infant death syndrome, miscarriages, and stillbirths), those without social support, and those who experience multiple losses in relatively short time periods. Finally, although the evidence is almost exclusively anecdotal or clinical, poor bereavement outcome seems to be associated with poor mental or physical health among the bereaved.

Obviously both normal and complicated bereavement occur throughout the life span. Each period of life, however, is associated with particular aspects of grief. In most cases, bereavement has been studied within particular life periods, often with respect to the kinship relations of the deceased and bereaved than across the life periods per se. Many of the responses during each life stage represent a continuation of the feelings and special issues already noted with regard to family members during the dying process, and at all ages the general reactions previously cited in the discussion of normal grieving are seen. The largest bulk of information on bereavement focuses on children as survivors of parental death, parents whose child has died, and adults who have lost a spouse (usually older adults).

As in other areas of the death and dying literature, much has been written and a large number of research investigations have been conducted about bereaved children and adolescents. Much of this work has focused on the loss of parents during these young periods. Research consistently shows that although most children do not show serious disturbance following a loss, negative immediate and long-term reactions among the bereaved young often are observed (see, e.g., Worden & Silverman, 1996). Among the special issues for grieving children and adolescents are a greater tendency than adults to identify with the deceased. Osterweis et al. (1984, p. 119) suggested that after the death of a parent three questions are typical: Did I cause this to happen? Will it happen to me? Who will take care of me now (or if something happens to my surviving caretaker)? These concerns about responsibility and guilt as well as vulnerability are also observed among children who lose a sibling. Identification and a feeling of continued presence in the life of the child have also been observed when children lose a sibling (e.g., Hogan & DeSantis, 1992). As with all issues of death and dying, the variables that might affect the child or adolescent's bereavement reactions and outcome include their age, developmental stage, their relationship to the deceased, the quality and availability of a supportive social system, and cultural background (including ethnic, religious, and social class). Osterweis et al. (1984) presented evidence that specific developmental groups at risk in bereavement include those where loss occurs before the age of 5 or in early adolescence, girls younger than 11 who lose their mothers, and adolescent boys whose fathers die.

Although negative consequences occur in children surviving parental deaths, the greatest negative impact of a death appears to occur in parents who have lost a child. Raphael (1983) suggested that because death in contemporary society is relatively rare in the young, the death of a child feels untimely, most often is unexpected, and often is associated with feelings of responsibility and guilt on the part of the family and even society itself. Children have a special emotional significance for their parents. They are supposed to grow to adulthood and outlive their parents, carrying on the family and parents' legacy, maintaining and furthering the interests and hopes of the society. Research findings have supported the greater intensity and duration of bereavement associated with the death of a child when compared to the loss of a parent or spouse (e.g., Sanders, 1989). Although not systematically studied in a comparative way, parents may lose children to death in several ways: miscarriages, abortions, stillbirths and deaths among newborns ("perinatal deaths"; see, e.g., Mander, 1994; Thomas & Striegel, 1994–95), deaths of preschool and grade-school children, and deaths among adolescent and even adult children. To the parents, deaths at all these ages are likely to seem untimely, with the parents losing the child, their relationship, and indeed a feeling of losing part of their self (see De Vries, Lana, & Falck, 1994; Osterweis et al., 1984; Rando, 1984).

Even though the loss of a child has been described as the greatest tragedy in life, the loss of one's spouse perhaps represents a more stressful event, requiring extensive readjustment (e.g., Holmes & Rahe, 1967). Although widowhood is a normative life event (compared to the non-normative loss of a child), especially for women, few find themselves prepared to face the consequences of their spouse's death and the grief that results. Responses to the loss of spouse commonly include difficult and protracted bereavement, increased susceptibility to illness, and, sometimes, even death, alterations in physical and emotional support, problems with economic stability and security, potential loneliness and isolation, difficulties with managing household affairs, difficulties associated with single parenthood (when young children survive), and sleeping and eating disruptions. The age of the widow and deceased spouse, the nature of their relationship, and the length of their marriage are important variables, affecting change in all arenas of life. Other factors observed by researchers that may particularly affect the outcome of bereavement include low income or socioeconomic status, the existence of life crises prior to the death, lack of preparation for the many losses accompanying the sudden death of the spouse, the presence of young children in the family, few family members and friends to provide emotional as well as various types of social and instrumental support, and sex (widowers experience greater suffering; Kastenbaum, 1991; Osterweis et al., 1984; Rando, 1984; Sanders, 1989; Stroebe & Stroebe, 1983).

Although not everyone needs formal assistance to confront and cope with their losses, interventions to aid the bereaved across the life span have been developed for those who do. Although traditional therapy and counseling techniques are employed, mutual and self-support approaches have become particularly widespread to assist healing and grieving. A variety of programs have been designed for those in specific circumstances (see Fitzgerald, 1994), such as widow-to-widow programs, programs for parents who have lost children (such as Compassionate Friends), and programs for those who have lost loved ones to suicide (see e.g., Dunne, McIntosh,

& Dunne-Maxim, 1987). Even though the precise approaches and ideologies of many of these intervention techniques vary, all are directed at confronting the loss, permitting normalization, allowing expression of the various normal and abnormal reactions to death of a significant other, and providing assistance with adaptation to the demands of continuing life (Osterweis et al., 1984; Worden, 1982).

CONCLUSIONS

Large clinical, anecdotal, and research literatures exist on death and dying. Although death and dying might be conceptualized as biomedical events, a more accurate representation recognizes them as complex processes. In addition to biomedical aspects, psychosocial and environmental factors interact and play prominent roles in the events and processes of death and dying as well as in the ways we grieve and conceptualize death throughout the life span.

Much about the end of life remains to be known and understood. There is a need for refinement, improvement, and clarification of factors in all areas. For instance, examples of some methodological issues that require additional attention from researchers and others include advancing the rigor and quality of existing research (while remaining mindful of the ethical issues involved; see, e.g., *Death Studies*, 1995), relying less often on clinical and anecdotal evidence and more often on sound research designs, improving measurement and sampling, conducting multivariate investigations to help sort out the complex factors involved, and committing to the use of longitudinal designs. Among the many other topics that should be high research priorities are expansion of knowledge on grieving to kinship relations and other groups for which we have little evidence, including particularly men's grieving; investigation of the dying process itself, especially addressing the adjustments and reactions of family members and friends of the dying individual; evaluation of the efficacy of intervention programs, including those for the dying and the bereaved. Improved and more precise evidence about death and dying are crucial to enhancing assistance at every life period.

All of us will die. To reduce premature death, however, it is necessary to address the many factors involved. Death by the leading causes (e.g., heart disease, cancer, etc.) can be reduced in several ways. Particularly important for both health enhancement and lessening unnecessary death is the promotion of lifelong habits of good health. Such habits and behavioral changes would include regular exercise, weight control, healthy dietary choices, regular breast and testicular self-examination, smoking cessation, moderating alcohol intake, and training in stress reduction and positive coping skills. In addition, other major causes of death such as accidents, suicides, and homicides would likely be reduced if proper use of air bags and seat belts were increased, helmets were worn by motorcyclists, poisons and other medications were stored properly, and firearms were less available and used responsibly (McIntosh, 1993). Some of these measures can be initiated by individuals, whereas others require societal-level efforts, but all have the potential to reduce premature, unnecessary deaths. Similar measures are needed to assist the other aspects of death and dying. Death education and encouragement of open communication about death might positively affect death attitudes, the dying process, and bereavement as well as normalizing them. Continuation and extension of present interventions for the dying and the bereaved should be encouraged in addition to the development of new approaches that might assist the dying and their loved ones.

Herman Feifel (1990), a pioneer in thanatology research, reminded us that our emphasis should be to improve the quality of individual living throughout the lifespan and particularly at the end of the life cycle. He noted:

> Refinement in the pursuit of our craft [understanding death and dying], however, will not be sufficient unless it is carried on in the context of healing the humanity of the dying patient and wounded mourner. Our model of understanding and treatment must be the humanity of the person. . . . The humanities, ethics, and the spiritual dimension must be in our ken along with biology and the behavioral sciences. Death and grief bring with them a preoccupation with a vision of life. (p. 542)

REFERENCES

Adams, D. W., & Deveau, E. J. (1986). Helping dying adolescents: Needs and responses. In C. A. Corr & J. N. Mcneil (Eds.), *Adolescence and death* (pp. 79–96). New York: Springer.

American Association of Suicidology. (1996). Report of the committee on physician-assisted suicide and euthanasia. *Suicide and Life-Threatening Behavior, 26*(Suppl.).

Anderson, R. N., Kochanek, K. D., & Murphy, S. L. (1997). Report of final mortality statistics, 1995. *Monthly Vital Statistics Report, 45*(11, Suppl. 2).

Butler, R. N. (1963). The life review: An interpretation of reminiscence in the aged. *Psychiatry, 26,* 65–76.

Cook, A. S., & Oltjenbruns, K. A. (1989). *Dying and grieving: Lifespan and family perspectives.* New York: Holt, Rinehart and Winston.

Critelli, T. (1983). Parental death in childhood—A review of the psychiatric literature. In J. E. Schowalter, P. R. Patterson, M. Tallmer, A. H. Kutscher, S. V. Gullo, & D. Peretz (Eds.), *The child and death* (pp. 89–103). New York: Columbia University Press.

Death Studies. (1995). [Special issue devoted to ethical issues in bereavement research]. *19*(No. 2), 103–181.

De Vries, B., Lana, R. D., & Falck, V. T. (1994). Parental bereavement over the life course: A theoretical intersection and empirical review. *Omega, 29,* 47–69.

Diekstra, R. F. W. (1995). Dying in dignity: The pros and cons of assisted suicide. *Psychiatry and Clinical Neurosciences, 49*(Suppl. 1), S139-S148.

Dunne, E. J., McIntosh, J. L., & Dunne-Maxim, K. (Eds.). (1987). *Suicide and its aftermath: Understanding and counseling the survivors.* New York: Norton.

Easterlin, R. A. (1987). *Birth and fortune* (2nd ed.). Chicago: University of Chicago Press.

Elkind, D. (1967). Egocentrism in adolescence. *Child Development, 38,* 1025–1035.

Epstein, G., Weitz, L., Roback, H., & McKee, E. (1979). Research on bereavement: A selective and critical review. In L. A. Bugen (Ed.), *Death and dying: Theory/research/practice* (pp. 55–65). Dubuque, IA: Wm. C. Brown. (Reprinted from *Comprehensive Psychiatry,* 1975, *16,* 537–546).

Erikson, E. H. (1963). *Childhood and society* (2nd rev. ed.). New York: Norton.

Farberman, R. K. (1997). *Terminal illness and hastened death requests: The important role of the mental health professional.* Washington, DC: American Psychological Association.

Feifel, H. (1990). Psychology and death: Meaningful rediscovery. *American Psychologist, 45,* 537–543.

Firestone, R. W. (1994). Psychological defenses against death anxiety. In R. A. Neimeyer (Ed.), *Death anxiety handbook: Research, instrumentation, and application* (pp. 217–241). Washington, DC: Taylor & Francis.

Fitzgerald, H. (1994). *The mourning handbook: A complete guide for the bereaved.* New York: Simon & Schuster.

Florian, V., & Mikulincer, M. (1997). Fear of personal death in adulthood: The impact of early and recent losses. *Death Studies, 21,* 1–24.

Gilbert, K. R. (1996). "We've had the same loss, why don't we have the same grief?": Loss and differential grief in families. *Death Studies, 20,* 269–283.

Gordon, A. K. (1986). The tattered cloak of immortality. In C. A. Corr & J. N. McNeil (Eds.), *Adolescence and death* (pp.16–31). New York: Springer.

Hoffman, S. I., & Strauss, S. (1985). The development of children's concepts of death. *Death Studies, 9,* 469–482.

Hogan, N., & DeSantis, L. (1992). Adolescent sibling bereavement: An ongoing attachment. *Qualitative Health Research, 2,* 159–177.

Holinger, P. C. (1987). *Violent deaths in the United States: An epidemiologic study of suicide, homicide, and accidents.* New York: Guilford.

Holmes, T. H., & Rahe, R. H. (1967). The Social Readjustment Rating Scale. *Journal of Psychosomatic Research, 11,* 213–218.

Hostler, S. L. (1978). The development of the child's concept of death. In O. J. Z. Sahler (Ed.), *The child and death* (pp. 1–25). St. Louis: Mosby.

Humphry, D. (1991). *Final exit: The practicalities of self-deliverance and assisted suicide for the dying.* Eugene, OR: Hemlock Society.

Jackson, J. J. (1981). *Minorities and aging.* Belmont, CA: Wadsworth.

Jenkins, R. A., & Cavanaugh, J. C. (1985/1986). Examining the relationship between the development of the concept of death and overall cognitive development. *Omega, 16,* 193–199.

Kalish, R. A. (1976). Death and dying in a social context. In R. H. Binstock & E. Shanas (Eds.), *Handbook of aging and the social sciences* (pp. 483–507). New York: Van Nostrand Reinhold.

Kalish, R. A., & Reynolds, D. K. (1976). *Death and ethnicity: A psychocultural study.* Los Angeles: University of Southern California Press.

Kamerman, J. B. (1988). *Death in the midst of life: Social and cultural influences on death, grief, and mourning.* Englewood Cliffs, NJ: Prentice-Hall.

Kastenbaum, R. (1978). Death, dying, and bereavement in old age: New developments and their possible implications for psychosocial care. *Aged Care & Service Review, 1*(3), 3–10.

Kastenbaum, R. (1991). *Death, society, and human experience* (4th ed.). New York: Merrill.

Kastenbaum, R. (1992). *The psychology of death* (2nd ed.). New York: Springer.

Kastenbaum, R., & Aisenberg, R. (1972). *The psychology of death.* New York: Springer.

Kastenbaum, R., & Costa, P. T. (1977). Psychological perspectives on death. *Annual Review of Psychology, 28,* 225–249.

Kevorkian, J. (1991). *Prescription—Medicide: The goodness of planned death.* Buffalo, NY: Prometheus.

Koocher, G. P. (1974). Talking with children about death. *American Journal of Orthopsychiatry, 44,* 404–411.

Kübler-Ross, E. (1969). *On death and dying.* New York: Macmillan.

Leming, M. R., & Dickinson, G. E. (1990). *Understanding dying, death, and bereavement* (2nd ed.). New York: Holt, Rinehart and Winston.

Lipton, H. (1978). The dying child and the family: The skills of the social worker. In O. J. Z. Sahler (Ed.), *The child and death* (pp. 52–82). St. Louis: Mosby.

Lonetto, R. (1980). *Children's conceptions of death.* New York: Springer.

Maglio, C. J., & Robinson, S. E. (1994). The effects of death education on death anxiety: A meta-analysis. *Omega, 29,* 319–335.

Mander, R. (1994). *Loss and bereavement in childbearing.* London: Blackwell Scientific.

Manton, K. G., Blazer, D. G., & Woodbury, M. A. (1987). Suicide in middle age and later life: Sex and race specific life table and cohort analyses. *Journal of Gerontology, 42,* 219–227.

McIntosh, J. L. (1992). Older adults: The next suicide epidemic? *Suicide and Life-Threatening Behavior, 22,* 322–332.

McIntosh, J. L. (1993). Risk to life through the adult years. In R. Kastenbaum (Ed.), *Encyclopedia of adult development* (pp. 414–421). Phoenix, AZ: Oryx Press.

McIntosh, J. L., Santos, J. F., Hubbard, R. W., & Overholser, J. C. (1994). *Elder suicide: Research, theory and treatment.* Washington, DC: American Psychological Association.

Nagy, M. H. (1959). The child's view of death. In H. Feifel (Ed.), *The meaning of death* (pp. 79–98). New York: McGraw-Hill. (Reprinted from *Journal of Genetic Psychology,* 1948, *73,* 3–27.)

National Center for Health Statistics. (annual volumes). *Vital Statistics of the United States, Volume 2— Mortality, Parts A & B.* Washington, DC: U.S. Government Printing Office.

National Center for Health Statistics. (1996). *Vital Statistics of the United States, 1992, Volume 2—Mortality, Part A* (DHHS Publ. No. PHS 96–1101). Washington, DC: U.S. Government Printing Office.

Noppe, I. C., & Noppe, L. D. (1997). Evolving meanings of death during early, middle, and later adolescence. *Death Studies, 21,* 253–275.

O'Donnell, C. R. (1995). Firearm deaths among children and youth. *American Psychologist, 50,* 771–776.

Osterweis, M., & Champagne, D. S. (1979). The U.S. hospice movement: Issues in development. *American Journal of Public Health, 69,* 492–496.

Osterweis, M., Solomon, F., & Green, M. (Eds.). (1984). *Bereavement: Reactions, consequences, and care.* Washington, DC: National Academy Press.

Parkes, C. M. (1980). The broken heart. In E. S. Shneidman (Ed.), *Death: Current perspectives* (2nd ed., pp. 222–233). Palo Alto, CA: Mayfield. (Reprinted from *Bereavement.* New York: International Universities Press, 1973).

Parkes, C. M., Laungani, P., & Young, B. (Eds.). (1997). *Death and bereavement across cultures.* London: Routledge.

Pattison, E. M. (1977). *The experience of dying.* Englewood Cliffs, NJ: Prentice-Hall.

Pollak, J. M. (1979–80). Correlates of death anxiety: A review of empirical studies. *Omega, 10,* 97–121.

Pollinger-Haas, A., & Hendin, H. (1983). Suicide among older people: Projections for the future. *Suicide and Life-Threatening Behavior, 13,* 147–154.

Preston, J. J. (1977). Toward an anthropology of death. *Intellect, 105,* 343–344.

Quill, T. E. (1991). Death and dignity: A case of individualized decision making. *New England Journal of Medicine, 324,* 691–694.

Quill, T. E., Cassel, C. K., & Meier, D. E. (1992). Care of the hopelessly ill: Proposed clinical criteria for physician-assisted suicide. *New England Journal of Medicine, 327,* 1380–1384.

Rando, T. A. (1984). *Grief, dying, and death: Clinical interventions for caregivers.* Champaign, IL: Research Press.

Raphael, B. (1983). *The anatomy of bereavement.* New York: Harper Collins.

Sanders, C. M. (1989). *Grief: The mourning after—Dealing with adult bereavement.* New York: Wiley.

Sanders, C. M. (1993). Risk factors in bereavement outcome. In M. S. Stroebe, W. Stroebe, & R. O. Hansson (Eds.), *Handbook of bereavement: Theory, research, and intervention* (pp. 255–267). New York: Cambridge University Press.

Schulz, R. (1985). Thinking about death: Death anxiety research. In S. G. Wilcox & M. Sutton (Eds.), *Understanding death and dying: An interdisciplinary approach* (3rd ed., pp. 16–31). Palo Alto, CA: Mayfield. (Reprinted from *The psychology of death, dying, and bereavement.* Reading, MA: Addison-Wesley, 1978)

Stambrook, M., & Parker, K. C. H. (1987). The development of the concept of death in childhood: A review of the literature. *Merrill-Palmer Quarterly, 33,* 133–157.

274   MCINTOSH

Stillion, J. M. (1985). *Death and the sexes: An examination of differential longevity, attitudes, behaviors, and coping skills.* Washington, DC: Hemisphere.

Stillion, J., & Waas, H. (1984). Children and death. In E. S. Shneidman (Ed.), *Death: Current perspectives* (3rd ed., pp. 225–249). Palo Alto, CA: Mayfield. (Reprinted from H. Wass (Ed.), *Dying: Facing the facts.* Washington, DC: Hemisphere Publishing, 1979)

Stroebe, M. S., & Stroebe, W. (1983). Who suffers more? Sex differences in health risks of the widowed. *Psychological Bulletin, 93,* 279–301.

Stroebe, M. S., Stroebe, W., & Hansson, R. O. (Eds.). (1993). *Handbook of bereavement: Theory, research, and intervention.* New York: Cambridge University Press.

Stroebe, M., van den Bout, J., & Schut, H. (1994). Myths and misconceptions about bereavement: The opening of a debate. *Omega, 29,* 187–203.

Taylor, S. E. (1991). *Health psychology* (2nd ed.). New York: McGraw-Hill.

Thomas, V., & Striegel, P. (1994–95). Stress and grief of a perinatal loss: Integrating qualitative and quantitative methods. *Omega, 30,* 299–311.

Tucker, J. S., Friedman, H. S., Schwartz, J. E., Criqui, M. H., Tomlinson-Keasey, C., Wingard, D. L., & Martin, L. R. (1997). Parental divorce: Effects on individual behavior and longevity. *Journal of Personality and Social Psychology, 73,* 381–391.

Waechter, E. H. (1971). Children's awareness of fatal illness. *American Journal of Nursing, 71,* 1168–1172.

Woodruff, D. S. (1984). Appendix B: Can you live to be 100? In A. N. Schwartz, C. L. Snyder, & J. A. Peterson, *Aging and life: An introduction to gerontology* (2nd ed., pp. 369–375). New York: Holt, Rinehart & Winston.

Worden, J. W. (1982). *Grief counseling and grief therapy: A handbook for the mental health practitioner.* New York: Springer.

Worden, J. W., & Silverman, P. R. (1996). Parental death and the adjustment of school-age children. *Omega, 33,* 91–102.

World Health Organization. (1991). *World health statistics annual, 1990.* Geneva, Switzerland: Author.

Zisook, S. (Ed.). (1987). *Biopsychosocial aspects of bereavement.* Washington, DC: American Psychiatric Press.

PART IV

Summary and Conclusions

14

Some Considerations on Integrating Psychology and Health From a Life-Span Perspective

E. Mark Cummings
University of Notre Dame

AN UNDERSTANDING of health, and the prevention of illness, requires consideration of psychological and environmental as well as of biomedical factors (Whitman, chapter 1, this volume). Thus, optimal models for understanding and predicting health and illness must be multifactorial. As if that challenge were not enough, models must also be rooted in a developmental perspective to account for variations in health. A life-span perspective is especially appropriate for the study of health, because health and risk for morbidity are fundamental parameters of the course of life, with relative health and risk for illness changing throughout the life span. That is, relations among health, illness, and psychological processes are dynamic and changing as individuals progress from infancy, to early childhood, to childhood, to adolescence, to early adulthood, to middle age, and to later life (chapters 5 to 11, this volume). Put another way, risk factors, stressors, coping resources, and protective factors vary in their relations to health and illness as a function of developmental status and individual differences in patterns of development. Furthermore, processes and events in early life are inevitably related to outcomes in later life (chapters 2 to 4, this volume), so that even if a perfect "snapshot" of biopsychoenvironmental processes were possible at a given age, it could yield no better than an incomplete picture of patterns and causes contributing to an individual's present health status.

This volume makes a unique and exciting contribution toward a life-span perspective on relations among psychological processes, health, and illness. The review is comprehensive: Psychological processes relating to health and illness are examined from the prenatal period to old age, including life-span perspectives on poverty (Bolig, Borkowski, & Brandenberger, chapter 4), caretaking for the elderly (Vachon, chapter 12), and death and dying (McIntosh, chapter 13). Each chapter adds a piece to the puzzle of understanding the etiology of health and illness across the life span.

However, a challenge for a life-span volume is to avoid a "piecemeal" appearance. In a volume addressing the numerous concerns of life-span development across multiple contributions, such a perception is a risk. The multidirectional and multidimensional nature of development makes difficult an integrated view of the life span.

Nonetheless, this integration must be the aim for a life-span perspective. The special purpose of life-span developmental science is the articulation of etiology of outcomes (e.g., psychological, biological, or medical) across the life span (Cairns, Elder, & Costello, 1996; Cicchetti & Cohen, 1995; Cummings & Cummings, 1988). However, achieving this end requires not only the consideration of multiple influences on development, and their interrelations, but also the processes and mechanisms that mediate or moderate relations between influences and outcomes, and the course of these relations over time and periods of development (Cairns et al., 1996; Cicchetti & Cohen, 1995; Cummings & Cummings, 1988; Fincham, 1994).

A commentary has the opportunity to examine the issues at a more general level of analysis, thereby perhaps contributing to a more integrated view. This chapter provides a framework for putting the contributions of this volume in a life-span developmental context and a way of thinking about the role of processes and mechanism in mediating or moderating relations between influences and outcomes. Specifically, this commentary (a) outlines a framework for a life-span perspective on health and psychology, (b) in that framework, illustrates how the various contributions of the chapters in this volume may be integrated around common themes, and (c) expands on notions of the mechanisms or processes accounting for development from a stress and coping perspective.

A FRAMEWORK FOR A PROCESS-ORIENTED PERSPECTIVE ON PSYCHOLOGY AND HEALTH

A framework for a life-span perspective on psychology and health is presented in Fig. 14.1. The left side of the figure outlines various factors that might influence health across the life span and the right side reflects the various health-related outcomes. The middle section of the framework represents the response processes of the individual over time that account for relations between influences on health and health-related outcomes (see Bergeman & Wallace, chapter 11; Whitman, chapter 1, for similar outlines). Notably, the time frame for the occurrence of coping processes and responses can vary from the immediate (e.g., the impact of traumatic events) to the life span (e.g., effects of diet on heart attack risk). Although direct paths among health-related outcomes and individual, family, and societal factors are recognized to occur (e.g., Down syndrome and health-related outcomes), it is posited that such purely direct pathways (i.e., not mediated or moderated by stress and coping mechanisms) are relatively rare.

Thus, according to this framework, individual factors (biological, genetic, or psychological), family and other social supports (marital, parent–child, siblings, extrafamilial, and peers), and societal and environmental factors (government, financial, community, and physical and health environment), each influence health-related outcomes. Moreover, these biopsychoenvironmental influences are interrelated and interdependent. That is, there might be links among the various antecedents (individual, family, and society). For example, genetic (e.g., reactive temperament) and family (e.g., parental insensitivity to children's needs; histories of high marital conflict) factors each might undermine children's coping with family stress, increasing the probability of adjustment problems (Cummings & Davies, 1996; Davies & Cummings, 1994).

Reflecting the life-span perspective, it is posited that different patterns of relations can occur at different points in the life span. The significance of age period, and age changes, to patterns of relations merits special notation, as indicated by the "Period of the Life Span" designation in Fig. 14.1. For example, Merluzzi and Nairn (chapter 10) report that lifestyle choices, which might be conceptualized as psychological aspects of individual functioning, are more important for men's health in midlife than during other periods of life. Thus, over time, and across life-span development, the various health-related factors are posited to contribute systematically, but in sometimes quite different ways at different ages, to health-related outcomes. Finally, health-related outcomes are conceptualized as not simply medical problems but might be manifested as physical illness or health or psychological adjustment or maladjustment.

However, an assumption of the model is that multiple, specific individual stress and coping processes, responses, and styles, which can be cognitive, social, biological or physiological, or emotional, account for the relations between specific health-related influences and specific health-related outcomes. In Fig. 14.1 health-related influences reflect current representations of individual, family and societal factors, which are typically measured at a relatively global level of analysis and in terms of relatively static characterizations (e.g., introversion–extroversion; "difficult" temperament; marital satisfaction; low socioeconomic status; large social support networks; low birthweight; Cummings & El-Sheikh, 1991). On the other hand, stress and coping processes, responses, and styles reflect relatively specific characterizations of response processes, often at a microanalytic level of analysis that is sensitive to, and might reflect, the possibilities of changing reactions to changing stimuli over time (e.g., emotional, cognitive, and behavioral reactivity during exposure to marital conflict; heart rate or skin conductance responses to family stresses; specific patterns of biological reactions over time to toxins). Moreover, these response dispositions are seen as dynamic and changing over time, reflecting transactional relations between health-related influences, stress and coping

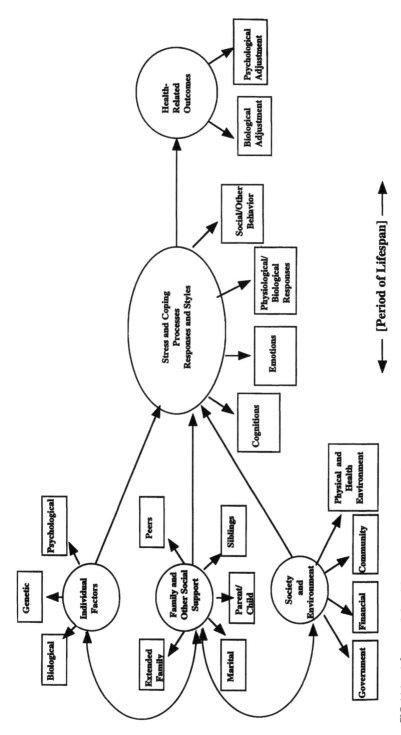

FIG. 14.1. A framework for a life-span perspective on psychology and health.

processes, and health-related outcomes. This focus on specifying precise relations-in-time between predictors and outcomes as mediated or moderated by dynamic processes or mechanisms of functioning reflects a *process-oriented* perspective on life span development (Cicchetti & Cohen, 1995; Cummings & Cummings, 1988; Cummings & El-Sheikh, 1991).

The study of processes of interaction among multiple intra- and extra-organismic and ecological factors over time promises to advance understanding of relations between life-span health and development. For example, this approach may account for inconsistencies that are sometimes reported (e.g., some foods are found to be healthful in some studies and harmful in others). Inconsistencies might reflect (a) an inadequate conceptualization of process relations, for example, examination only of the bivariate correlations, without assessing important third variables; (b) a sampling of too few of the multiple variables influencing outcomes, so that even relatively complex models have gaps; or (c) measurements that are too global and not sufficiently precise, so there is slippage on critical dimensions of individual variables. Thus, further advances in understanding of process relations necessitate (a) broader, more inclusive models of health-related influences and their interrelations in the context of life-span development, and, at the same time, (b) more precise and delineated specifications of individual variables in multivariate models.

Moreover, multiple risk factors increase the risk for health-related problems (see Fig. 14.1) additively, or even multiplicatively, increasing risk for medical or psychological disorder (Hauser, Vieyra, Jacobson, & Wertlieb, 1985; Rutter, 1980, 1981). Different health-related influences also might affect the same processes in predicting risk for health-related problems (Cummings & Davies, 1994; Jaffe, Wolfe, & Wilson, 1990). For example, similar disturbances of emotional regulation have been reported in children exposed to parental depression, marital conflict, or physical abuse, respectively, with heightened risk for problems in children exposed to two or more of these factors (Cummings & Davies, 1994; Jaffe, Wolfe, Wilson, & Zak, 1986). In addition, in some instances variables might act as mediators of health-related outcomes (e.g., depressive cognitions), whereas in other instances variables might serve as moderators (e.g., gender is a common example; see Holmbeck, 1997, for extensive treatment of the distinction between mediators and moderators in predicting health-related outcomes; also see Braungart-Rieker & Guerra, chapter 7). That is, in some instances the influence of antecedent factors on health-related outcomes might be explained by various stress and coping processes (i.e., a mediated relation), whereas in other cases different antecedent factors may have quite different overall patterns of relations with health-related outcomes (i.e., a moderated relation).

As noted earlier, the period of the life span and change across age are also significant to health-related outcomes (see Fig. 14.1). The conceptualization of what is meant by life-span development, that is, development over time across the life span, merits consideration. Development can be conceptualized in terms of pathways that emerge over time, with specific pathways probabilistically, but not certainly, related to health-related outcomes (Cicchetti & Cohen, 1995; Cicchetti & Richters, 1997; Sroufe, 1997; Sroufe & Rutter, 1984). In other words, disorder can be viewed as a deviation over time, with the possibility of multiple pathways leading to the same manifest outcome. However, there is also the possibility of dispersion of pathways from similar early risk trajectories (Egeland, Pianta, & Ogawa, 1996). Although change is possible at many points in a pathway, it is also constrained by prior adaptation. Earlier structures of the individual's organization are incorporated into later structures; thus, early vulnerability tends to predict later vulnerability. Moreover, there is also an interplay between nature and nurture in development of these structures (Rutter et al., 1997). In other words, development is a series of successive adaptations of persons to their environments, with structural organizations and reorganizations in and among the biological and behavioral systems of the individual underlying developmental continuity and change.

Ultimately, a person-oriented level of analysis focusing on groupings of individual styles or patterns, as opposed to a less integrative variable-oriented approach, might hold the most promise for predicting health-related outcomes (Bergman & Magnusson, 1997; Cummings & Cummings, 1988).

The framework in Fig. 14.1 thus provides bases for conceptualizing multiple pathways of effect between biopsychoenvironmental factors and health associated with life-span development. The model also assumes that both past and present health-related influences are related to current health. Health-related influences are examined next, focusing on the contributions of this volume toward understanding the roles of these factors.

INFLUENCES ON RELATIONS BETWEEN HEALTH AND PSYCHOLOGY ACROSS THE LIFE SPAN: ILLUSTRATIONS FROM THIS VOLUME

Three main categories of influence on relations between health and psychology are outlined in Fig. 14.1: individual factors, family and other social supports, and society and environment. Each domain contributes multiple factors. Many of these influences are treated in this volume.

Individual Factors

Intra-organismic influences can be biological, genetic, or psychological. These processes might interact with each other and with extra-organismic factors to affect the processes and mechanisms of development. However, these factors are not outcomes in themselves. For example, genetic influences are propensities or tendencies, not main effects, resulting from the interaction of multiple genetic and environmental influences (Braungart-Rieker & Bergeman, chapter 3).

Biology. As Kolberg (chapter 2) indicates, processes of biological develop-ment are particularly important causes of mortality at either end of the life span, that is, during the early prenatal, birth, and infancy periods, and among the elderly. On the other hand, biological development at every point in the life cycle relates to present and subsequent health and longevity (see Fig. 14.1). Biological develop-ment is also influenced by behavior; some developmental problems even might be reversible when behavior changes appropriately. For example, although bone loss and loss of muscle mass (sarcopenia) typically occur with increasing age, this de-cline can be minimized or reversed by strength training, even among the very eld-erly (Kolberg, chapter 2). Furthermore, the importance of stimulation to healthy neural functioning is particularly important among the very young and the very old. In early life, stimulation lays the neural foundation for healthy later develop-ment, whereas among the elderly stimulation slows declines in neural functioning. Although the upper limit of life expectancy remains at about 120 years, lots of ex-ercise, reduced exposure to toxins (e.g., cigarettes), and healthy diet might increase health and the average life expectancy (Bergeman & Wallace, chapter 11; Merluzzi & Nairn, chapter 10; McIntosh, chapter 13).

Another example of biological influence concerns the effects of chronic illness on adjustment (Miceli, Rowland, & Whitman, chapter 9). Although the severity of illness affects adjustment, these relations are not necessarily linear, and they also depend on the nature of the illness. Child characteristics, family, and other social supports might be more predictive of psychological adjustment than illness char-acteristics and generally interact with illness characteristics in predicting outcomes (Miceli et al., chapter 9). However, at this point, relatively little is known beyond the fact that there are associations or correlations among variables. Accordingly, support for theoretical or explanatory models about causality and the direction of effects pertaining to chronic illness in children is weak; thus, conclusions about which are the most important predictors of adjustment remain uncertain (Miceli et al., chapter 9).

In reporting the effects of death and dying on psychological adjustment, McIn-tosh (chapter 13) provides yet another perspective on how biological processes may affect health-related concerns. Perhaps counterintuitively, death anxiety does not increase with age, and, in fact, death attitudes and fears are lowest among older adults, and, according to some research, is highest among younger individuals. These findings again call attention to the need for more process-oriented study of mechanisms accounting for causality in health-related outcomes. Death also has negative ramifications for the living, that is, loved ones of the deceased, with long-term consequences for children of their parents' death, and for parents of their children's death. However, McIntosh reports that the most negative outcomes of death on the living might be for the spouses of the deceased, particularly among older adults; death or sharp declines in health frequently follow after the loss of a spouse.

Genetics. The contributions of genetic factors to health were considered in several of the chapters. For example, Whitman, White, O'Mara, and Goeke-Morey (chapter 6) report that genetic analomies are responsible for many of the birth defects in the 3% to 5% of infants born with these problems, and most babies born with chromosomal or genetic analomies have health-related problems. Maturational status at birth (e.g, prematurity) also affects susceptibility to health problems.

Braungart-Rieker and Bergeman (chapter 3) describe genetic influences on a variety of health-related outcomes, including obesity, cardiovascular disease, diabetes mellitus, longevity, and self-rated health (see also Braungart-Rieker & Guerra, chapter 7). Genetic influences are conceptualized as affecting propensities or tendencies rather than being deterministic. Moreover, the influence of genetics is a complex interaction of multiple genetic and environmental influences, which might contribute additively or even interchangeably. Heritability across the life span varies as a function of specific illnesses. Some illnesses have increased heritability with age, partly due to "niche picking" (i.e., individuals with similar genetics seeking similar environments), whereas for others decreased heritability across the life span is reported. Furthermore, changes in environment may affect heritability; for example, changes in diet affect the probability that certain genetic predispositions will develop into actual disorders. As Braungart-Rieker and Bergeman point out, longitudinal studies are needed to sort out the nature of these relations and interactions over time. For genetic influences, as with other factors that affect health, questions remain about the complex processes and mechanisms that cause outcomes, and these types of questions are next steps for research.

Finally, temperament, which reflects biological and genetic factors, also influences health. For example, Braungart-Rieker and Guerra (chapter 7) report that children with active, intense, negative temperaments are at greater risk for accidental injuries. Children's temperament is also related to adjustment to chronic illness, with children with more difficult temperaments having greater adjustment problems (Miceli et al., chapter 9; see also Whitman et al., chapter 6).

Behavior and Psychology. Relations among psychological and behavioral variables and health are featured throughout the volume; therefore, due to limitations of space, I only survey some of the highlights across the life span (see Fig. 14.1). Even before birth, sensory stimulation (e.g., touch, light, sounds) derives from interaction with the mother, with evidence of implications for the later course of neural development (Kolberg, chapter 5). After birth, the bright lights and high noise levels associated with traditional newborn intensive care unit settings may interfere with infants' sleep patterns and physiological functioning (Whitman et al., chapter 6). On the other hand, the availability of sensitive, individualized nursing care, rooming-in, and other aspects of family-centered care, optimizes infant behavioral and physiological status (Whitman et al., chapter 6). Touch, active handling, close contact, and affection, is also significant to infants' optimal self-regulation and development, including early growth, immune system functioning, physiological regulation, and sleeping (Kolberg, chapter 5; Whitman et al., chapter 6).

Childhood is a period of relatively good health from a biological perspective; accidental injuries are the greatest cause of death (Braungart-Rieker & Guerra, chapter 7). Parenting and environmental factors (e.g., low socioeconomic status [SES]), in addition to children's temperament, are predictors of likelihood of accidents. Obesity in childhood, which is predictive of higher mortality later in life, is also linked with psychological and environmental risk factors (single parents, lots of TV watching, low SES), as well as genetic predisposition (Braungart-Rieker & Bergeman, chapter 3; Braungart-Rieker & Guerra, chapter 7).

Surprisingly, juvenile diabetes is a greater health risk in childhood than all forms of cancer. Interestingly, the onset and course of juvenile diabetes is related to both genetic and environmental factors (Braungart-Rieker & Bergeman, chapter 3). Although the contributions of the environment to the etiology of juvenile diabetes are little understood, the control and treatment of the disease, which are highly predictive of relative mortality, are associated with family factors (parental involvement; low family conflict; Braungart-Rieker & Guerra, chapter 7).

Adolescence is also a period of life marked by high potential for good health from a biological perspective (Gondoli, chapter 8). Behavioral and psychological factors are especially important for predicting health; accidents, homicides, and suicides, and lifestyle choices are the major causes of morbidity. With regard to biological factors, pubertal development predicts psychological health in girls; early maturing girls have more problems, especially in coed schools. Interestingly, pubertal development is a much less significant factor for adjustment for girls attending all-girls schools (Gondoli, chapter 8). Dissatisfaction with body image, especially concerns about body fat increases, appear to underlie girls' dissatisfaction, whereas early maturing boys are more satisfied with their increases in height and muscle development during this period. Contrary to the conventional wisdom, adolescents' risky behavior is not due to an inability to make adult decisions, or their supposed perceptions of invulnerability (e.g., the personal fable); risky behavior is more closely related to needs to succeed socially, assert autonomy, and have fun (Gondoli, chapter 8).

Personal habits are important for health in midlife, especially among men (Merluzzi & Nairn, chapter 10). Lifestyle (not smoking, moderate alcohol intake, regular physical activity, maintaining appropriate weight) and health consciousness (weight loss, cholesterol reduction, controlling blood pressure) are more important to the health of men between 50 and 74 years of age than for younger or older men. Psychological factors are also closely related to health, with personal control beliefs, self-efficacy expectations, and personal characteristics of hardiness (commitment to one's goals, perceptions of stress as changeable, and perception of change as a challenge rather than primarily a threat) each contributing to the probability of health.

Similarly, control beliefs, self-efficacy, and hardiness are related to resiliency in later life (Bergeman & Wallace, chapter 9). Older people are more diverse in health

286 CUMMINGS

than younger people, with wider variations than in earlier life periods. Psychological characteristics are important for the course of aging. For example, control beliefs affect the actions older people take with regard to health. Hardiness is related to the ability to mobilize resources, with possible implications even for the functioning of the neuroendocrine system. However, Bergeman and Wallace (chapter 9) underscore the lack of knowledge concerning the mechanisms and processes underlying plasticity, resiliency, and reserve capacity among older adults.

Family Relationships and Social Supports

Good family relations and social support are also important to an individual's health (see Fig. 14.1). A vast literature supports the role of family relations in the adjustment and physical health of children (Bolig, Borkowski, & Brandenberger, chapter 4; Braungart-Rieker & Guerra, chapter 7; Kolberg, chapter 5; Miceli et al., chapter 9; Whitman et al., chapter 6). Family and social relationships are also potential buffers against the negative effects of stress in midlife (Merluzzi & Nairn, chapter 10) and older age (Bergeman & Wallace, chapter 9; Vachon, chapter 12). Even older people turn first to family members for assistance in times of crisis, and recent research suggests that the attachment relationships older adults form with their adult children predict mental and physical health (Barnas, Pollina, & Cummings, 1991). Interestingly, beyond childhood, not only do children rely on their parents for support and emotional security, but parents also rely on children, with substantial implications for the mental and physical health of the parents under certain circumstances (e.g., illness or disability; Vachon, chapter 12).

However, support from family is not always beneficial. Excessive support reduces autonomy and leads to feelings of helplessness; support may also be inappropriate or ineffective (Bergeman & Wallace, chapter 11). Moreover, support provision can have high costs for the caregiver, particularly when substantial and continuing care is required for relatives developing chronic illnesses or disabling conditions (Vachon, chapter 12). Interestingly, caregiving for older adults is not rare but, in fact, is relatively common (Vachon, chapter 12). For spouses it may be assumed as part of the marital commitment. As there are phases in coping with loss (McIntosh, chapter 13), there are also predictable phases in coping with caregiving for an adult in later life (Vachon, chapter 12). How an individual copes with these stages of adjusting, or failing to adjust, to caregiving is related to the impact of caregiving on the caregiver's health.

In general, caregiving for disabled or elderly family members is linked with increased marital discord and depression, increased feelings of burden and stress, job or parenting problems, and medical problems, but it also might be rewarding and enriching (Nixon & Cummings, 1998; Vachon, chapter 12). Characteristics of the care recipient, personal factors of the caregiver's cognitive appraisal, psychological functioning, health, and spiritual/philosophy of life are linked with the effects of caregiving on the caregiver. Provision of household services and social support networks help caregivers cope with the demands of caregiving (Vachon, chapter 12). However, making causal relations is difficult, especially given the relative absence of longitudinal studies, sampling problems (e.g., a bias toward sampling more distressed caregivers), and measurement limitations (e.g., overreliance on self-report; neglect of measurement of caregiver gain; Vachon, chapter 12).

As Fig. 14.1 illustrates, a variety of different aspects of family functioning and social support are related to adjustment or other health-related outcomes, but, as the reviews in this volume indicate, examinations of these variables are incomplete. Moreover, multiple family systems are interrelated in their effects on development. For example, qualities of marital, parent–child, and sibling relations are interrelated and mutually influential, each with implications for stress and coping processes, responses and styles, and, ultimately, children's adjustment (Cummings & Davies, 1994; Cummings, Davies, & Simpson, 1994). Illustrating interrelations between individual and family factors (see Fig. 14.1), psychological problems in marital partners have been related to the psychological functioning of spouses and to the functioning of marital, parent–child, and sibling systems (Cummings, 1998). Moreover, interrelations between the functioning of nuclear and extended family are reported (Hall & Cummings, 1997), as are relations between patterns of interacting in the family and with peers (Beach, 1995). More systematic and differentiated investigation of the impact of family on health as a function of periods of the life span is thus a promising direction for future research.

Society and Environment

Another major class of influence on health is the social and physical ecology in which an individual develops, that is, society and environment (see Fig. 14.1). Prenatal development is particularly affected by chemical agents, toxins, and infectious agents, including alcohol, tobacco, radiation, and rubella (Kolberg, chapter 5; Whitman et al., chapter 6). Illustrating interrelations among biological factors, environment, and health, prenatal stages of development and genetic susceptibility influence the impact of environment agents on health. Thus, exposure to physical and chemical agents (a) might be lethal in the first few weeks; (b) might cause structural malformations in the embryonic stage, and (c) might lead to functional deficits (e.g., mental retardation) during the fetal stage (Kolberg, chapter 5). Some teratogens exert influence throughout development (e.g. alcohol), whereas others (e.g., the rubella virus) are most damaging in specific periods of development (Whitman et al., chapter 6). Moreover, reflecting interrelations among psychological factors, family influences, and prenatal health, maternal stress can directly translate into elevated exposure to toxins and teratogens, or indirectly increase exposure to toxins and teratogens when stress increases negative maternal behaviors (e.g., high levels of alcohol consumption; Kolberg, chapter 5). Although the effects on health are much less understood, it also appears that positive inputs (e.g., provision of appropriate patterns of maternal movement and other sources of stimulation), as well as the avoidance of negative factors, are important to optimal prenatal health and development (Kolberg, chapter 5).

Poverty is an index of the availability and allocation of governmental, financial, and community resources. Bolig et al. (chapter 4) provide a review of the negative health consequences of poverty across the life span (Bergeman & Wallace, chapter 9; Merluzzi & Nairn, chapter 10). More children than adults are poor, and poverty is associated with more medical health and other problems, particularly among children. These outcomes might be exacerbated by lack of health care; abuse, neglect, and maltreatment; exposure to crime and violence; overcrowding; and exposure to negative environmental agents (e.g., toxic chemicals, insufficient heat, damp conditions, rats and mice). Poverty is associated with violence, which is the leading cause of death for African Americans between the ages of 15 and 34. In adolescence and adulthood, poverty is also linked with a lack of positive future orientation, sexually transmitted diseases, and mental health problems (Bolig et al., chapter 4). In addition, shorter life expectancy is associated with poverty. Governmental and societal responses to poverty include Head Start, health insurance, and Medicaid, and programs to help adolescents make healthier behavioral choices. However, as Bolig et al. note, much more coordinated and multidimensional governmental planning is needed; despite the responses of government, community, and society, poverty remains a pervasive risk factor for health-related problems across the life span.

Finally, community support is implicated in the health of the elderly (Bergeman & Wallace, chapter 11). Because some older individuals refuse family support out of concern about being unable to reciprocate, community supports can provide an essential complement to other forms of social support. In particular, community support can foster a sense of social integration outside of the family (e.g., church, voluntary organizations; Bergeman & Wallace, chapter 11).

STRESS AND COPING PROCESSES, RESPONSES, AND STYLES

Next we further consider the conceptualization of stress and coping processes, responses, and styles as elements of a life-span perspective on health and psychology (Fig. 14.1).

Impetus for a Process-Oriented Explanatory Model

Although important advances have been made in demonstrating associations among psychological, biological, and environmental factors, and their relations to health, questions remain. Interrelations among these variables and development across the life span are highly complex, posing a significant challenge for scientific understanding. At this stage in the development of biopsychoenvironmental models, demonstrating that variables are correlated has reached a point of diminishing returns (Whitman, chapter 1). Accordingly, increasingly, calls are made to move beyond the identification of simple correlations to the study of processes and mechanisms, including the identification of risk and protective factors (Vachon, chapter 12), the testing of explicit multivariate models (e.g., Braungart-Rieker & Bergeman, chapter 3), and the explication of causal relations (Braungart-Rieker & Guerra, chapter 7; Merluzzi & Nairn, chapter 10).

The limitations of current models for understanding health and psychology are noted by many of the chapters in this volume. For example Miceli et al. (chapter 9) indicate that available models for understanding children's adaptation to chronic illness were only descriptive and do not address the reasons relations exist or operate. Consistent with the framework outlined in Fig. 14.1, Bergeman and Wallace (chapter 11) stressed that (a) development is "as a dynamic and continuous interplay between growth [gain] and decline [loss]" and (b) research should move "beyond simply demonstrating that there is a link between various resilience mechanisms and not-optimal outcomes, to examining [more explicitly] the processes that underlie the link." As we have seen, the chapters in this volume strongly support the influence of individual, familial, and ecological factors, and the value of a process-oriented approach for explaining relations between health and psychology across the life span.

The urgent need for process-oriented explanations is evident in how health and psychology are treated in the popular media. For example, drinking is presented as problematic in some media stories and healthy in others. As has become apparent, these differences in outcomes might depend on many factors, including differences in sex, weight, alcohol intake, and family history, which might vary widely across the stories reported in the news. Moreover, these effects are mediated by differences in the stress and coping processes of individuals (e.g., biological reactions, social behavior changes, or cognitive or appraisal changes). Similarly, as the complex patterns of findings in these chapters indicate, a "sound bite" approach to health and psychology is not consistent with the evidence, and much more research is needed to explicate interrelations at a process level of analysis.

The Stress and Coping Approach

The stress and coping approach offers one useful heuristic for conceptualizing interrelations among complex biopsychoenvironmental factors at a process-oriented level of analysis. A process-oriented approach reflects a concern with more than charting simple relations among risk factors (e.g., biological, psychological, environmental) and health-related outcomes (e.g., physical illness and psychological disorder). The assumption is that risk factors and health related outcomes are interrelated due to the actions of underlying mechanisms and processes (e.g., specific behavioral, biological, or social response patterns), and that the understanding of causality obtains from articulating how the risk factors set these processes and mechanisms in motion, and, further, how these processes and mechanisms result in diagnoses or classifications of health-related outcomes.

Thus, for example, high exposure to the sun does not immediately cause skin cancer; rather, over time, high exposure to the sun probabilistically increases the likelihood of changes the action of the skin at a cellular level which, ultimately, and in interaction with other factors (e.g., genetic predispositions towards cancer or vulnerability to the sun; social behavior, such as the application of sun blocks), result in cancerous cellular functioning. Similarly, exposure to social environments characterized by high psychosocial stress does not immediately result in mental health disorders, rather, over time, high exposure to such environments increases the likelihood of behavioral, cognitive, or social dysregulations that ultimately, in interaction with other factors (e.g., genetic predispositions toward depression or aggression; social environments, such as supportive family), results in adjustment problems.

The process-oriented perspective outlined by stress and coping models offers one useful way for thinking about underlying processes and mechanisms. Lazarus and Folkman (1984) defined *stress* as "a particular relationship between the person and the environment that is appraised by the person as taxing or exceeding his or her resources or endangering his or her well-being" (p. 19). *Coping* is conceptualized as a dynamic process, that is, "the changing thoughts and acts that the individual uses to manage the external and/or internal demands of a specific person-environment transaction that is appraised as stressful (Folkman, 1991).

When coping is viewed in this way, emphasis is placed on the specific thoughts, acts, biological reactions, and other responses that the individual uses to cope with specific contexts, as guided by personal biological, genetic, behavioral, and psychological dispositions (e.g., behavioral habits, cognitive response patterns) or predispositions (e.g., genetic influences). The notion of specificity and precise definition is critical to a process-oriented perspective. For example, in assessing the impact of alcohol on an individual, it is important to know how much an individual drinks and other multidimensional aspects of functioning (body weight and sex), not simply whether he or she drinks, to predict whether consumption of alcohol will be related to healthy or harmful consequences. Individual differences also figure prominently in outcomes, and it is important to a process-oriented perspective to be as specific as possible about individual difference factors in attempting to explain or predict outcomes. Individual difference dimensions include, for example, personal dispositions or habits, biological functioning, family history, age, and sex. Interactions among the individual and specific environmental contexts find expression in multidimensional coping processes and strategies that develop into patterns that contribute over time to health or illness, adjustment or maladjustment.

Put another way, adversity, stress, and exposure to risk factors do not lead directly to diagnoses of health-related problems. The development of health-related problems reflects a series of microsocial processes that occur interactively over time, typically reflecting gradual adaptations by individuals to circumstances, although, in the case of traumatic events, effects might be virtually immediate. That is, the interval of time needed to induce health-related outcomes varies, for example, immediate consequences might occur from serious accidents, whereas effects might be more gradual with some environmental hazards (e.g., smoking). Nonetheless, even a stressor that typically induces relatively immediate health-related consequences does so by inducing complex patterns of change at a microsocial level; that is, specificity and multidimensional characterization of response processes remain important to the possibility of causal explanation. In summary, stress and coping processes, responses, and styles that occur in specific biopsychoenvironmental contexts account for relations among risk factors on the one hand and health-related outcomes on the other.

A point that merits emphasis from a life-span perspective is that relations among risk factors, stress and coping processes, and health might change significantly, or even dramatically, during the life course. This point is evident for several of the topics considered in this volume. For example, the impact of toxins (e.g., chemical or infectious agents) varies considerably even during the relatively brief period of prenatal development (Kolberg, chapter 5). As another example, the long-term implications of bone loss due to dietary inadequacies is particularly significant in adolescent girls (Kolberg, chapter 2).

On the other hand, age per se is not the best index of period of life-span development. Individuals age at different rates, with these differences "fanning out" with age, so that dissimilarity among individuals in aging is considerable in later life (Bergeman & Wallace, chapter 11). In other words, because aging itself is a process, periods of life-span development are better conceptualized in terms of processes of biopsychological functioning than in terms of chronological age.

Finally, although the stress and coping perspective is offered as useful heuristic for outlining a process-oriented perspective in this chapter, many questions still remain with regard to how best to conceptualize the study of processes and mechanisms and how best to describe causality and etiology in terms of multivariate, longitudinal models. Moreover, other approaches describe similar notions (e.g., developmental psychopathology, Cicchetti & Cohen, 1995; developmental science, Cairns et al., 1996), and these might add important concepts about the nature of developmental processes, enhancing the explanatory power of life-span models (e.g., resiliency, protective and vulnerability factors; see Whitman, chapter 1; Bergeman & Wallace, chapter 11; Egeland, Carlson, & Sroufe, 1993).

HEALTH-RELATED OUTCOMES

Stress and coping processes, responses, and styles might influence biological adjustment, psychological adjustment, or both. That is, outcomes are not mutually exclusive; biological and psychological adjustment might be affected simultaneously (Whitman, chapter 1).

Numerous specific illnesses and other health-related outcomes are noted in this volume, but issues of how to diagnosis or classify disorders are not treated in depth. Notably, the mission of life-span developmental science as a discipline is not the articulation of nosologies for medical or psychological disorders. The procedures and practices for the diagnosis and classification of various illnesses and disorders is in the realm of practice-oriented disciplines and is beyond the scope of this commentary and this volume. Life-span developmentalists (as well as developmental psychopathologists and developmental scientists) are concerned with etiology, and the processes and mechanisms that contribute to etiology, rather than the important but also distinctly sophisticated and complex matter of diagnosis.

Thus, life-span developmentalists might properly rely on the procedures and practices of clinicians and physicians or other health care providers and professional for the assessment of outcomes (e.g., paper-and-pencil tests with excellent psychometric support, clinical interviews, or medical testing). Clearly, numerous illnesses and disorders can be differentiated, and, again, consideration of these matters in depth is beyond the scope of this chapter and this volume.

However, some questions recently have been raised about the adequacy of traditional, static classification schemes for biological and psychological disorders (e.g., Jensen & Hoagwood, 1997; Rutter et al., 1997; Sroufe, 1997). As explanatory models become more complex, a question is whether traditional means for assessing outcomes will remain sufficient. Are notions of biological or psychological syndromes as static, well-defined entities fundamentally inadequate? In particular, arguments can be made for incorporating considerations of context in making psychological diagnoses (e.g., Sroufe, 1997). For example, depending on the context, an individual who sits in one place for 10 hours a day obsessively repeating certain small motor movements might be classified as obsessive–compulsive or a university professor (or both!). One must await the further debate on these matters.

CONCLUSION

The chapters in this volume provide a review of numerous exciting developments in understanding of relations between psychology and health across the life span. Furthermore, many of the chapters address issues toward developing a more adequate explanatory model, that is, a process-oriented understanding of life-span relations among health-related influences and health-related outcomes. The life-span approach offers many advantages for advanced understanding of health-related outcomes, including its ability to address sensitive and critical period issues regarding health (e.g., the different effects of toxins during different prenatal stages), and changes in predictors of health at different stages of development; the advance in understanding afforded by a dynamic rather than static model of development. As noted at the outset of this chapter, a life-span perspective is especially appropriate, even essential, for the study of health, because relative health and risk for illness change throughout the lifetime, with each stage of life influenced by past events and affecting future outcomes. However, although some of these issues are described in the chapters in this volume, these concerns need to be more systematically incorporated into health research. This commentary outlines some of the issues articulated and provides a framework for a process-oriented, life-span perspective on health-related outcomes. We hope that these chapters and this framework will stimulate broader, even more sophisticated, future study of relations between health and psychology across the life span.

REFERENCES

Barnas, M., Pollina, L., & Cummings, E. M. (1991). Life-span attachment: Relations between attachment and socio-emotional functioning in adults. *Genetic, Social, and General Psychology Monographs, 117,* 175–202.

Beach, B. (1995). *The relation between marital conflict and child adjustment: An examination of parental and child repertoires.* Unpublished manuscript.

Bergman, L. R., & Magnusson, D. (1997). A person-oriented approach in research on developmental psychopathology. *Development and Psychopathology, 9,* 291–320.

Cairns, R. B., Elder, G. H., & Costello, E. J. (1996). *Developmental science.* Cambridge, England: Cambridge University Press.

Cicchetti, D., & Cohen, D. (1995). Perspectives on developmental psychopathology. In D. Cicchetti & D. Cohen (Eds.), *Developmental Psychopathology* (pp. 3–22). New York: Wiley.

Cicchetti, D., & Richters, J. E. (1997). Examining the conceptual and scientific underpinnings of research in developmental psychopathology. *Development and Psychopathology, 9,* 189–192.

Cummings, E. M. (1998). Children exposed to marital conflict and violence: Conceptual and theoretical directions. In G. Holden, B. Geffner, & E. Jouriles (Eds.), *Children and family violence* (pp. 55–93). Washington, DC: American Psychological Association.

Cummings, E. M., & Cummings, J. S. (1988). A process-oriented approach to children's coping with adults' angry behavior. *Developmental Review, 3,* 296–321.

Cummings, E. M., & Davies, P. T. (1994). *Children and marital conflict: The impact of family dispute and resolution.* New York: Guilford.

Cummings, E. M., & Davies, P. T. (1996). Emotional security as a regulatory process in normal development and the development of psychopathology. *Development and Psychopathology, 8,* 123–139.

Cummings, E. M., Davies, P., & Simpson, K. (1994). Marital conflict, gender, and children's appraisal and coping efficacy as mediators of child adjustment. *Journal of Family Psychology, 8,* 141–149.

Cummings, E. M., & El-Sheikh, M. (1991). Children's coping with angry environments: A process-oriented approach. In M. Cummings, A. Greene, & K. Karraker (Eds.), *Life-span developmental psychology: Perspectives on stress and coping* (pp. 131–150). Hillsdale, NJ: Lawrence Erlbaum Associates.

Davies, P., & Cummings, E. M. (1994). Marital conflict and child adjustment: An emotional security hypothesis. *Psychological Bulletin, 116,* 387–411.

Egeland, B. Carlson, E., & Sroufe, L. A. (1993). Resilience as process. *Development and Psychopathology, 5,* 517–528.

Egeland, B., Pianta, R., & Ogawa, J. (1996). Early behavior problems: Pathways to mental disorders in adolescence. *Development and Psychopathology, 8,* 735–750.

Fincham, F. D. (1994). Understanding the association between marital conflict and child adjustment: An overview. *Journal of Family Psychology, 8,* 123–127.

Folkman, S. (1991). Coping across the lifespan: Theoretical issues. In E. M. Cummings, A. Greene, & K. Karraker (Eds.), *Lifespan developmental psychology: Perspectives on stress and coping* (pp. 3–20). Hillsdale, NJ: Lawrence Erlbaum Associates.

Hall, E., & Cummings, E. M. (1997). The effects of marital and parent-child conflicts on other family members: Grandmothers and grown children. *Family Relations, 46,* 135–144.

Hauser, S. T., Vieyra, M. A., Jacobson, A. M., & Wierlieb, D. (1985). Vulnerability and resilience in adolescence: Views from the family. *Journal of Early Adolescence, 5,,* 81–100.

Holmbeck, G. N. (1997). Toward terminological, conceptual, and statistical clarity in the study of mediators and moderators: Examples from the child clinical and pediatric psychology literatures. *Psychological Bulletin, 65,* 59–610.

Jaffe, P. G., Wolfe, D. A., & Wilson, S. K. (1990). *Children of battered women.* Newbury Park, CA: Sage.

Jaffe, P., Wolfe, D., Wilson, S. K., & Zak, L. (1986). Family violence and child adjustment: A comparative analysis of girls' and boys' behavioral symptoms. *American Journal of Psychiatry, 143,* 74–77.

Jensen, P. S., & Hoagwood, K. (1997). The book of names: DSM-IV in context. *Development and Psychopathology, 9,* 231–250.

Lazarus, R. S., & Folkman, S. (1984). *Stress, coping, and appraisal.* New York: Springer.

Nixon, C. L., & Cummings, E. M. (1998). *Sibling disability and children's reactivity to conflicts involving family members.* Manuscript submitted for publication.

Rutter, M. (1980). *Changing youth in a changing society.* Cambridge, MA: Harvard University Press.

Rutter, M. (1981). Stress, coping, and development: Some issues and some questions. *Journal of Child Psychology and Psychiatry,* 323–356.

Rutter, M., Dunn, T., Plomin, R., Simnoff, E., Pickles, A., Maugham, B., Ormel, J., Meyer, J., & Eaves, L. (1997). Integrating nature and nurture: Implications of person-environment correlations and interactions for developmental psychopathology. *Developmental Psychopathology, 9,* 335–364.

Sroufe, L. A. (1997). Psychopathology as an outcome of development. *Development and Psychopathology, 9,* 251–268.

Sroufe, L. A., & Rutter, M. (1984). The domain of developmental psychopathology. *Child Development, 55,* 17–29.

Author Index

298   AUTHOR INDEX

Cradock-Watson, J. E., 95, 103
Craighead, J. E., 58, 63
Crandall, R.C., 193, 204
Creasia, J. L., 242, 245
Cresanta, J. L., 130, 142
Criqui, M. H., 251, 274
Critelli, T., 251, 271
Crnic, K., 174, 184
Crockett, L. J., 72, 81
Cromwell, R. L., 212, 223
Cross, J. L., 96, 102
Cruickshanks, K., 133, 143
Cummings, E. M., 286, 278, 279, 281,
    282, 287, 293, 294
Cummings, J. 30, 44
Cummings, J. S., 278, 281, 282, 293
Cunningham, W., 134, 143
Curry, J. J., 212, 223
Cutrona, C., 215, 223
Czajkowski, S. M., 215, 225

D

Dadds, M. R., 176, 186
Dahlen, G., 56, 64
Dahlquist, G., 58, 63
Damiata, M., 154, 162
Dannefer, D., 207, 223, 224
Davies, P.T., 279, 287, 293
Davis, K., 74, 81
Davis, W., 153, 163
Death Studies, 270, 271
Debanne, S. M., 239, 247
Decker, S., 236, 238, 239, 240, 247
deFaire, U., 55, 56, 63
DeFries, J. C., 54, 65
DeGuire, M., 135, 143
Deimling, G. T., 235, 245
Dekel, A., 121, 123
DeMaso, D. R., 170, 172, 173, 181, 184
Dempsey, N. P., 238, 247
Den Boer, D. J., 198, 205
DeSantis, L., 268, 272
Desmond, K., 74, 82
Despres, J-P., 53, 63
Deveau, E. J., 263, 271
DeVries, B., 269, 271
DeVries, H., 198, 205
Diamond, M., 29, 30, 44
Diaz-Cintra, S., 70, 82
Dickinson, G. E., 250, 251, 261, 263, 266,
    267, 272
DiClemente, C. C., 202, 205
Diekstra, R. F. W., 265, 271
Dietz, W. H., 126, 130, 143
DiGuiseppi, C. G., 127, 142

Dillihay, T. C., 73, 81
Disney, E. R., 69, 82
Dolcini, M., 154, 162
Dolcini, M. M., 157, 158, 160, 161
Donaldson, C., 231, 232, 234, 235, 246
Doraiswamy, P., 36, 44
Dore, M. M., 71, 73, 81
Dornbusch, S. M., 136, 143
Dorris, M., 94, 102
Douglas, J. W. B., 126, 130, 144
Downs, W. R., 157, 160, 161
Drake, C.,128, 144
Drotar, D., 120, 123
Dubow, E. F., 168, 172, 185
Dubowitz, H., 69, 80
Duffy, F., 29, 31, 43
Duffy, M.,E., 211, 223
Dunlap, W. P., 134, 144
Dunn, L. M., 177, 184
Dunn, T., 282, 292, 294
Dunne, E. J., 269, 270, 271
Dunne, R. G., 130, 142
Dunne-Maxim, K., 269, 270, 271
Dura, J. R., 231, 232, 236, 239, 246
Durham, D., 29, 45, 99, 103
Dyson, L., 174, 184

E

Earls, F. J., 129, 142
Earp, J. L., 234, 247
Easterlin, R. A., 254, 271
Eastham, J., 234, 237, 239, 247
Eaves, L., 220, 223, 282, 292, 294
Ebina, Y., 59, 65
Edelman, M. W., 75, 77, 81
Eff, C., 135, 141
Egeland, B., 282, 293
Ehrlich, R., 135, 144
Eiberg, H., 137, 142
Einhaupl, K. M., 32, 45
Eisdorfer, C., 242, 247
Elder, G. H., 278, 291, 293
Elizur, E., 137, 143
Elkind, D., 153, 260, 271, 161
Elliot, R. B., 58, 64
Elster, A. B., 147, 161
Emlen, A. C., 232, 247
Emmanaul, J., 198, 206
Endriga, M. C., 177, 186
Engel, G. L., 211, 223
Engeland, B., 75, 81
Enstrom, J. E., 196, 204
Epstein, G., 251, 271
Erickson, E. H., 262, 263, 271
Erickson, S., 69, 81

Subject Index

311

Milton Keynes UK
Ingram Content Group UK Ltd.
UKHW022102141024
449569UK00031B/1741